Power Nutrition
for your
Chronic Illness

D0003550

KRISTINE NAPIER

Power Nutrition
for Your Chronic Illness

*A Guide to Shopping, Cooking and Eating
to Get the Nutrition Edge*

Macmillan • USA

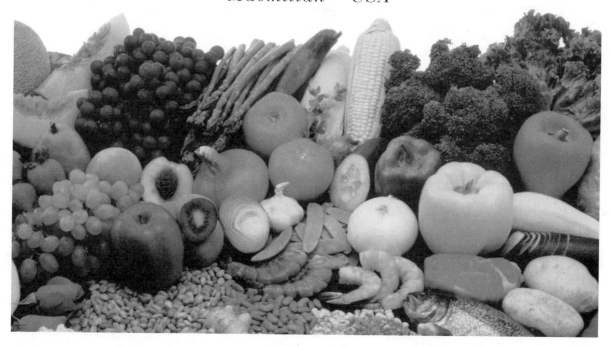

MACMILLAN

A Simon & Schuster Macmillan Company

1633 Broadway

New York, NY 10019

Text and illustrations copyright ©1998 by Kristine Napier

Macmillan Publishing books may be purchased for business
or sales promotional use. For information please write:
Special Markets Department, Macmillan Publishing USA,
1633 Broadway, New York, NY 10019.

All rights reserved. No part of this book may be reproduced or
transmitted in any form by any means, electronic or mechanical,
including photocopying, recording, or by any information storage
and retrieval system, without permission from the Publisher.

Library of Congress Cataloging-in-Publication Data available

ISBN: 0-02-862059-3

10 9 8 7 6 5 4 3 2 1

Printed in the United States of America

In the midst of winter, I finally learned that there was in me an invincible summer.

—Albert Camus

P9-BBP-760

Contents

Foreword

Believe it or not, nutrition is largely absent from most medical school curricula these days and still relegated to obscure courses within some nursing schools. Doctors therefore are not likely to be the ones to transmit valuable dietary information of any sort to any patients, never mind those with chronic illness. Nevertheless, times of chronic illness are exactly the times when the body's breakdown of vital nutrients and exceedingly increased demands for others is obvious. In essence this process called catabolism must be stopped if patients are to maintain a healthy weight, have healthy immune function, and maintain all of their vital bodily processes. Unless the spiral to bodily dysfunction is aborted, your chronic illness will be worse and your life miserable.

There are specific illnesses that require good nutrition, some that can be overcome with good nutrition, and probably a few that research will show can be cured with good nutrition. This book read cover to cover may be a resource that will allow the patient to conduct his or her own research, in the privacy of his or her own kitchen.

Heart disease can be prevented with good nutrition and existing disease can be improved. Nutrients like B vitamins can prevent clogged arteries, while vitamins C and E might eventually be the preventive compounds that keep arteries clear. Elements like selenium and others may also be important to such processes and increase life span. Calcium and vitamin D, found in many foods, could strengthen immune function, bone structure, and cell function in all organs. Most recently certain vegetables have been shown to prevent breast cancer within families and decrease the incidence of autoimmune disease. These are but a few examples. It makes absolutely no sense to ignore the substances which we ingest daily, because these are the medicines which predated the pharmaceutical substances later developed for use in chronic disease. Age-old remedies are based on nutrients found in various foods. One needs only to read this important book and use it as a guide to see improvement.

The key to living to old age—chronic illness or not—is a good diet. We know this from data in experimental animals that those fed diets similar to those described in this book simply lived longer. While it is true that we all have to die someday, I prefer to eat well and live well on the road to old age. Most of us will eventually get a chronic illness while we age because it is the nature of life. Read this book to maximize the good quality of life by being smart about your diet.

Robert G. Lahita, M.D., Ph.D., FACP, FACR
Columbia University, New York, NY

Acknowledgments

I am indebted to the many people who inspired me to write, revise and improve this book. First, to my husband, who has always buoyed me up yet pushed me forward through so many difficult health moments—who would never let me give up when the going was so tough. I am grateful to Mrs. Henrietta Aladjem, a dear friend and lupus patient for over forty years, who taught me to take charge of my life and my illness. And to my physician and friend, Dr. Larry Kent, who has taught me how to get on with life despite the constraints of a chronic illness.

I am very grateful to the many experts who took the time to review this book and offer their comments and support: Dr. Robert G. Lahita, Dr. Michael Lockshin, Dr. Helen Gartner Martin, Mary Anne Saathoff, Dr. Daniel J. Wallace and Dr. Bianca Weinstock-Guttman. In good health, many thanks to all of you.

A profound thank you to my culinary and research assistants: Bethann Barry, Nancy Morgan, Susan Napier, Sara Stuhan, Ruth Savchuk and Sara Wilson.

Introduction

If you want to live a long life, get a chronic disease and learn how to take care of it.

—Sir William Osler

My daughter, Susie, four at the time, marched proudly into my bedroom with a sandwich (sans plate) and a glass of milk in one of her plastic Disney cups. "I made it myself, Mommy, and I didn't even make a mess on the counter."

I had been in bed for several weeks with a flare-up of the chronic disease with which I live, systemic lupus erythematosus. It was very difficult, as I not only couldn't take care of my precious daughter, but I couldn't even make it up and down the steps from the bedroom to the kitchen to fix myself a meal. I was both proud and touched by Susie's display of affection and her desire to help. "I'm so proud of you, Susie, and it doesn't even matter if you did make a mess," I said as I bit into the peanut butter and jelly sandwich that was particularly heavy on the jelly—her favorite part of these sandwiches.

"Do you want to know why I didn't make a mess, Mommy?" she asked. "I made the sandwich on the floor!" I couldn't remember the last time the kitchen floor had been washed, but I didn't have the heart to reject the sandwich. Figuring that a little dirt and dust wouldn't hurt me, I ate the sandwich as if it were a gourmet meal from a fine restaurant. Susie watched, pleased at my enjoying her culinary skills and obviously appreciating her love and affection.

For many of us with chronic illness, eating healthy is an incredible challenge. For some, it's very difficult to shop for groceries. For others, standing in the kitchen for any length of time is painful or too exhausting, or nearly impossible because they need to use crutches, a walker or a wheelchair. Still others have hands disabled by arthritis or other diseases, hands that are able only to perform limited tasks in the kitchen. And even on days when we have enough energy to prepare a meal (beyond just opening a can or box), cleaning up the aftermath of cooking is another formidable task. Nearly everyone with chronic illness goes through times when appetite is poor to nonexistent. Many people face all these challenges.

I, too, have experienced every one of these challenges. I also know, though, that it is during these times of disease flare-ups that good nutrition is even more important.

As a registered dietitian, I have been acutely aware of the importance of good nutrition as an asset in fighting my disease. I have been frustrated, though, at my inability at times to get healthy food into my body. Knowing that supplements are only a crutch—that they can't possibly provide all the fabulous nutrition in food—I have long sought ways to simplify the task. I have experimented for years with easy ways to get healthy, good-tasting food into me without using up my energy allowance for the day—and without leaving a mess for the next day.

Turning to convenience foods isn't the answer, I know, because **if** they taste good, they are often loaded with sodium and fat. While many people can handle a sodium overload, a majority of people with chronic disease cannot—either because of their condition or due to the side effects of the medication they take. The same is true of many take-out foods—not only are they expensive, but they are often fat and sodium overloaded as well.

I know I am not alone in my frustration, nor in my desire to eat healthy food. That's why I wrote this book. I want to share the secrets of making life in the kitchen manageable for even the most physically and energy challenged (people with lupus are often very challenged when it comes to energy).

When I decided to write this book, I had no idea that I would be further challenged, nor that I would have to work in the kitchen in a wheelchair to perfect my recipes. But that was the case. Shortly after starting this project full time, I found out that I had a complication caused by the steroid medication I must take to calm the lupus—prednisone, a cortisone medication. Although cortisone is indeed a lifesaver for many people, it has many undesirable and potentially serious side effects. I, unfortunately, was suffering from one of those serious side effects, avascular necrosis. Both of my hip joints had been destroyed by the cortisone medication, and I could not walk unassisted. On top of that, I needed surgery to restore blood flow to the hips and to reconstruct them. I had the first surgery shortly into this project, and faced a long, difficult recovery. Because bone was taken from the lower leg to reconstruct the hip and also because the bone graft had to "take," I needed to be in a wheelchair or use a walker (or crutches) to avoid putting any weight on my leg for six weeks. Then, I still had to use crutches or a walker for another six weeks to allow complete healing. As if all that weren't enough, the other hip was exceedingly painful, as it bore the brunt of all my weight during that healing process as it awaited surgery.

The point of sharing all this with you is that I developed and perfected all the recipes in this book from a wheelchair, a kitchen chair pulled over to the sink, stove or counter (or sometimes one at each location to facilitate food preparation). It was the rare day that I could stand for more than a few minutes when I was creating these recipes. **Be reassured that no matter how disabled you are, you, too, can get back into the kitchen and warm up your tummy, your family and your home with delicious and fabulously nutritious home cooking again.**

Good nutrition during chronic illness is important for four chief reasons. First, a body that is well nourished is stronger to fight the illness. Second, getting all critical nutrients may help you avoid the potentially serious side effects of some of the medications used to treat chronic illness. Third, every body, sick or well, needs good quality fuel to perform optimally every day (see "Eat to Energize," page 7). That fuel needs to be composed of the right kind of calories, as well as an appropriate amount of protein and generous amounts of vitamins and minerals. Finally, people with chronic illness need to think about an eating plan that fights other diseases—cancer, heart disease and osteoporosis being prime among them.

To give you the nutrition advantage, this book has several types of information in it that you will find useful:

➤ Information about many chronic diseases, and how each impacts your nutritional status and how good nutrition can fight your disease.

➤ Important facts about many of the medications used to treat chronic disease and how they can affect nutrition and/or how they interact with nutrients.

➤ Detailed information and countless tips on how to make shopping, cooking and cleaning up easy.

➤ A chapter on how to entertain again if you have limited physical ability and/or energy.

➤ Guidance on how to gain or lose weight in the face of illness, limited physical movement and medications that impact appetite and metabolism and therefore body weight.

➤ Critically important information about preventive health maneuvers you can take. Although this sounds odd, I am firmly convinced that most people with chronic disease don't take the steps they *can* take to prevent heart disease, cancer, osteoporosis and other chronic conditions because they (and often their physicians) are so focused, and understandably so, on treating the disease.

➤ Information on using nutritional supplements and herbs. While many of us with chronic disease would do just about anything to feel better and be more active, going overboard with nutrition supplements and even so-called "normal" use of herbs can be very dangerous.

➤ Advice on how to use nutrition to help you recover from additional health insults piled on top of those you face daily; namely, how nutrition can help you recover from infections and surgery.

I want you to take charge of your life and to be in the best possible position to fight your disease and live as energetic and active life as you possibly can. I am convinced that good nutrition can put you on the winning side of your disease.

Kristine Napier

Nutrition Basics

1

Unraveling nutrition science has gotten to be a tough job. It seems that we hear new nutrition advice just about every week. For example, one week you hear that a diet high in carbohydrates is the healthiest; the next week, that high protein is the way to go. Perhaps you've heard the confusing information about giving up butter for margarine, only to later hear that margarine is full of dangerous transfatty acids (what are they, anyway?). Indeed, it's no wonder that most people are perplexed and don't know what to eat.

In this chapter I'd like to simplify the basics of nutrition and explain some of the current nutrition buzzwords you're hearing. This should be a big help as you read on and learn how to use nutrition to help fight disease.

What Is in Food?

Nature has loaded up food with several categories of substances we need to live, including:

➤ MACRONUTRIENTS. There are three of these calorie-providing nutrients: carbohydrates, protein and fat.

➤ MICRONUTRIENTS. The thirteen vitamins and twenty-four minerals in this category don't contribute any calories, but they are necessary to live and to fight disease.

➤ FIBER. Composed of the indigestible portion of plants and vegetables, fiber doesn't contribute any calories. But this "bulk" is absolutely necessary for the intestinal tract to function normally. In addition, there's mounting evidence that fiber helps fight off other diseases, including cancer and heart disease.

➤ PHYTOCHEMICALS. The latest substances in food to be discovered, phytochemicals show great potential in fighting cancer, heart disease and other maladies.

➤ MYSTERY CATEGORY

Let's look at each of these categories, beginning with the last one, Mystery Category.

Mystery Category

It probably seems odd to start this discussion with an undefined category. But this category is the most important reason to eat a balanced diet. Don't worry, this will make sense in a minute.

The science of nutrition is a relatively new one, barely a century old. Vitamins themselves weren't discovered until the late nineteenth century.

Early nutrition scientists learned which nutrients were essential to life; in the process they identified vitamins and minerals. Gradually they learned how much of these substances our bodies need to function normally. Nutritionists then discovered that some of these essential nutrients might have other roles in the body, that they might help prevent diseases other than nutrient deficiencies—diseases such as cancer and heart disease.

One compelling example is folic acid. The discovery that getting 400 micrograms of folic acid daily in the very earliest days of pregnancy can prevent spina bifida and other neural tube defects (birth defects of the spinal column) has been heralded as one of the greatest nutrition discoveries of the twentieth century. (Nutrition experts now recommend that all women of childbearing age consume that much folic acid because it is so essential in the earliest days of pregnancy—before most women know they are pregnant.)

In the most recent phase of nutrition research, scientists have discovered phytochemicals (see below), naturally occurring plant chemicals with a wide range of health benefits. Although these substances have been in food for literally millions of years, it's just in the last decade that food scientists have realized these substances have benefits to humans.

The question remains: if we've just discovered phytochemicals, what else haven't we discovered that may be necessary for good health and disease prevention? No doubt there are other substances in food that are yet to be found. How can you get these substances? *Eat a balanced, varied diet,* one that supplies all the macronutrients, micronutrients and phytochemicals we know about (you'll learn how below). Most importantly, realize that using supplements instead of food to meet known nutrition needs means cutting out unknown potentially beneficial substances.

Macronutrients

Three types of nutrients, called macronutrients, supply the body with the energy it needs to keep going. The three macronutrients are carbohydrates, protein and fat.

CARBOHYDRATES Carbohydrates, often called starchy foods, include breads, grains, vegetables, fruits and legumes; they also include sugar, syrup, candy, soda pop and other highly refined, sugary foods. Carbohydrates are the body's number-one fuel choice; that's why you should get no less than 50 percent of your calories as carbohydrates, and possibly as much as 60 percent. The great majority of these carbohydrates should be as complex carbohydrates rather than the simple counterpart.

All carbohydrates are made up of sugars, either simple sugars or more complex sugars or of some combination of the two. You've probably heard that foods made up of complex sugars, often called complex carbohydrate foods, are much healthier than simpler sugars (or simple carbohydrates). Think of it this way: complex carbohydrates are fruits, vegetables and grains close to how they come from nature. The more refined these foods are, the fewer complex carbohydrates and the less of nature's goodness they have. For example, squeeze the juice out of an apple and you have a simple sugar instead of the complex carbohydrate you would have had by eating an apple. The same is true of refining wheat into white flour and of stripping rice of its outer coats and ending up with white rice.

PROTEIN   While protein is another source of fuel for the body, our bodies don't use it for pure energy. Rather, bodies depend on protein to support growth and tissue repair. It also drives the complex set of never-ending chemical reactions that make us breathe, keep our heart beating and stimulate every other action vital to life. Without protein, our hormones, antibodies and genes, the body's code for making any tissue or cell, could not function.

FAT   Although we mostly hear about how bad fat is, the truth is we can't live without it. Each of the body's millions upon billions of cells could not form properly or regulate the entry and exit of nutrients, hormones and other life-essential chemicals. Vital internal organs might suffer serious injury in its absence. Hormones couldn't form or function, nor could the body harness, transport and use certain vitamins without it.

Fat is the most compact source of energy available to us. While each gram of protein and carbohydrate has four calories, a gram of fat has nine calories, more than twice as many, making it very easy to overeat fat calories. Indeed, fat is as overconsumed as it is necessary to life and good health.

Avoid the Low-Fat Trap

Too many Americans are gaining weight on nonfat and low-fat foods. What confuses people is one very basic fact: low fat does not mean low calorie— not even nonfat foods are automatically low in calories. Reduced-fat cookies and coffee cakes, for example, make up their calories in sugars, and often have just as many calories as their higher fat counterparts. Seeing the reduced-fat label, however, lulls many people into a false sense of security. Researchers at Penn State University studied this recently, giving groups of women three different types of yogurt with their lunch: low fat, low calorie; low fat, high calorie; and high fat, high calorie. They labeled half the women's yogurt as either low or high fat, but didn't label the other half.

The results are very telling about the effects of the low-fat label. Women eating yogurt labeled low fat took in more calories at lunch than women eating yogurt that was unlabeled— even though in many cases the yogurts were equal in calories. The researchers speculated that women eating yogurt labeled as *low fat* allowed themselves to indulge at lunch, while those eating unlabeled yogurt listened to their bodies' internal signals of when they'd eaten enough.

The bottom line? Reduced-fat foods aren't a license to eat unlimited quantities. Instead, use them as substitutes for their higher fat counterpart, limiting yourself to a healthy serving size.

Striking an appropriate balance is critical. Fat calories should claim no more than 30 percent of all the calories you eat in a day. To be healthy, you can safely go down to around 15 percent of calories, although that is very difficult to achieve. Sliding in around 20 to 25 percent is probably best, as well as healthiest.

CREATING THE OPTIMAL FUEL MIX While most people aren't aware of it, human bodies function best when they have the right fuel mix. Here's an analogy to help put this into perspective. To run properly, your lawnmower has to have just the right mix of gas and oil. Add too much oil, and it will stutter to a stop; the same is true if you skimp on oil. While bodies don't have such a dramatic response to the wrong fuel mix, they certainly don't function as efficiently and as energetically as they would with the right fuel mix.

The best fuel mix for human bodies derives about 55 to 60 percent of calories from carbohydrate, 15 to 20 percent from protein and 20 to 30 percent from fat. Let's translate that into how to eat. An easy way is to figure how to divide up your plate. Have you ever used the type of paper plate that is divided into sections? They're a great visual aid in figuring out how to fill your plate to derive the best fuel mix for the body. Fill the big portion (the one most people fill with the meat part of a meal) with vegetables; in other words, vegetables should take up about half your plate. Put your meat in one of the small portions (which makes it about a two- to three-ounce portion) and a starch in the other small portion. This is a great way to picture how you should divide your daily calories.

Micronutrients

The body needs at least twelve vitamins and twenty-four minerals that are called _essential_. They're called essential because while we need them to live, we can't make them from "scratch" inside the body using other ingredients. Instead, we have to eat them in food, or we can suffer the symptoms of deficiency. Not getting enough vitamin C, for example, can result in sore, bleeding gums. The Recommended Dietary Allowance (RDA) is the amount of nutrients we need to live—with a generous margin of safety built in. For example, while the RDA for vitamin C is sixty milligrams for adults, we need less than that to live. Note that soon you'll be seeing an alternative term for RDA—DRI, for Dietary Reference Intake.

Pay attention to one very important point when it comes to nutrients and how much to get: just because some is good, it doesn't mean that a whole lot more is better. Loading up on one or another nutrient in hopes that it will cure or prevent a malady may throw the body out of kilter. Taking doses of vitamins or minerals that are more than the RDA can have disastrous consequences. Upsetting the balance by taking a supplement with many times the RDA of one or several nutrients often has more negative than positive effects.

For example, getting too much folic acid can mask the signs of a vitamin B_{12} deficiency, which could lead to permanent nerve damage. Note that many times the symptoms of vitamin/mineral excess are so vague that you may never pin them on the fact that you're taking too much of any particular nutrient. Many nutrition experts agree that taking a vitamin at doses beyond the RDA is like taking a prescription medication. It should only be done under a physician's watchful eye. Refer to the chapter on supplements for more information on the potential danger in taking too many supplements.

Fiber

Fiber is that portion of plant foods (fruits, vegetables and grains) that the human intestinal tract cannot digest. As a result it adds bulk to the diet, and therefore to the intestinal tract. That's why fiber helps prevent constipation, keeping wastes moving through the intestinal tract quickly and easily. There's also evidence that fiber may help in lowering blood cholesterol levels and reducing cancer risk, especially the risk of colon (intestinal) cancer.

Unfortunately, most Americans come up grossly deficient on dietary fiber. As discussed earlier, if people consumed more complex carbohydrates—whole fruits, vegetables and grains—they would consume enough fiber. But most Americans consume more refined (or simple) carbohydrates than complex ones, which also means they come up quite short on fiber, too.

The consequences of not getting enough fiber go beyond constipation. The excessive straining that accompanies chronic constipation can lead to hemorrhoids and diverticular disease. In people with diverticular disease, potentially painful pockets develop in the intestine wall when tissues are rendered weak from repeated and excessive straining associated with constipation. These pockets can also be very dangerous, as they can rupture or become infected.

Phytochemicals

Although it sounds very complicated, phytochemicals are simply plant chemicals—*phyto* is the Greek word for plant.

Going back million of years to the beginning of life on earth, we know that plants were anaerobic. In other words, they lived in a world devoid of oxygen. As time progressed, plants evolved to meet the changing milieu of their surroundings. They began to turn carbon dioxide into oxygen. But they weren't equipped to deal with the by-products of oxygen production; indeed, producing oxygen actually meant polluting their own environment.

In order to survive, plants had to evolve once again—and indeed they did. They were forced to develop defenses against these oxygen byproducts, which are unstable forms of oxygen, commonly called oxygen-free radicals or free radicals. Left unchecked, free radicals become stray, high-energy particles that ricochet wildly, scarring and punching holes in cells. Phytochemicals became key warriors in protecting plants against oxygen-free radicals—we now refer to these warriors as antioxidants. As antioxidants, they capture and disable those wildly wandering free radicals (see sidebar, page 6).

Phytochemicals also give fruits and vegetables their rainbow range of brilliant colors. But the phytochemicals have even more roles in protecting the health of plants. They also guard plants against an array of adversities including viruses, insects, harsh weather and even handling. That's because many, but by no means all, of these substances have very strong odors and tastes. The phytochemicals called *indoles* and *isothiocyanates,* for example, account for some of the "bite" or strong taste in cruciferous vegetables, that large category of vegetables that includes broccoli, cabbage, Brussels sprouts, cauliflower and mustard greens. Indoles and isothiocyanates are produced when parent chemicals in cruciferous vegetables, glucosinates, are broken down by an insect or an animal chomping down on them (they're meant to act as a repellent) or when we cook them. Not selective in when they release their odor, these phytochemicals do their skunk trick when a person breaks off part of the plant, cuts into it or cooks it. That's why the kitchen smells so foul when you cook broccoli; it's also why you cry when you cut into an onion.

To use an analogy, phytochemicals are to plants what the immune system is to the human body: they're meant to defend plants against foreign invaders.

Although phytochemicals have been in food for millions of years, we're just now discovering what they are and how intriguing and powerful they are. Phytochemicals are classified as nonnutrient constituents of foods because they have no calories and aren't essential for the body to function normally, unlike essential vitamins and minerals. Although we don't need them to function normally, we probably do need them for good health. There's rapidly accumulating evidence that phytochemicals help us fight cancer, heart disease and even infections; there's very limited and preliminary evidence that one type might help fight systemic lupus erythematosus, one chronic disease discussed in this book.

Free Radicals, Antioxidants and Phytochemicals

In humans, free radicals can cause cellular damage that can progress to cancer, set the stage for artery-clogging heart disease—or worsen—and possibly affect the early development or progression of other diseases. While the body has natural antioxidants, it needs help from the outside, especially when someone is exposed to cancer-causing substances such as cigarette smoke (including passive smoke) or too much sun. Phytochemicals seem capable of acting as critical antioxidants in people as well as in plants. (Some nutrients, including vitamin C, vitamin E and selenium, also have antioxidant powers in the body.)

But their power seems to go far beyond their antioxidant capabilities, fighting cancer in other ways, too. Phytochemicals may also boost the immune system, relieve the symptoms of menopause, and offer protection against artery-clogging heart disease. Researchers at the National Cancer Institute are keenly interested in many of these chemicals and their ability to prevent cancer. They're studying, for example, green tea, garlic and soybeans to assess their role in cancer prevention. In 1991 alone, the National Cancer Institute allocated nearly $3 million to study the anticancer effect of soy.

Eat to Energize

2

Fuel up before putting your engine to work. Refuel before the tank reads empty.

No, it's not your car's engine we're talking about, but your body's engine. This food-is-fuel philosophy is how athletes regard food. To them, food is a source of energy and good health. Used properly, it helps them perform better and longer.

As someone with a chronic illness, you can benefit from the same philosophy. You, too, can turn food into energy, to feel the best you can, concentrate better, accomplish more and manage your disease.

Eating to energize involves several key steps: balancing the three food fuels, optimally timing food intake and drinking plenty of water.

The C-P-F Balance

Athletes who have learned to make food work for them consistently balance the three food fuels—carbohydrate, protein and fat—to supply a mix of short-, moderate-, and long-term energy. At each meal, they include plenty of complex carbohydrates for fast efficient fuel; some protein for moderate and long-term fuel; and limited amounts of fat for palatability and more long-term fuel. I call this the C-P-F balance.

While it's not wrong, nutritionally speaking, to eat the bulk of your protein at dinner as many people do, you'll put that protein to work to maximize energy if you include some throughout the day. In particular, eating high-quality protein at breakfast and lunch helps energize you through a long day. True, you generally don't think of protein as an energy food, but as a tissue builder, which is its main purpose. But because about half of it is eventually broken down into fuel, it also supplies critical moderate and long-term fuel, long after the fuel from carbohydrates has been burned.

Eating a high-sugar meal, especially at breakfast, can be energy robbing. Such a meal causes blood sugar to rise sharply and then plummet midmorning, leaving you in an energy crisis. Yet another reason to follow the C-P-F balance rule!

Time Meals and Snacks

One key maneuver is to eat enough during the day, when calories can be burned as fuel. Many people, either because they are weight-conscious or just don't have time, skimp on food all day and load up on food at dinner. Think about it, though. When you awaken in the morning, your fuel tank is literally on empty after some eight to twelve hours of not eating. It makes sense that that's when you need a fuel boost the most—not at the end of the day. Try to change your habits to eat at least one-third of your daily calories at breakfast and in a morning snack, one third at lunch and in an afternoon snack and the final third later in the day.

Eating every three to six hours is a great way to boost energy. That means eating several small, frequent meals. Just as an athlete who doesn't eat enough won't have enough fuel to complete a race, a person who starves during the day feels sluggish and has a hard time concentrating. This may be even more true for people with chronic illness who must fight pain and the actual disease process all day long—energy-gobbling tasks, indeed!

Worried that you'll gain weight if you eat three meals and two snacks daily? The key is to keep meals and snacks small, and to know serving sizes. Most people who eat more of their food early in the day actually lose weight. Because they aren't starving at the end of day, they don't binge, and therefore end up eating less.

Timing food around exercise is also key to maximizing energy. Eat one to three hours before a workout to feel most energetic during exercise. Fruit, a bagel, or low-fat yogurt are great preworkout fuels, and the amount you should eat depends on the intensity of the workout and how much before the workout you snack. The more time between your snack and the exercise session, the more you can eat. If you exercise after work, for example, have a carton of yogurt midafternoon.

Stay Well Hydrated

Getting enough fluid is just as important as practicing good nutrition habits. Water, in fact, is one of the most vital compounds to human life. Although athletes readily acknowledge the critical importance of staying well hydrated, many others do not. While the consequences of dehydration are very apparent when the body is exercising and working hard, there are also problems associated with walking around slightly dehydrated. Each cell of the body contains countless chemicals, minerals and vitamins, and they function best when they're diluted in just the right amount of fluid.

The body is also dependent on the bloodstream to transport nutrients and other substances from one part of the body; this, too, depends on optimal fluid conditions in the blood. Although research has focused on the consequences of severe dehydration, it stands to reason that when vital components are in a less than optimal fluid concentration, cells are handicapped. Fatigue is a very likely consequence.

Dehydrating during an intense workout packs a double punch: you'll be less able to tolerate the heat strain of heavy exercise, and you'll feel yet more fatigued.

How much should you drink? Unfortunately, you can't rely on thirst to tell you; the thirst mechanism doesn't kick in until dehydration becomes serious. You can, in fact, lose up to 2 percent of your body weight as sweat before you feel thirsty; for a 135-pound woman, that's nearly three pounds of sweat! Drink at least sixty-four ounces daily (about two quarts), and more when you exercise.

Try this eat-to-energize eating plan. Note that calories are concentrated early in the day, and dinner is on the light side. While you may think this is a lot of food, it's actually less than most women need, which means you may lose weight slowly if you adopt this style of eating. This plan supplies 1,800 calories, is low in fat, has plenty of fiber and supplies at least 100 percent of all essential nutrients except calcium. See page 25 for information on calcium supplements. It's also big on variety, a cornerstone of good nutrition. But serving size is key. Take out your measuring cups and food scales occasionally to fully appreciate a half-cup or three-ounce serving.

DAY ONE

Breakfast
1 cup high-fiber cereal
1 banana
1 cup skim milk

Morning Snack
½ whole wheat bagel
1 tablespoon low-fat cream cheese
1 orange

Lunch
Turkey sandwich: 2 ounces turkey breast, 2 slices whole wheat bread, 3 leaves romaine lettuce, 1 tablespoon low-fat mayonnaise

10 baby carrots
1 cup strawberries
2 small chocolate chip cookies
1 cup skim milk

Afternoon Snack
1 large apple
1 carton low-fat, fruited yogurt

Dinner
2 ounces roasted beef eye of round
1 medium baked potato
2 tablespoons low-fat sour cream
8 asparagus spears

1728 calories, 15% fat (30.5 g total fat, 11.2 g saturated), 65% carbohydrate (294 g), 19% protein (86.5 g), 44.6 g fiber

DAY TWO

Breakfast
1 poached egg
1 slice whole wheat toast
1 teaspoon tub margarine
1 cup grapefruit juice

Morning Snack
1 whole wheat bagel
1 tablespoon low-fat cream cheese

Lunch
1 fast-food hamburger (3 ounces ground beef on bun) with ketchup

1 fast-food tossed salad, with 1 tablespoon low-fat French dressing
1 low-fat chocolate frozen yogurt cone

Afternoon Snack
2 small oatmeal raisin cookies
1 cup skim milk

Dinner
Chicken-barley casserole: 2 ounces skinless chicken breast, ½ cup green peas, ½ cup carrot slices, 1 cup cooked barley
1 cup skim milk

1833 calories, 24% of calories (50.2 g total fat, 16.9 g saturated), 55% carbohydrate (258 g), 21% protein (98.2 g), 35.5 g fiber

DAY THREE

Breakfast
- 1 large waffle
- 1 tablespoon pancake syrup
- 1 cup skim milk

Morning Snack
- 1 banana
- 1 cup low-fat fruited yogurt

Lunch
- 2 slices cheese pizza (8 slices to a 15-inch pizza)

Salad: 1 cup chopped romaine lettuce, 10 cherry tomatoes, ¼ cup grated carrots, with 1 tablespoon low-fat salad dressing

Afternoon Snack
- ½ whole wheat bagel
- 1 tablespoon peanut butter

Dinner
- ½ roasted skinless chicken breast
- ½ cup brown rice
- 1 cup broccoli

1833 calories, 21% fat (43.4 g total fat, 13.6 g saturated), 58% carbohydrate (273 g), 21% protein (100 g), 22 g fiber

DAY FOUR

Breakfast
- 1 whole wheat English muffin, toasted, spread with ½ cup 1% low-fat cottage cheese
- 1 cup orange juice

Morning Snack
- 1 banana
- 1 cup low-fat fruited yogurt

Lunch
- Garbanzo bean salad: 1 cup garbanzo beans, ½ cup canned green beans, 5 quartered cherry tomatoes, 2 table-spoons low-fat Italian dressing; served on ½ cup chopped romaine lettuce
- 1 cup vegetable juice cocktail

Afternoon Snack
- 1 Pumpkin Muffin (page 260)
- 1 cup skim milk

Dinner
- 1 broiled pork loin chop
- 1 cup pasta
- 1 cup cauliflower/broccoli mix
- 4 ounces red wine

1797 calories, 15% fat (30.8 g total fat, 9 g saturated), 59% carbohydrate (274 g), 22% protein (99.4 g), 28.5 g fiber

DAY FIVE

Breakfast
- 1 cup high-fiber cereal, with 3 sliced figs and 1 cup skim milk

Morning Snack
- 1 ounce low-fat cheese
- 5 crackers

Lunch
- Roast beef sandwich: 2 ounces beef eye of round, 2 slices whole wheat bread, 3 leaves romaine lettuce, and 2 slices of tomato with mustard
- 1 cup low-fat fruited yogurt
- 2 kiwis

Afternoon Snack
  Fruited Cottage Cheese (page 12)

Dinner
  3 ounces grilled salmon

1 cup couscous (prepared with
  1 teaspoon olive oil per cup)
½ cup corn kernels
4 ounces wine

1781 calories, 18% fat (35.4 g total fat, 12 g saturated), 57% carbohydrate (257 g), 22% protein (99.2 g), 39 g fiber

Day Six

Breakfast
  1 whole wheat bagel
  1 tablespoon peanut butter
  2 teaspoons jam
  1 cup skim milk

Morning Snack
  1 banana

Lunch
  Chili: 1 cup red kidney beans,
    1 ounce lean ground beef,
    ½ cup canned stewed tomatoes,

½ cup celery, ½ cup onions,
  ¼ cup tomato paste
1 cup fruited yogurt

Afternoon Snack
  1 cup blueberries
  1 cup nonfat skim milk

Dinner
  2 ounces roasted turkey
  1 medium sweet potato
  1 teaspoon tub margarine
  ½ cup green peas
  1 pear

1825 calories, 14% fat (29.3 g total fat, 8.2 g saturated), 66% carbohydrate (316 g), 20% protein (94.7 g), 48 g fiber

Day Seven

Breakfast
  Oatmeal: Mix ½ cup oats with 1 cup
    skim milk. Microwave on high 2 min-
    utes; stir and microwave for 2 minutes
    more. Or combine in heavy pot and
    simmer 7 minutes.
  2 tablespoons raisins

Morning Snack
  1 cup low-fat fruited yogurt

Lunch
  Peanut butter and jelly sandwich:
    2 tablespoons peanut butter, 1 table-
    spoon jam, 2 slices whole wheat bread

Spinach salad: 1 cup chopped raw
  spinach, ½ tomato, 1 tablespoon
  Italian salad dressing

Afternoon Snack
  Power Shake (page 12)

Dinner
  Lentil soup: 1 cup cooked lentils,
    1 cup diced celery, 1 cup carrot slices,
    ½ cup chopped onion
  1 cup skim milk

1798 calories, 15% fat (30.8 g total fat, 7.6 g saturated), 67% carbohydrate (316 g), 18% protein (86.6 g), 40 g fiber

Fruited Cottage Cheese

SERVES 4

1 cup 1% low-fat cottage cheese

1 cup raspberries

1 cup light frozen whipped topping
   (such as Cool Whip)

1 cup canned mandarin oranges (drained)

1 package raspberry gelatin

Mix gelatin powder with frozen whipped topping until blended well; fold in fruit. Refrigerate 3 to 4 hours, or until mixture has jelled.

Per Serving: 119 calories, 9.5 g protein, 2.7 g fat, 7.6 g fiber.

Power Shake

SERVES 1

½ cup nonfat vanilla yogurt

1 banana

½ cup frozen strawberries

2 tablespoons wheat germ

Place all ingredients in blender and puree.

Per Serving: 295 calories, 12 g protein, 2.3 g fat, 5.6 g fiber.

Preventive Health

3

If you have a chronic illness, the title of this chapter might seem a little odd to you. But it's not! Whether you have multiple sclerosis, lupus, arthritis or some other chronic condition, it is important to protect yourself against heart disease, cancer and osteoporosis.

Unfortunately, many people who have a chronic illness don't get the routine preventive health checks that others do. That's because they and their doctors are so attentive to the care the chronic condition needs that routine things often go by the wayside. In some cases, these cancer and heart disease preventive maneuvers may be even more important in people with chronic disease. Due to medications needed to control the disease, a lack of activity because of the illness, or another reason, the risk of developing cancer, heart disease and osteoporosis may be even greater in some people with chronic disease than it is in people who don't have chronic illness. It is known, for example, that women with systemic lupus suffer earlier and more serious heart disease than do other women.

Preventing Heart Disease

Preventing heart disease begins with understanding the process by which arteries become clogged, choking off the life-giving blood supply to the heart.

Every cell of the body needs oxygen to function. After we breathe in oxygen from the air around us, it dissolves in the blood and is carried to each cell. The cells that form the heart, though, need oxygen for one additional, and critical, reason. The heart is a muscle whose main job is to collect blood as it returns from the body, replenish it with oxygen and then send it out to the body again. If the heart muscle cannot perform this function, no other cell in the body can receive oxygen. That's why it is so critically important to keep the blood vessels in the heart clear: they feed the heart with oxygen-rich blood and enable it to pump blood out to the rest of the body.

More than thirteen million Americans have some form of artery-clogging heart disease, also called atherosclerosis. Atherosclerosis can cause chest pain (angina pectoris), heart attack and/or stroke. According to the American Heart Association (AHA), an American suffers a heart attack every twenty seconds and one dies about every minute. On average, says the AHA, someone suffers a stroke every minute, and someone dies of one about every

3.5 minutes. Preventing artery-clogging heart disease remains key in stopping these two common killers.

How Blood Vessels Become Clogged

There are several risk factors for developing atherosclerosis, *many within your control*. Among the factors within your control are:

➤ HIGH BLOOD PRESSURE. When blood pressure remains high, the inside surfaces of the vessels take a beating. In response, the blood vessels can become scarred, which contributes to the artery-clogging process. Even if the blood vessels don't become scarred and clogged in response to high blood pressure, continued high blood pressure can increase stroke risk.

➤ BLOOD CHOLESTEROL LEVELS. This is one of the most important ways to prevent atherosclerosis.

➤ EXERCISE. Incorporating regular exercise, if you're able, can be a huge help in reducing blood pressure and cholesterol levels.

➤ SMOKING. Heart disease experts estimate that about one-fifth of deaths from heart disease are caused largely by smoking.

Because lowering blood pressure and cholesterol are such important and complicated points, let's take a closer look at each of them and what you can do to achieve healthier readings.

LOWERING BLOOD PRESSURE Some fifty million Americans, or one of every four adults, have high blood pressure, also called hypertension. It is the single most significant risk factor for stroke and a major contributor to heart disease and kidney failure. Blood pressure is expressed as one number over another. The top number is the systolic pressure, or the pressure on arteries as the heart beats, and the bottom number is the diastolic pressure, the pressure on arteries between beats of the heart. Someone is said to have hypertension when the blood pressure is at or above 140/90mm Hg (or millimeters of mercury, the unit for measuring blood pressure).

Eating too much salt is one risk factor for developing hypertension—this is especially true for people who take glucocorticosteroid medications and certain other drugs. There are two ways that the sodium part of salt raises blood pressure. First, all people experience some elevation in blood pressure with too much sodium. In addition, some people are called "salt sensitive." This means that they experience even greater increases in blood pressure when they eat too much salt. Fortunately, they also experience more significant drops in blood pressure when dietary sodium is reduced. Experts believe that about 30 to 50 percent of people who have high blood pressure are salt sensitive, as is a much smaller percentage of the general population.

To lower blood pressure, there are several dietary maneuvers you can make:

➤ Reduce dietary salt.

➤ Lose excess weight.

➤ Exercise regularly, to the best of your ability.

➤ Increase the fiber in your diet.

➤ Increase intake of these three minerals: potassium, magnesium and calcium.

Let's take a look at a couple of these in more detail; in particular, how other minerals work to lower blood pressure.

Potassium may exert more than one effect on the body to lower blood pressure. We know that potassium helps the body flush out extra fluid. When fluid levels are normal, or there is no fluid retention, there is a greater chance that blood pressure will be normal. Potassium may also help keep artery walls relaxed. Relaxed arterial walls do not contract as strongly as more "taut" or rigid arterial walls, which means the pressure created with each heartbeat is not as great. The result: blood pressure is lower.

Calcium helps lower blood pressure by much the same mechanism as potassium. It also helps keep artery walls from contracting too strongly.

Magnesium most likely helps keep blood pressure at a normal low reading by moderating the strength of the contractions on the artery walls.

LOWERING CHOLESTEROL READINGS If you've had your cholesterol checked lately, you may be confused about what you learned. Your doctor may have told you, for example, that your total cholesterol reading was okay, but that your *good* cholesterol was too low and your *bad* cholesterol too high. Just what does all of this mean?

Before explaining each of these cholesterol numbers—or fractions, as doctors officially call them—let's run through a few cholesterol basics. Because cholesterol is a fatty substance, it cannot travel in the blood as it is. That would be like trying to mix oil into water, which is impossible. To overcome this problem, the body packages cholesterol into balls that do dissolve in the watery contents of the blood. These microscopic balls are called lipoproteins: *lipo* means fat, and stands for the fatty cholesterol that forms the interior of the ball. The outside layer or shell of these microscopic balls is made up of proteins. Unlike cholesterol, protein does mix well with watery substances; stuffed into protein-coated balls, the cholesterol can then travel through the blood.

There are two main types of lipoprotein balls: low-density lipoprotein (LDL) and high-density lipoprotein (HDL). Shells light in weight have relatively less protein, leaving

---

Truly, no substance is as misunderstood as cholesterol. Here are two important myths clarified with the facts. **Myth 1: Cholesterol is synonymous with fat**. Cholesterol isn't fat at all, but a waxy lipid substance without calories. **Myth 2: All cholesterol is bad.** Contrary to popular belief, we couldn't live without cholesterol in our bodies— that's why our livers churn out about 1,000 milligrams each day of the waxy white stuff. Without it, we couldn't make new membranes or manufacture such vital hormones as estrogen and cortisol. It's only when there is too much cholesterol in the blood, or when the bad version (LDL) becomes particularly abundant that we get into trouble.

Cholesterol Myths

more room for cholesterol on the inside; these are the low-density lipoproteins. Shells with heavy protein coats have just a little cholesterol stuffed into their thick or dense protein coats; they are the high-density lipoproteins. As you can imagine, LDL cholesterol, with its heavy cholesterol load, is much more likely to lodge in arteries—that's why doctors like you to keep this cholesterol fraction on the low side.

For reasons not entirely understood by heart disease experts, HDL cholesterol helps shuttle excess fatty substances from the bloodstream and back to the liver, from where they can be excreted in waste products that leave the body. Hence, it is often called good cholesterol, and that's why it's desirable to have a high HDL cholesterol reading.

The situation is more complicated than that, though. As you may know, people with normal cholesterol readings can develop atherosclerosis. Also, some people with high cholesterol readings are more likely to suffer chest pain or a heart attack than others with equally high cholesterol readings. One of the reasons this may happen has to do with oxidation of the LDL cholesterol particles.

Manufacturing Dietary Fat

Mother Nature constructed fats, proteins and carbohydrates from the same basic building blocks of life: carbon, hydrogen and oxygen. What makes them fascinatingly different is the proportions and patterns of these elements. The major difference between fat and its lower calorie counterparts, protein and carbohydrates, is the amount of oxygen: there's far less oxygen in fat. Giving this a visual image, you might even say that the air has been squeezed out of fats, making them compact little calorie packages.

All dietary fats have a basic backbone, called a triglyceride. To it is attached a segment that distinguishes one type of fat from the other; that segment is called a fatty acid. Some fatty acids are saturated, some are monounsaturated and others are polyunsaturated. Saturation, as complicated as it sounds, describes how much hydrogen a fat contains. Saturated fatty acids are saturated with hydrogen, or contain as many as they possibly can. You know saturated fats by their appearance: they're solid at room temperature. No doubt you've seen the drippings from a roast beef after they've cooled: they become a solid white greasy mess; butter is also high in saturated fat, which makes it solid at room temperature. Fats missing just one pair of hydrogen atoms are monounsaturated and those missing more than a pair are called polyunsaturated. Both poly- and monounsaturated fats are liquid at room temperature.

If margarine is high in poly- and monounsaturated fats, why is it solid at room temperature? To make margarine hard, vegetable oil has been hydrogenated, or beefed up with hydrogen atoms—some of the missing hydrogen atoms have been added artificially. This process, which also keeps fats from becoming rancid at room temperature, creates something called transfatty acids. As you may have read, transfatty acids are thought to function somewhat like saturated fats, which means they raise the LDL cholesterol fraction. Some nutrition experts, in fact, think that transfatty acids are just as dangerous as saturated fats.

While all LDL cholesterol is prone to depositing on and blocking the inside of arteries, LDL cholesterol that is oxidized is even more likely to plop itself on the wall of an artery. Oxidation, or free radical oxidation, is caused by free radicals that wander wildly around the body. While the body needs oxygen to live, in the process of burning the oxygen for fuel, unwanted by-products are formed—the main one being oxygen free radicals. These free radicals become stray, high-energy particles that ricochet wildly, scarring and punching holes in cells and instigating all sorts of damage throughout the body. They can damage LDL cholesterol particles, turning them rancid. While LDL cholesterol is already bad enough on its own, rancid LDL becomes swollen. As a result, oxidized and swollen LDL particles are more likely to lodge in and block arteries.

While all of this cholesterol information is rather complicated, the most important things to remember are what you can do to lower your total and LDL cholesterol levels, prevent LDL cholesterol particles from becoming oxidized and raising your HDL reading—and thereby reduce your risk of having chest pain, a heart attack and a stroke.

What You Can Do to Lower Total and LDL Cholesterol

➤ Reduce total fat in the diet, especially saturated fat.

➤ Reduce dietary cholesterol.

➤ Achieve and maintain a healthy body weight.

➤ Incorporate a regular form of exercise into your lifestyle.

Let's take a closer look at each of these.

REDUCE FAT IN THE DIET While reducing total fat is important to keep blood cholesterol readings at healthy levels, reducing saturated fat is even more important. Saturated fat is the main dietary culprit in raising blood cholesterol levels—both total and LDL levels. Here's how. In addition to making cholesterol, our liver is responsible for filtering LDL cholesterol from the blood. It does this via thousands of proteins (called LDL receptors) that jut from the surface of each liver cell, snaring LDL particles as they flow by. Saturated fats somehow gum up the works, by either reducing the number of LDL receptors or impairing their efficiency. The result: LDL cholesterol isn't removed, and blood cholesterol levels (both total and the LDL fraction) rise.

On the other hand, unsaturated fats can lower blood cholesterol levels (in fact, they lower total cholesterol and LDL cholesterol while leaving healthfully high the HDL cholesterol fraction). That doesn't mean, however, that you should load up on monounsaturated fats such as olive and canola oils. Eating too much fat of any kind, even healthier fats, will cause blood cholesterol to rise. In addition, eating too much fat means you have a greater chance of gaining weight, which will also cause blood cholesterol levels to rise

Remember, though, that decreasing fat may not be easy at first. Beyond that fatty foods are among the most favorite and irresistible, and people are more likely to overconsume fats as opposed to carbohydrates and proteins for other reasons. Because fats are more calorically dense than carbohydrates and proteins—each gram of protein and carbohydrate has just four calories, while one gram of fat has nine calories—it takes far less volume to consume excessive amounts of fat calories. As a result, people often passively overeat fat calories, or eat them without even knowing they are exceeding a healthy limit of calorie intake. It's no wonder that fat is the most overconsumed nutrient, which, in turn, makes it the most potent dietary enemy.

The Three Types of Fat

Is there a healthier fat?

While an excessive amount of any fat quickly slides anyone into trouble, there are healthier types of fat that you should use when you must use some fat. The most important change you can make for heart health is to cut saturated fat as much as you can, substituting mono- or polyunsaturated fats wherever possible. For example, in recipes that call for butter for sautéing, use olive or canola oil, both high in monounsaturated fatty acids.

Should you choose poly over mono, or vice versa? The answer is a qualified *maybe.* Until the mid-1980s, heart and nutrition experts believed that poly was the healthiest fat, saying it lowered serum cholesterol when used in place of saturated fat. Monounsaturated fats, when substituted for saturated varieties, simply had no effect—or so they thought.

Advice changed in 1985 when a highly publicized study reported that monounsaturated fat was better than polys because it not only lowered LDL cholesterol as much as polys, but that it left alone the good HDL cholesterol fraction (at the time, researchers thought that polys lowered both LDLs and HDLs).

That's when olive oil became so popular—a notoriety that has lasted to today. But then in 1995 researchers at Stanford University Medical School analyzed fourteen studies comparing the effects of monos and polys on both HDL and LDL cholesterol fraction, reporting that both types of unsaturated fats have indistinguishably similar effects on HDL and LDL cholesterol, leaving alone the helpful HDLs and lowering the sinister LDLs.

While most heart disease experts support this latest analysis, some say there is another variable to factor into the equation. Test tube research shows that monounsaturated fats, but not polys, stop the process that turns bad cholesterol (LDL) rancid and even more dangerous: free radical induced oxidation.

What's the best heart-healthy advice for now? Cut down on all fat, limiting total fat to 20 to 30 percent of calories. Also, limit saturated fat to just 8 to 10 percent of calories—possibly even less if your blood cholesterol level is too high. As for what to do with polys and monos? Split the difference between the two of them, perhaps leaning a little heavier on monos. Practically speaking, that means using olive or canola whenever possible. While you should cut down on all forms of margarine, when you must use one, choose a soft tub margarine over stick varieties to limit transfatty acids.

If you remember nothing else from all of this, just remember this little rule when it comes to dietary fat: subtract and substitute, never add dietary fats. In other words, think about reducing all dietary fat and substituting unsaturated for saturated forms.

REDUCE DIETARY CHOLESTEROL Are you puzzled over why reducing dietary cholesterol wasn't listed before reducing total and saturated fat? Most people are. But it is true that reducing fat and saturated fat is far more important to lowering cholesterol levels than is reducing dietary cholesterol. In most people, dietary cholesterol is relatively insignificant to your final blood cholesterol reading, as a small proportion of it is absorbed—the rest just travels through the body unabsorbed. What most people don't realize is that the great majority of cholesterol is made in the body, in the liver, to be exact. In addition, it is a little appreciated fact that dietary cholesterol is distinct from blood cholesterol. In order to become blood cholesterol, dietary cholesterol has to be absorbed and processed. Since so little is absorbed, it is rarely an issue. Most people have an amazing ability to regulate cholesterol levels, employing one or all of the following strategies in response to eating a meal high in cholesterol (such as a plate of eggs):

➤ The body will turn down its cholesterol absorption machinery, thereby allowing a larger percentage of the dietary cholesterol to pass through the body unabsorbed.

➤ The liver will turn down its production of cholesterol, thereby producing less to account for the greater intake.

➤ The body will turn up the machinery that removes cholesterol from the bloodstream, and thus achieve fairly stable levels in the bloodstream.

Even though the body has an amazing ability to regulate how much cholesterol it makes, absorbs and excretes, it is still a good idea to limit dietary cholesterol intake to about 300 milligrams per day. For most people, that means that consuming around four eggs per week is perfectly fine. This is good news if you have a limited appetite or ability to cook, as eggs are easy to prepare and digest, as well as high in protein.

Preventing Cancer

According to the American Cancer Society (ACS), the World Cancer Research Fund (WCRF) and the American Institute for Cancer Research (AICR), about one-third of the 500,000 cancer deaths that occur in the United States each year are caused by inappropriate diet. Worldwide, that means that some three million to four million cases of cancer per year could be prevented by eating a better diet (which includes staying leaner).

What You Can Do

According to the ACS, WCRF and AICR, there are many dietary maneuvers you can make to slash your risk of cancer, including:

➤ Choose more plant foods than animal foods.

➤ Be physically active and maintain a healthy, lean body weight.

➤ Avoid alcohol.

CHOOSE MORE PLANT FOODS THAN ANIMAL FOODS For Americans, this is one of the most difficult pieces of advice to follow. We're so accustomed to planning our meals around meat, and then adding, almost as an afterthought, a vegetable and a starch. It is indeed the rare American who has more than one vegetable per meal (many have none), and also the rare American who eats whole grain foods (such as barley, whole wheat pasta, brown rice). But these simple acts can significantly reduce cancer risk.

A significant body of research provides very strong evidence that eating more fruits, vegetables and whole grains lowers cancer risk, particular cancers of the gastrointestinal and respiratory tracts. Additional strong evidence finds that eating lots of fruits and vegetables can lower colon cancer and lung cancer, with slightly weaker evidence that fruits and vegetables lower breast and prostate cancer. All plant foods are good bets when it comes to lowering cancer risk, with certain fruits and vegetables showing greater promise in fighting certain types of cancer. That's why it's so important to eat a variety of fruits and veggies.

Eat at least five to ten servings of fruits and veggies, where a serving is about one-half to one cup. This action alone may slash cancer risk by 20 percent. Produce should supply about 7 percent of your day's total calories.

Cancer experts believe that there are a multitude of factors in fruits and vegetables that may help lower cancer risk—no less than a hundred beneficial vitamins, minerals, fiber, phytochemicals and other substances. They don't yet know what combination is best, or which factors play the most significant role—just that nature knows best. Eating the widest variety possible is also key. One easy way to tell if you're eating enough variety is to assess the color of fruits and vegetables in your diet. The wider the rainbow range of colors, the more variety, and thus the health benefits, you gain. One other note: try to get five to ten different fruits and vegetables today and a different five tomorrow.

Eat at least seven servings of whole grains and legumes daily, where a serving is about one-half cup or one slice.

Whole grains may be the most underappreciated—as well as underconsumed— food in America. While most people eat plenty of white bread, white rice and white flour products, few people eat whole grain versions of these foods, anemic in both color and nutritional benefit. In addition to a good complement of vitamins, minerals and phytochemicals, grains also have lots of fiber, which seems to be an important aid in fighting cancer. But don't take the easy way out and opt for fiber supplements: research is most convincing that when consumed in real foods such as whole grains, fiber is the far more beneficial in fighting off cancer.

The same is true for legumes, or what you might call "beans," which includes pinto beans, lentils, soybeans and other dried beans. These foods are also high in certain nutrients, fiber and phytochemicals that add more cancer protection power.

Limit red meat to three ounces daily. Limiting red meat translates into limiting the amount of saturated fat we take in, which may be a help in reducing cancer risk. There may be other benefits in preventing cancer, say cancer experts. Instead of red meat, emphasize poultry, fish and vegetable sources of protein such as legumes (dried beans and peas).

Limit fats and oils to 15 to 30 percent of calories. An easy way to do this is to cut back on the amount of fat you add to your food—butter, margarine, sour cream, mayonnaise, salad dressing and oils. Also, cook with less oil—steaming, broiling and baking food.

➤ Plan a fresh fruit for each breakfast and lunch meal, and one piece for between meals—and try to make each of the three pieces different choices.

➤ Plan one vegetable for lunch (such as ready-to-eat baby carrots) and two for dinner. Try to plan three different colors of vegetables each day, as certain nutrients and phytochemicals tend to be found in vegetables of the same color.

➤ Plan a whole grain breakfast cereal for at least five days of the week—ideally all seven. For example, plan oatmeal, barley or brown rice with raisins for breakfast. If you love oatmeal, have it every day—it's a great whole grain.

➤ Plan some form of legume for at least five days of the week. You might sprinkle garbanzo beans (chick peas) on your salad two days during the week (it's a great protein source; see the recipes on pages 382–83, 393). Include a lentil or split pea soup at least one day during the week. Finally, try a stir-fry vegetable dish with tofu (made from soybeans); try the recipe on page 391. Remember, tofu takes on the flavor of what you cook it with, meaning you make it taste like your favorite flavors.

➤ Instead of white bread, switch the family to whole grain varieties, such as nine-grain bread and bagels.

BE PHYSICALLY ACTIVE AND MAINTAIN A HEALTHY BODY WEIGHT

I'm the first to admit that this is a tall order for people with chronic illness. But as much as you are able, try to burn a few more calories each week—whether it's taking a quiet, slow stroll each day; propelling yourself an extra distance in your wheelchair; swimming or doing gentle water exercises regularly; or following easy, isometric exercises every day. Remember, just because you can't go out for a daily jog doesn't mean you can't try to do some type of exercise.

If you're at a loss on how to exercise because of your unique health situation, ask your physician if you can consult a physical therapist once or twice for ideas that will work for you. It may be one of the best actions you've taken. In addition to cancer protection, keeping your body strong and active and your stamina as high as possible means a greater independence for you as well as less chance of falling.

As with the other advice you read above, scientists don't yet know why too little exercise and being too heavy raises cancer risk—they just know that an imbalance of caloric intake with energy output leads to overweight and an increased risk for cancers at several sites, including colon, rectum, prostate, endometrium, breast (in postmenopausal women) and kidney cancers.

AVOID ALCOHOL If you do drink, limit alcohol consumption. Are you confused about alcohol intake and its effect on your health? With good reason! You probably have heard some news reports about the benefits of alcohol, particularly red wine, in reducing the risk of heart disease, but have also heard that alcohol increases cancer risk. Actually both are true.

Cancer experts know that cancer risk begins to rise with any alcohol at all. If you do drink, limit alcohol to two drinks (for men and one for women) A drink is defined as 12 ounces of regular beer, 5 ounces of wine and 1.5 ounces of 90-proof distilled spirits.

Preventing Osteoporosis

If your chronic disease makes you inactive and unable to exercise properly, or if you take certain medications (see sidebar), you may be at increased risk for developing osteoporosis, a bone-thinning disease that causes bones to break with a simple sneeze. Even if you don't have any other risk factor, though, you are still at risk of developing osteoporosis, just by virtue of the fact that you grow older each year. And compared to men, women have a greatly exaggerated risk of osteoporosis. Let's take a look at why, but first let's develop a better understanding of this potentially devastating disease.

A Life-Changing Disease

At least twenty-five million Americans have dangerously thin bones, which causes 1.5 million fractures yearly, commonly of the hip, spine (vertebrae) and wrist. Hip fractures are the most devastating. Up to a quarter of people who suffer hip fracture and were living on their own before the fracture, lose their independence for at least a year, remaining in rehabilitative residential facilities. Hip fractures are also deadly in 20 percent who suffer them. Many people with osteoporosis become so disabled that they need help in dressing; some need so much assistance that they must enter a long-term care facility. *Maintaining strong bones is one of the most important ways to remain active and vibrant throughout life.*

Why Women Are at a Special Risk

Eighty percent of osteoporosis victims are female. A woman's unique hormonal milieu accounts for her increased risk. At menopause, a woman's body nearly stops producing estrogen, causing symptoms such as hot flashes and night sweats. Among other jobs, estrogen helps bones hold on to cells that make them strong (see "Understanding Your Bones," below). In the first five to seven years following menopause, estrogen loss can cause a woman to lose up to 20 percent of her bone mass—if she does nothing to prevent it. While the normal loss of estrogen at menopause is enough to cause osteoporosis, other factors further predispose women to osteoporosis, including:

➤ Lack of regular periods (called amenorrhea), which can be caused by excessive exercise or eating disorders such as anorexia. Just six months of amenorrhea can cause osteoporosis.

➤ Early menopause. Because an earlier menopause means that a woman loses her estrogen earlier, she has fewer years of estrogen-fueled bone protection. And that translates into more years when osteoporosis is more likely.

Understanding Your Bones

Think of your skeleton as the steel framework of a skyscraper: it supports body tissues just as steel upholds the building. But the bones forming your skeleton are distinctly different from lifeless metal. Like other tissues, those forming bones are very much alive and constantly changing in a process called remodeling. Just as skin continually sloughs off old cells and lays down new ones, old bone is constantly broken down and new bone tissue brought in.

Two types of cells are critical to this process. Osteoclasts break down and carry away old bone, while osteoblasts are new bone cells. In women, estrogen plays an important role in regulating osteoclast and osteoblast function. Before menopause, estrogen keeps osteoclasts and osteoblasts functioning in balance. As a result, new bone formation keeps up with the rate at which old bone is broken down (provided you meet the other needs of maintaining healthy bone; see below). But when estrogen production drops off at menopause, the balance is upset, and old bone is lost more quickly than the rate at which new bone can be brought in.

Surprisingly, bones grow well into the third decade of life. Although they stop growing in length during adolescence, bones bulk up, or increase in density, until somewhere between the ages of twenty-five and thirty-five. Getting enough calcium throughout this entire bone-building process is critically important. Calcium intake, in fact, is the single most important predictor of bone strength. After age thirty-five, the bones start giving up calcium, just as a normal part of the aging process. People who don't get enough calcium in their first thirty-five years of life arrive at this time with thinner bones. Translation: bones have less mass to give up, which means they approach the point of osteoporosis much sooner.

For women, arriving at menopause with the densest bones possible is especially critical. Estrogen-related bone loss accelerates into osteoporosis much sooner. According to surveys, the average American woman consumes less than half of the calcium she needs to

---

Medications That Can Cause Osteoporosis

When it comes to your bones, the most devastating medications are the glucocorticoid steroids, such as prednisone, methyl-prednisolone and solumedrol. More than any other, this class of medication, when used long-term, greatly increases the chances of developing osteoporosis.

Other medications that can cause osteoporosis include:

➤ Excessive thyroid replacement medication.

➤ Certain seizure medications.

build and maintain strong bones. Don't forget: calcium is critically important no matter what your age. After menopause, calcium is amazingly effective: taking at least 1,000 milligrams of calcium daily decreases postmenopausal bone loss by as much as 50 percent.

Bone health is also determined by other factors. After calcium and estrogen, two other factors play approximately equal roles in building stronger bones:

➤ Vitamin D. This fat-soluble vitamin is necessary to absorb and use calcium properly. Because the intestinal tract becomes less efficient as we age, vitamin D needs increase with age (see sidebar, page 25).

➤ Weight-bearing exercise. Exercise that makes you work against gravity, such as walking, tennis and dancing, helps bones bulk up in adolescence and also into old age. In one study, postmenopausal women who did weight-bearing exercise for twenty-two months bulked up spine bone density 6.1 percent; women who didn't lost bone.

When it comes to things that cause bones to thin, various factors play approximately equal roles:

➤ Cigarette smoking. Premenopausal women who smoke have 5 to 10 percent less bone mass when they reach menopause than women who don't smoke. Also, smoking can cause an earlier menopause—up to two years earlier—which translates into an earlier loss of bone and a greater risk of osteoporosis.

➤ Excessive use of alcohol.

➤ Being too thin.

➤ Prolonged use of certain medications (see sidebar, page 23).

The Power of Prevention

Fortunately, every one has within her control several excellent strategies for preventing osteoporosis. Whether you're fifteen, thirty-five or sixty, it's not too late to strengthen your bones and stop further bone loss—and reduce your risk of life-changing fractures. For every 10 percent loss of bone, the risk of spine fracture increases by 50 percent. If you can stop that bone loss, the risk of fractures does not compound so dramatically. More good news: while prevention remains the most powerful strategy, medical advances have yielded various methods to restore bone strength.

Your strategy to prevent osteoporosis should begin today, no matter what your age (see sidebar, page 25).

Although you should embark on a bone-strengthening plan without delay, you may want to determine just how strong your bones are. This may be especially important if you have increased risk factors for osteoporosis, such as the need to take glucocorticoid medications, an early menopause or a strong family history. One test remains the standard: the bone density test. This painless test detects low bone mass long before a regular X ray can. Doctors may also use the bone density test to monitor the progress of your osteoporosis treatment program.

If you're a woman concerned about bone health and are approaching, at, or after menopause, one of the most critical issues you face is estrogen replacement therapy. Whether you're just beginning menopause or long past, estrogen remains the most powerful osteoporosis prevention and treatment strategy. Granted, beginning estrogen therapy at the onset of menopause is most effective, preventing early, accelerated bone loss. This translates into reducing overall fracture risk by about 50 percent. But even if you begin estrogen replacement therapy after osteoporosis has already set in, you can still increase bone mass and reduce fracture risk.

To protect bones, estrogen therapy must be continued indefinitely. Women who still have a uterus are advised to take another hormone, progesterone, to reduce uterine cancer

At Every Age

- ➤ Perform weight-bearing exercise regularly (walking, dancing, tennis, jogging).

- ➤ Avoid smoking.

- ➤ Avoid excessive use of alcohol.

- ➤ Avoid being too thin.

- ➤ Ask your doctor about having a bone density test if you have special risk factors, including a strong family history, early menopause, or the need to take glucocorticoids or certain seizure medications.

Age 11 to 19

- ➤ Get enough calcium: 1,200 to 1,500 mg daily.

- ➤ Get enough vitamin D: 200 IU.

Age 20 to 24

- ➤ Get enough calcium: 1,200 to 1,500 mg daily.

- ➤ Get enough vitamin D: 400 IU.

Age 25 to Menopause

- ➤ Get enough calcium: 1,000 mg daily.

- ➤ Get enough vitamin D: 400 IU.

Beginning at Menopause

- ➤ Discuss estrogen replacement therapy with your doctor.

- ➤ If you cannot or choose not to take estrogen, discuss other treatment options with your doctor.

- ➤ Get enough calcium: 1,200 mg daily.

- ➤ Get enough vitamin D: 400 before age 60 and 800 IU after age 60.

- ➤ Continue weight-bearing exercise and also exercise that develops flexibility, coordination and cardiovascular fitness, all of which help reduce the risk of falling.

Osteoporosis Prevention: Age-Appropriate Strategies

A Special Note if You Take Glucocorticoids

If you must take glucocorticoids (cortisone, prednisone, Medrol) for any length of time, boosting calcium and vitamin D intake may help counter the bone-thinning tendency of this medication. Some evidence suggests that people on long-term glucocorticoids should take 2,000 mg of calcium and 800 IU of vitamin D daily. Check with your doctor to make sure there is no medical reason that you should not do so.

risk. Many women object, however, to the associated monthly bleeding. Although it is unpleasant, a woman should weigh the great advantages of estrogen therapy, not only for her bones, but also for the powerful protection it affords against coronary artery disease.

For women who cannot or will not take estrogen, there are several other options. Ask your physician about the following choices, which may or may not be appropriate for you and your unique medical condition:

➤ ESTROGEN DERIVATIVES

➤ VITAMIN D DERIVITIVES

➤ BIPHOSPHATES

Shopping Made Easier

4

The first time I entered the grocery store in a wheelchair was memorable.

My children, ages nine and fifteen at the time, accompanied me to help me retrieve items from shelves I couldn't reach and also to push the grocery cart. The first stop should have been the produce section, where I tend to linger the longest and that has the foods that generally fill my cart at least halfway to the top. The kids, however, had different plans!

"We're just going to skip the produce, Mom, except for the bananas," said Susie (the fifteen-year-old), "and you can't really do much about it." She and her brother delighted in commandeering the grocery cart, and heading for the snack aisle, alias the junk food section. I realized that letting them get away with purchasing sugar-coated cereal, chips, sticky fruit snacks (that really didn't have much fruit in them) and ice cream, to the exclusion of produce, wasn't the end of the world, and let them enjoy their little joy ride through the grocery store.

But the event gave me a newfound understanding of how difficult it is for people who are dependent on wheelchairs, crutches or walkers to get through the grocery store—*in charge* and able to gather independently the healthy food that is so important to helping them achieve the nutrition advantage to fight their disease and boost their energy.

Here are some suggestions to make shopping easier:

➤ Choose the right store.

➤ Choose the right time.

➤ Enlist some help.

➤ Make every trip count, shopping for several days.

If shopping is too hard, consider two alternatives:

➤ Find a grocery store with telephone service.

➤ Find someone who can shop for you.

Choose the Right Store

Many grocery stores make shopping easier for people who have limited energy or mobility. Choose your store based on:

- The availability of handicapped parking. Is the handicapped parking area close enough to the store? Is the handicapped parking area well shoveled and deiced in the wintertime?

- The presence of electric carts. My favorite grocery store has several electric carts, allowing disabled customers to sit down and "drive" through the grocery store. Well designed, these carts are an appropriate height so that items on the higher shelves are accessible. The basket for groceries is within easy reach, both in terms of placing items in it and unloading items from it.

- Is the size of the store manageable for you? While a discount market may save you a few grocery pennies, the size of many of these markets is so monstrous that it is difficult for someone with limited energy and/or mobility to get through the store.

- Does the grocery store have grocery packers? In many grocery stores, customers are expected to pack their own groceries. This is difficult for people with limited mobility.

- Similarly, does the grocery store have someone to load your groceries into your car, and without too much trouble? While some grocery stores offer loading services, it is often difficult to find someone to help you—many times, you just end up loading the groceries yourself after a futile search for help.

- Does the grocery store have a salad bar? Standing and preparing salad is a time- and energy-consuming job. Choosing fresh salad for the two to three days following your trip to the market is a tremendous help in saving energy and eating healthfully. It costs a bit more, but the trade-off is worth it.

- Does the grocery store have other convenience items that will save you a trip to another store? For example, is there a greeting card section and/or enough drugstore items?

Once you choose the market that best suits your needs, stick with it. After learning where things are in one particular grocery store, you'll save an incredible amount of energy (and time) by shopping there on a regular basis. Although you may save a little bit by "shopping the specials" at several grocery stores, you may use up so much energy that it may not be worth it. Instead, buy items on special at the market where you shop, gearing your shopping list around what is on special there.

Choose the Right Time

You'll want to time your trip to the grocery store according to three factors; specifically:

- When your energy and mobility are best. Do you generally feel most energetic during the morning hours? Whenever it is, seize the opportunity and shop at that time of the day.

➤ When the grocery store is not crowded. Try to avoid shopping in the after-work hours, especially between 5 and 7 P.M. These are often the busiest hours in grocery stores. While weekend shopping may be necessary because that's when you have help, try to shop early or late in the day. These are the least busy hours on the weekend. If you shop late on Sunday, though, be aware that the produce is often least abundant at this time. Similarly, the fish and meat are also the least fresh.

➤ When someone can help you unload the car, unpack the groceries and put the items away. While the first two factors are critical to timing your trip to the grocery store, so is this one. If you need help in unloading the car and putting away items, make sure you time your trip accordingly.

Other Tips

Shop with a List

Arriving at the grocery store with a plan is critical to saving energy and getting through the store quickly. The basis for your plan should be your weekly menu. After you plan your menu, determine what items you need from the grocery store. Shopping with a list not only gets you through the store faster, but also saves you repeated trips to the grocery store during the week. Another payoff: shopping with a list generally saves you money, as you're less likely to buy impulse items.

As you prepare your grocery list, organize it by section of the grocery store. For instance, put all of the fresh produce items under one column; the yogurt, margarine, milk, cheese and other dairy items under another column, and so forth.

If you're thinking that preparing a menu and shopping list is time consuming, you're right. But being so organized saves you critical time and energy, and is well worth the time you spend on it. Incidentally, planning a menu and shopping list generally turns you into a healthier eater, yet another reason to take the time to do it. Because it is time consuming, you might want to compose your menu and shopping list the day before you shop.

Choose the Right Size

Faced with the option of purchasing one 2-pound can or two 1-pound cans of kidney beans for the chili on your weekly menu, consider choosing two of the smaller cans. They'll be easier to load into the cart, and then unload and pack away in the cabinets when you arrive home. In addition, they're less strain on tired, sore hands, wrists and elbows. Although you may pay a few more pennies, you'll be saving energy and discomfort now and down the line. The same is true for large versus small boxes of laundry detergent and dishwasher soap: although you'll save a few cents with the larger size, the fatigue and discomfort that occurs with hauling, storing and then using them may not be worth it.

Choose Healthy Convenience Foods

Whether you are tight on time or limited on energy and strength, one of the keys to eating healthy is stocking your kitchen with healthy convenience foods. And that means redefining convenience foods.

Like most Americans, you think of convenience foods as prepared, complete frozen dinners or a complete meal in a can, such as chili. But many of these convenience items are exceptionally high in fat and sodium. While an occasional high-sodium/high-fat meal is okay, a regular diet of these types of food leads to weight gain and possibly to problems with blood pressure and blood cholesterol levels.

Instead, think of convenience items in a new light, such as:

➤ Cleaned and sliced vegetables and prepared salad from the produce section. Concerned that these foods are lower in nutrients? Don't be. Remember that they are far healthier than chips, cookies and other such convenience items.

➤ Cleaned and cut fruit from the produce section. This is an especially great idea during melon season—cutting and cleaning melons is a particularly difficult task.

➤ Sliced and shredded cheese from the dairy section. If you're making lasagna or another recipe that calls for shredded cheese, you might skip it if you're low on energy. But using already shredded cheese makes the job a snap. You can freeze the extra for several weeks.

➤ Frozen vegetables. If cleaning broccoli, cauliflower, green beans or other vegetables is too difficult for you, don't hesitate to buy the frozen versions. In many cases, they are even more nutritious than the fresh varieties. That's because they are picked at their peak of freshness (which means they were at their peak of nutritional goodness, too) and then flash frozen to preserve that nutritional goodness. Don't forget to pick up frozen chopped green peppers, a great addition to many recipes. Also, spend a few minutes in the frozen produce section to study the many varieties of vegetable medleys now available: these make fabulous and very easy additions to stir-fries, casseroles and many other recipes. Just a reminder: choose those without added sauces, as most of those sauces are exceptionally high in salt and fat.

➤ Meat cut into strips or chunks for stir-fry. I love these packaged meats, and always keep chicken, beef and pork chunks on hand for easy, fast stir-fry meals.

➤ Individual yogurts in the dairy section. Change the way you think about snack foods, making yogurts and other healthy foods your prepared snack foods instead of chips and cookies—the latter two of which are generally very high in salt and fat.

Choose Healthy Microwavable Foods

There will be times when you'll have to depend on prepared foods. Although you don't want to make a steady diet of them, you can choose fairly healthy frozen meals that just require a zap in the microwave. Incidentally, if you have the option of microwaving or baking (in a traditional oven) your frozen meal, always opt for the microwave: you'll preserve more nutrients. Here are some guidelines for choosing healthy microwavable meals:

1. Check the front label to eyeball the vegetable portion, which is often the limiting factor on dinners that are otherwise healthy. The picture is your only clue (although you're looking for at least one-half cup of vegetables, the label doesn't include this information), so it should suggest a decent-sized vegetable portion. In sampling many frozen meals, I found the label pictures fairly representative of what's inside.

2. Turn to the "Nutrition Facts" label on the back, checking for the following:

    ➤ SERVING SIZE: Listed directly under the "Nutrition Facts" heading, you'll find one or two facts. If the package is intended as one serving, just "Serving Size: 1 meal or 1 package" is listed. If the package is meant for multiple servings, you'll find the measured "Serving size" and "Servings per container." It's important to understand serving size, as the nutrition information that follows is for just one serving. If, for example a package contains two servings, and you eat the whole thing, double figures to tally what you've really eaten.

    ➤ CALORIES: Choose a meal with just enough calories: not too many but not so few that you're rummaging in the refrigerator an hour later. As a general rule of thumb, look for frozen meals with 300 to 600 total calories. Whatever your size or age, choose a meal containing no more than one-third of your daily calorie allotment; better to aim 80 to 150 calories under this one-third figure so that you have calories left for a glass of nonfat milk and a salad or fruit to round out the frozen dinner.

    ➤ FAT: Food labels describe fat content in so many ways that you're often confused. As a quick guide, choose a meal with no more than 20 fat grams total, preferably 15 fat grams (especially if you're eating on the lighter side).

    ➤ SODIUM: As a general rule, don't exceed 750 milligrams per serving, and preferably not more than 500 milligrams (while an occasional meal exceeding this, 1,000 milligrams or so, is just fine for most people with normal blood pressure and not on medications, it's pretty high for people on medications that affect blood pressure or who have high blood pressure). Convenience foods such as frozen meals are among the highest contributors to sodium intake. While 750 milligrams seems high, it's okay to use up such a large chunk of your sodium allotment in one fell swoop if you eat fewer convenience foods during the rest of the day, even if you're following a moderately sodium restricted diet for hypertension or for another reason. If you have a health condition that requires quite stringent sodium restriction, follow those guidelines instead.

    ➤ PROTEIN: As a quick rule of thumb, choose a dinner with at least 15 grams of protein. Most adults (and even most children) don't need to worry about protein content, simply because it's the nutrient we commonly get too much of (average adult intakes are around 100 grams; we need only 45 to 60 grams of protein daily).

Grocery Packing

Ask the person who packs your groceries to pack all perishable items in the same bags, and all the frozen items together. I generally ask them to put these refrigerator and freezer items in the plastic bags with handles, and the nonperishable items in paper bags. This way, if I am tired when I get home, I can just pop the bags with the freezer items right into the freezer without unpacking them, and then put them away properly later or even the next day when I'm not so tired. I can easily sit on a chair in front of the refrigerator and unpack the refrigerator items into their appropriate compartments with little effort. If I'm too tired, I can just leave the nonperishable items on the kitchen counters until later.

Incidentally, ask the packer to pack all the bags lightly. This is easier on your joints (if you have arthritis) and on your energy, which is important for everyone.

Telephone Service

If grocery shopping is just out of the question for you, call the grocery store chains in your area and ask if they have a home delivery service. Many do, and they even have a home shopping list. You can call in your order one day and have it delivered later that day or the next day. Generally, there is a charge associated with this service, but it is often well worth it if you don't have the ability to shop.

Pantry and Freezer Items

One of my greatest challenges is having foods on hand to put together a meal when my energy is limited and I'm not able to get to the grocery store for several days. Over the years, fortunately, I've learned what items I need to keep in stock that make meal preparation possible when I don't have fresh, perishable items *and* my energy is especially limited.

Canned Items

I tend to skip canned vegetables, because they are too high in salt and I also find their taste far inferior to fresh or frozen. However, many canned items are perfectly fine and very helpful, including:

➤ CANNED FRUITS: Canned in fruit juice when possible, canned fruits are excellent pantry items to keep on hand for desserts or as additions to gelatin dishes.

➤ CANNED SOUPS: If you have to watch your salt intake, canned soups may not work well into your eating plan. However, used in casseroles or creamed dishes, where you'll get a much smaller proportion, canned soups can make meal preparation a real breeze.

➤ LOWER SODIUM CANNED SOUPS: If you read labels carefully, you can find canned soups with acceptable sodium levels. Look for one with 500 milligrams of sodium (or less) per serving—just make sure you understand what the serving size is.

➤ CANNED BEANS: There are many varieties, such as kidney beans, pinto beans, white beans (such as navy) and garbanzo beans. Although these are generally are moderately high in salt, you can drain and rinse them to substantially lower the salt level. These make easy, instant additions to soups, stews, casseroles and salads.

Other Pantry Items

Additional staples to keep in your pantry include:

➤ PASTA: Keep several varieties of pasta on hand, choosing what your family likes best and what you'll use in casseroles or as a side dish.

➤ RICE: Opt for brown rice as much as possible. You'll be pleasantly surprised to find that brown rice isn't strong tasting; its light, slightly nutty flavor is gentle and interesting, and the rice is more nutritious.

➤ VINEGARS: Keep several varieties of vinegar on hand to make interesting recipes and salad dressings. Balsamic vinegar and raspberry wine vinegar, for example, are among my favorites and those I use most often. If you haven't used balsamic vinegar, do give it a try. It's a lot milder than most vinegars, and interesting in flavor.

Frozen Meat

Keeping a good supply of frozen meats allows you to put together a meal in no time at all. Try to keep enough meat on hand for five meals. Here are some excellent choices to keep on hand; I've chosen them because they're the cuts lowest in fat (see table, page 34):

➤ PORK: tenderloin, sirloin, center loin. Try to keep some on hand in regular cuts or cut for stir-fry. Although you may think pork is too high in fat, you'll see in the chart below that when chosen properly, pork is just as low fat as lean beef, and it's even close to chicken in terms of fat content.

➤ BEEF: tenderloin, top sirloin, sirloin strip steak, top round, eye of round, round tip, flank steak. Again, keep some on hand as roasts, some as small steaks and some cut for stir-fry or stew.

Frozen Vegetables

Browse through the frozen vegetables section, and choose several varieties that you and your family like. A good rule of thumb is to have enough on hand for at least an entire week. For each family member, you'll need one cup of frozen vegetables per dinner meal.

Lean Cuts of Meat*

Cut of Meat	Calories	Protein (g)	Total Fat (g)	Saturated Fat (g)	Cholesterol (mg)
Pork					
Tenderloin	159	26	5.4	1.9	80
Sirloin	181	24	8.6	3	72
Center loin	199	22	11.5	3.2	68
Beef					
Tenderloin	179	24	8.5	3	71
Top sirloin	166	26	6	2.4	76
Strip steak	176	24	8	3	65
Top round	153	27	4.2	1.4	72
Eye of round	149	25	4.9	1.8	59
Round tip	157	24	5.9	2	69
Flank steak	176	23	8.6	3.7	57

Nutrition information, per 3-ounce serving of cooked meat (trimmed of fat)

Another way to figure is a quarter pound of frozen vegetables per person per dinner meal. For example, a one-pound of bag of frozen broccoli stir-fry vegetable medley would serve four people at one meal. If you think this is more than you generally eat—you're definitely right. But splitting a one-pound bag of frozen veggies between four people at a meal is what everyone should be eating.

Creating an Energy-Saving Kitchen

5

How long has it been since you enjoyed being in your kitchen? Since you whipped up something for yourself or for your family to enjoy?

If you're like a lot of people with chronic illness, you probably look at your kitchen and sigh with fatigue at the thought of cooking. But it's time to look through different eyes. You can reclaim your kitchen, and make it user-friendly, no matter how great your disability. The information in this chapter will help you do that.

There are several ways to make your kitchen user-friendly, all of which fall into two major categories:

➤ Stock the kitchen with energy-saving items.

➤ Create a convenient work space.

Stock the Kitchen

Although I acknowledge that your budget may be limited, I am firmly convinced that equipping your kitchen with the right tools considerably extends your energy and capabilities and allows you to prepare the nutritious meals you need with greater ease. Here are some of the items that I find absolutely essential, and why. Remember, having the simplest version, which is also the most inexpensive style, is worlds better than not having it at all.

Microwave. Having a microwave opens up worlds of possibilities in your kitchen. You can cook a whole meal on the dinner plates on which you'll serve the food, eliminating pots, pans and serving platters—and the task of washing them. In addition, a microwave makes it easier for you to warm up leftovers and the extra batches of food you cook up and freeze when you feel better and have more energy.

Toaster oven. Although you can use the broiler in your oven for everything you can use the toaster oven for, the toaster oven has a distinct advantage. Whether you're feeling weak, or you are unsteady on your feet, or are in a wheelchair and have a tough time reaching inside the oven, the toaster oven is much easier to use. I remember trying to broil a hamburger for my husband after I had just spent several weeks in bed with a flare-up of my disease. Very weak and shaky (because of the high-dose cortisone medication), I brushed my hand against the side of the oven as I pushed the broiler pan back in after turning his hamburger, suffering a second-degree burn on the back of my hand. Because of all the medication I was taking, the burn took several weeks to heal and required fastidious care. If I'd had a toaster oven, I probably would have avoided the burn. I highly recommend the toaster oven over a regular toaster, as the toaster oven will double as an ordinary toaster.

Food processor. I would be lost without my food processor. Chopping, grating, slicing and mincing are very difficult for people with arthritis, and also challenging for people with energy limited by disease. The food processor, though, makes these common kitchen tasks accessible to just about anyone. This piece of equipment allows me to chop up ingredients in just seconds, and extend my energy many times over. As a result, I can prepare fairly complicated (and energy-consuming) recipes with relative ease. I can also use chopped or minced fresh onions for any recipe. I have tried to use dried onions when energy is limited, but that is one ingredient that is just not acceptable, at least to my taste buds. If I had to choose between a food processor and a blender, the food processor would win hands down. While you can use a food processor for many jobs a blender can do, the reverse isn't as true.

An extra tip: rinse the food processor (and the blade) immediately after using it—you'll avoid a dried-on mess that requires lots of cleanup care later on.

Food miniprocessor. Although it seems like an optional piece of equipment, a food miniprocessor is an essential. It's great for those small chopping jobs—such as chopping an onion or mincing garlic—that are too small for a regular food processor but too large for tired and/or sore hands. It's well worth the $25 to $35 it costs.

Nonstick cookware. Investing in three high-quality nonstick pans is a must for at least two reasons. First, nonstick pans allow you to prepare healthy, low-fat meals much more easily. Another great reason: good quality nonstick pans make cleanup a breeze. Purchase a small one, appropriate for steaming two eggs; a medium one, just right for cooking two to three grilled cheese sandwiches; and a large one, the size that could can hold four to six chicken breasts. When you're shopping for nonstick cookware, lift the ones you are considering purchasing, remembering that they'll be heavier with food in them. When you purchase covers, opt for the glass variety. They allow you to see how things are progressing without having to continually lift the lid.

Nonstick cookie tins and pans. If you like to bake anything at all, you know well how much work it is to scrub muffin tins and/or cookie sheets if they're not nonstick. Put the few extra pennies into nonstick baking ware—it will be well worth it.

KitchenAid mixer. Although I'm not in the habit of using brand names, this piece of equipment (a free-standing mixer) is so fabulous, it's hard not to. I consider this another kitchen essential. Even when I'm dead tired, I can mix up a cake, brownies or quick bread with very little effort. Because it's so easy to use and to clean up, I also use the mixer for mashed potatoes. Even the large mixing bowl fits in the dishwasher, making cleanup especially easy.

As with all electric appliances, select those with levers or push buttons so that operation is easy if you have tired, sore hands.

Knives in a knife block. Leaving commonly used kitchen items such as knives out on the counter and readily accessible is a great idea. The knife block accomplishes this; it also helps keep knives sharp, which makes your cutting jobs easier.

Ergometric knives. These knives have specially designed handles that allow you to cut with your wrist in a neutral position (in other words, without placing a strain on the wrist). You'll find them in many sizes and styles.

Slow cooker such as a Crock Pot. Whether your time in the kitchen is limited because of low energy or a busy schedule, you should invest in a slow cooker. You can cook a whole dinner (without having to continually check it) by placing all the ingredients in it early in the day when your energy is highest.

Mixing bowls with nonskid bottoms. Whether you're tossing a salad or mixing cookies, you shouldn't be without bowls with nonskid bottoms (there's a permanently attached rubber ring on the bottom of the bowl). They allow you to keep your hands free to accomplish your mixing job. If you can't find them, purchase a rubber-type material called dycem (see catalog resources, page 403 for availability), or suction cups to hold bowls and pans in place while you use both hands to stir or mix, or one hand to steady yourself. Alternatively, place the mixing bowl on a wet dishcloth to hold it in place while you mix. Yet another possibility: secure the bowl in place by putting it in a kitchen drawer.

Incidentally, avoid ceramic bowls, opting instead for plastic or aluminum varieties—they're much lighter and require less of your energy.

Electric can opener with an electric knife sharpener feature. Invest in a better model that works smoothly and with very little of your effort.

Jar opener. Install a jar opener under one of your hanging kitchen cabinets. This wonderful gadget, which grips the lid of the jar as you use both hands to turn the jar itself, allows you to open jars even if you are weak or have arthritic hands.

Kitchen stools. Depending on the size of your kitchen and your ability to move things around, purchase one or two kitchen stools, placing one in front of the kitchen sink and one by the kitchen counter where you'll accomplish most of your food preparation. If your kitchen is smaller and/or you don't have trouble moving the stool around, you may need just one. Choose a height that is comfortable for you, and also one that is lightweight. Instead of standing at the sink, you can sit down to wash dishes; the same is true for food preparation.

Rolling cart. Unless your kitchen is quite small, a rolling cart is a tremendous help in food preparation, serving and cleanup; it's a great addition to parties and cookouts. Choose one with a "lip" all around the shelves, which helps prevent things from slipping off. At mealtime, make one trip to the refrigerator and pantry, loading up the cart with everything you'll need to prepare that meal. This not only saves you steps if you can walk on your own, but it also allows you to move things around the kitchen even if you use a wheelchair, walker, crutches or a cane.

Cutting board with nails. To hold food to be cut, leaving both hands for the knife (or one hand to steady yourself). Also, place dycem (rubbery material) under the cutting board to hold it in place. This is especially helpful if you're using the cutting board from a sitting position (such as from a wheelchair) and don't have the normal leverage.

Metal pot supports. These wonderful gadgets hold pots on the burners, freeing both hands for stirring and mixing, and saving your energy.

Door handle loops. To place on your cabinet and refrigerator handles, through which you can slip your wrist or forearm to ease doors open.

Dishwasher. This, too, is a kitchen essential, if you have the room for it. Not only does a dishwasher save you energy, but it also sterilizes the dishes, an important detail for the chronically ill, whose immunity is often low.

Create a Convenient Kitchen

Many of the energy-eating tasks of food preparation are just taking out and putting away food preparation tools. You can eliminate these energy-consuming tasks—saving your energy for the more fun parts of food preparation—by setting up a convenient kitchen.

The key to this is in creating a food preparation area fully equipped with the tools you use most often within easy reach.

First, choose an area of the kitchen that is close to the sink and the stove; ideally, you have a section of counter that stands between the two. Designate this as your food preparation area. Purchase three to four ceramic flowerpots (in a pretty design to match your kitchen decor), and fill them with the utensils you use most: measuring spoons, spatulas, mixing spoons, whisks. Set up your utensil-holding flowerpots there, as well as your wooden knife block.

Also set up your food processor, KitchenAid (free-standing) mixer, can opener and cutting board. Even though I don't like clutter, I find that if I put these items away, I am more likely, on low-energy days, to skip a recipe that requires their use. If you'd like, cover your appliances with pretty fabric covers that match the ceramic flowerpots. In the drawers and cabinets in this location, place all items you use in food preparation: measuring cups, spices, mixing bowls, strainers, and so on. Finally, place one of your kitchen stools at this location.

If there's room, also place canisters with sugar and flour at this location. Again, although the clutter may bother you, remember the chore it can be to lift out large containers, or even just the bag, of flour and sugar. Make sure the canisters you choose allow you to scoop out what you need without having to lift the container.

Short on room? This is where your rolling cart comes in handy for another task: if you need more counter space during food preparation, roll the cart over to your work area.

Other Tips

Timing kitchen tasks appropriately can also save you precious energy. If you have a dishwasher, try to unload it at mealtime, transferring the plates, cups, bowls and eating utensils you need for that meal right to the table. This way, you save the energy required to put the dishes away and then take them out again at mealtime.

Other ways to save energy in the kitchen and increase the tasks you can do there if your mobility is limited include:

➤ Keep a bent coat hanger in the kitchen, and use it to pull out oven shelves.

➤ When you have to fill large pots with water (such as for cooking pasta), place them on the counter between the sink and the stove. Use the spray hose to add the water and then slide the pot over to the burner. This is a tremendous energy saver. (If this setup doesn't work in your kitchen, place the empty pot on the burner and then fill with water using smaller containers.)

➤ If your hands are sore or unsteady and you have to peel vegetables, place the vegetables on a cutting board, and hold them in place with the palm of your nondominant hand. Then, use the peeler, turning the vegetable as necessary.

➤ Line baking dishes and broiler pans with aluminum foil, which you can toss. Cleanup is incredibly easy.

➤ Choose cookware in which you can mix food, bake, serve and even freeze. Having one container from start to finish saves cleanup time and energy.

➤ As often as possible, cook a double or triple batch of what you're preparing and freeze the extras. This way, you can always have a few meals in the freezer for when you don't feel well.

➤ Find one-pot meals that you and your family love. This makes cooking, serving and cleanup many times easier. The great majority of recipes in this book are one-pot meals, and exceptionally delicious.

Entertaining:
Yes, It Is Possible!

6

Like many people with a chronic disease, you probably haven't tried to entertain for quite some time. Dust off the ice bucket and pull out the hors d'oeuvre tray, because you *can* entertain. I firmly believe that anyone can entertain, even those who depend on a wheelchair or a walker. It's such a boost to your self-esteem and sense of normalcy to entertain family, friends and colleagues in the warmth of your own home.

No doubt you remember trying to entertain in the past. By the time you cleaned the house, polished the sliver and set the table, you couldn't even imagine planning the menu, let alone shopping or cooking the meal. You'd like to crawl into bed just thinking about the formidable jobs typically associated with serving a meal to guests.

I remember the first dinner party I tried after my diagnosis of lupus. Before my diagnosis, entertaining a crowd for dinner had been not only great fun, but terribly easy. Our home had always been the gathering place for friends, and we always loved it. But the fatigue and pain of living with lupus had brought all that to a grinding halt. It was six years before I finally got up the nerve to entertain again. And I did it all wrong that first time.

It was just fifteen minutes before ten guests would arrive for dinner. I couldn't get my shoes onto my swollen, painful feet. I'd been racing around since sunrise, scrubbing the bathrooms, cooking the entire meal and cleaning a colossal mess in the kitchen—to say nothing of all the grocery shopping and housecleaning I'd done the day before. But I couldn't cancel the party at the eleventh hour. I applied a bit more blush to hide my sallow cheeks, shoved my feet into my moccasins and eased myself down the steps to the beckoning doorbell.

That party was a social success but a medical disaster. I had failed to plan ahead, leaving the bulk of the work for the forty-eight hours before the party. I hadn't practiced my "rule of optimal health": resting frequently and listening to my body's barometer. I pushed my health to the brink, teetering on the edge of a serious flare, requiring strict rest for several days to recover.

As I soaked in a hot bath, I was convinced there was still a way I could entertain, perfect health or not. I wouldn't believe that I was out of the entertaining league, and I wasn't. By using these ideas, entertaining was not only possible, but much easier:

➔ Time your party to your health.

➔ Revise your standards, accepting help from people who offer to bring a salad or dessert, and using disposable items whenever possible.

➔ Keep the menu simple, choosing items that you can make ahead and freeze or store.

➔ Organize yourself with a countdown calendar.

➔ Choose clothes to match your most comfortable shoes.

➔ Whenever possible, hire a helping hand.

➔ Be prepared to leave the mess overnight.

Time Your Party to Your Health

Choose the season, as well as the day and time of day, when your health is generally best. During the summer and fall, for example, you may be less likely to suffer a cold or other virus that is particularly taxing for you. Or perhaps it is during the summer that your arthritis calms down the most. If you work outside the home, maybe Saturday afternoon is the time when you're most rested and able to take on a project like entertaining (and still have another day to rest and recuperate). Or, perhaps a Sunday brunch is the best time for you to entertain friends—it's still relatively early in the day when your energy is at a peak. Don't forget to take into account when family or friends are available to help you put things together and take them apart—always time your event around their ability to help, too.

Revise Your Standards

Before my diagnosis, I never imagined using disposable plates or cups for guests, or even paper napkins. All through my twenties, I was an old-fashioned hostess, polishing the crystal, china and silver for every guest who came into my home. I couldn't imagine having company without washing the light fixtures, cleaning the garage, dusting the blinds and scrubbing the kitchen floor just hours before they came. But by relaxing my standards for all aspects of entertaining, I can enjoy having family and friends in my home more often, and don't suffer the consequences of wearing myself out each time I entertain.

Here are some of the important ways to revise your standards and save precious energy:

➔ Consider using disposable items, at least in some aspect of entertaining. The bigger the crowd, the more sense it makes to choose disposable items. Chronic illness or not, many people use disposable items when entertaining a crowd, so don't hesitate to make this choice. If you want to use your china and crystal, something I love to do, then use disposable items for hors d'oeuvres, beverages and dessert. If I decide to use my china and crystal, I compromise by relaxing with the mess for a day or two after the party as I take my time washing and putting away a few pieces at a time.

➤ Don't insist on serving something that must be cooked fresh just before the guests arrive, or after they gather. Instead, choose menu items that can be prepared ahead, frozen, or at least refrigerated, and reheated.

➤ Accept the offers of your guests to bring an appetizer, salad beverage or dessert. Many guests, in fact, feel better if they can bring something.

➤ Don't worry about a little dust here or the odd piece of postvacuuming lint there. Clean your house a couple of days ahead (saving a *few* last-minute jobs for the day of the party), and then don't worry about the little bit of dust and dirt that accumulates. If you can afford it, hire a cleaning service, scheduling them for the morning of your party.

Countdown Calendar

Four weeks ahead. Choose your date and your guests. How many can you comfortably entertain in your home, given your physical limitations? If writing is a problem for you, extend your invitations by phone.

Two weeks ahead. Plan your menu and how you will serve, choosing a menu that allows you to do as much ahead as possible. Remember, your guests won't enjoy watching you struggle if they know you work your life around a chronic illness.

Hours d'oeuvres should be simple. Even using convenience items, you can still keep the appetizers delectable and pleasing to the eye; here are some suggestions to help:

➤ Several types of cut-up vegetables, most of which you can purchase already sliced and ready-to-serve at the grocery store and others that require only washing before serving. Choose lots of different colored items to lend visual appeal to the tray, such as red, gold and green peppers; baby carrots; cherry tomatoes; cucumbers; celery sticks. Although it's not necessary, add a fat-free dip by blending a dried soup mix into nonfat sour cream. Create another easy, great-tasting dip by mixing equal portions of salsa and nonfat plain yogurt.

➤ Several types of berries: depending on the season, buy, wash and arrange strawberries, raspberries and/or blueberries on a platter. Out of berry season, arrange red and green grapes on a platter, adding some whole wheat crackers and low-fat cream cheese dip, which you can buy in many great flavors.

➤ Prepared hummus is available in a variety of flavors. Simply serve with cut-up pita bread and some grapes or other fruit. As for the main menu, consider a buffet-style menu, as it is generally less taxing for you. Choose items that can be prepared one or several days ahead and frozen (or at least stored in the refrigerator). Examples of items that can be frozen are lasagna (try the exceptionally easy and fabulously delicious recipes on pages 288–89), chalupas, chicken or veal Parmesan, twice-baked potatoes, sweet potato pie, chili (see the recipe on page 375) and spaghetti (other great recipes on pages 286–87). Some items are actually better when prepared and allowed to sit for a day or two in the refrigerator. Try, for example, the jambalaya on page 363.

Try to include prepared foods in your menu planning. Grated cheese, for example, costs just pennies more per pound than chunk cheese. Already-cut vegetables, bagged and prewashed lettuce and fruits make salads a snap. You also have the option of purchasing your entrée from a caterer. In addition, some frozen products—such as lasagna or spinach soufflé—are more than acceptable; they're delicious and welcome additions to your menu.

Plan your menu with serving bowls and platters in mind. If you haven't entertained for a while, you may have forgotten how heavy that crystal bowl is. You might think about using disposable, lightweight aluminum foil pans for cooking, storing, reheating and serving.

As for the dessert, choose one that can be made ahead and frozen. Many iced cakes, ice cream pies and cheesecakes freeze well. Alternatively, purchase a dessert or accept the offer of one of your guests to bring one.

Twelve days ahead. Choose your attire, paying attention to comfort and function first. Wash and press or dry clean your outfit and put aside with accessories and hose. Although this seems like a minor detail, getting it (and other minor details) out of the way far ahead saves precious energy on the day you entertain.

Eight days ahead. Shop for dessert ingredients and beverages, and disposable cups, if that's what you're planning to use, as part of your regular grocery trip. Instead of putting the beverages away, only to have to take them out later, place these items where you'll set up the beverage bar later on.

Six days ahead. Make and freeze the dessert. If you've made an iced cake, freeze totally unwrapped until the icing is hard. Remove from freezer, cover with plastic wrap and then foil and return to freezer until the day of the party. When you remove it from the freezer, unwrap it before it defrosts—this will prevent the icing from sticking to the plastic wrap.

Five days ahead. Shop for dinner items, except perishables. Don't put away those items you'll use the next day in food preparation.

Four days ahead. Prepare any easily frozen main course items, such as twice-baked potatoes, chicken Parmesan, and so on. But sure to rest before cleaning the cooking mess. Better yet, ask your spouse or other family members to clean up, if possible.

Three days ahead. Clean the house. Make a list of all cleaning tasks and how you will tackle them. If you have regular housecleaning help, try to schedule it appropriately before your party. Frequent rests will keep you going longer. It is much better to work thirty minutes, rest ten, and begin again, than to try to do the job start to finish without a break. Although it doesn't sound like it, you'll actually accomplish more in a shorter period of time and won't put excessive, prolonged strain on weak or sore joints, legs and arms.

Don't do jobs three days in advance that you know you'll only do again the day of the party, like wiping out bathroom sinks and sweeping the entryway floor. Relaxing your standards is the ticket to an enjoyable and successful party.

Two days ahead. If you have a dining room table that you don't use every day, set it with a cloth, silverware and glassware.

Set up the beverage bar in a location where guests will feel free to serve themselves. Disposable glasses and paper napkins are real work-savers here. Place a plastic-lined trash bin next to the bar and you'll be surprised how cleanup of this area will be finished without an energy drain.

Shop for perishables, such as fresh fruits and vegetables. If you're going to serve a fresh vegetable and fruit tray as hors d'oeuvres, you might want to call the day before and ask the produce department to set aside all the cut vegetables and fresh berries you'll need. Also include fresh flowers from the grocery store on this list. If you've ordered prepared items from the grocery store, plan on picking them up (make sure you have storage for them).

The day of the party. Sleep late. Remove dessert and dinner items from freezer. I always plan my dessert as a centerpiece, accented on either side by two small floral bouquets. This saves several trips to the kitchen to serve dessert.

Finish the few last-minute tidy-up jobs.

Treat yourself with a long midday rest, getting up just in time to dress and place dinner items in the oven for reheating. Lay out hors d'oeuvres with disposable plates and napkins, again in an accessible spot with a lined trash bin nearby. Prepare the coffee pot; just don't plug it in or turn it on.

As guests arrive, make the coat drop a self-service job, and then direct them to the drinks and hors d'oeuvres.

Because everything is done, you are free to chat with your guests. Take advantage of this time to rest, sitting whenever possible. When it's time to serve, enlist the help of family or friends to remove heavy pans from the oven to buffet area or table. A roller cart is great for this step, whittling five trips to one (see chapter 5, "Creating an Energy-Saving Kitchen" on user-friendly kitchens). I always plan to have all food items in the buffet or on the table, absolving me from repeated trips to the kitchen. As you sit down to dinner, switch on the coffee pot.

Pouring coffee may be particularly difficult, especially if your hands are shaky or sore and stiff from arthritis, or if you are in a wheelchair or use a walker. This job should be passed on to someone with strong, steady hands and who is steady on his or her feet. Better yet, set up a self-service coffee bar. And, if you don't use your dessert as a centerpiece, make it a coffee and dessert bar. This is a great place to use disposable items, including paper plates, plastic forks and spoons, paper coffee cups, and paper napkins. Placing the trash bin next to this area encourages people to dispose of their dessert and coffee items when they have finished.

After the party. This may be the most difficult aspect of giving a party: go to bed and leave most of the mess. By now, you're probably tired. Rather than push yourself way beyond your physical abilities, retrain yourself to just refrigerate the leftover food and live with the rest of the mess until the morning. When you awake in the morning, you'll be fresh and your battery will be recharged—and you'll be able to tackle the mess with greater ease.

Maintaining a Healthy Weight

7

In this chapter we'll take a look at two common weight problems that people with chronic illness often face: gaining weight and losing too much weight.

Battling Excessive Weight

There are many reasons why people with chronic illness tend to gain weight. First, some conditions dictate a sedentary or relatively inactive lifestyle. Oftentimes, it is difficult to figure out how to eat to get enough nutrients yet cut back on calories to prevent gaining weight during sedentary times. Also, not able to get around very well, some people with chronic illness often turn to frozen and other convenience foods, which are heavy on fat and calories. As a result, although they aren't eating that much volume (fat is a very concentrated source of calories), they often eat far too many calories without even realizing it.

In addition, it is often during these times of greatest disease activity, dictating physical inactivity, that people with chronic illness must be on medications that can cause weight gain. For example, when asthma, multiple sclerosis, lupus and other diseases flare, some people must go on or increase their dose of prednisone or other cortisone medications. And that wreaks absolute havoc with trying to limit food intake (see chapter 11 for more information on how prednisone and other cortisone medications affect appetite and weight).

And if these two problems aren't bad enough on their own, people with chronic illness often turn to food for comfort, companionship and for an extra spark of interest in their lives. Take Martha, for example.

Martha was thirty-three years old when she was diagnosed with multiple sclerosis; her children were just toddlers. Over the next ten years, Martha became less and less mobile, gradually becoming totally dependent on a wheelchair for mobility. She resigned from many volunteer responsibilities, and left the house only on rare occasions.

Lacking enough stimulation and diversity in her life, Martha turned to food for comfort and amusement, although she really didn't make the connection—at least until she had gained enough weight to make moving from bed and chairs into her wheelchair and back again difficult.

Martha's situation, unfortunately, is common for many people with chronic illness. Immobilized, or at least greatly limited by the physical dictates of a chronic illness, many people fall into the trap of using food to relieve boredom, loneliness, frustration and depression. Food, after all, is a comfort.

Just stop and think about it for a moment. From the time we were little, food often was given nearly magical powers to solve problems and assuage negative emotions, as well as to create a celebratory atmosphere. Happy times, like birthdays and hitting a home run, were often acknowledged by a favorite treat: cake or ice cream (or even both!). Disappointments, too, were healed and tranquilized by food: there was nothing better than Mom's scrumptious chocolate cake or her fried chicken and gravy to help us forget a black eye and the fight that caused it, or a bad grade on a test.

So, it's no wonder that as adults, we turn to food to help us manage negative emotions, including those that often accompany living with a chronic illness. For people with chronic illness, food might be the only interesting thing in the whole day, the only decision to make. Mealtimes often become the focal points of the day, as they are the only things that break up long, monotonous days when a person with chronic illness is homebound, or at least greatly restricted in activity. In a sense, food becomes a therapist that helps chronic illness sufferers cope with their disease, at least temporarily.

As a result of developing such a close relationship with food, many people with chronic illness gain weight. To further compound the situation, these close relationships with food are often formed when being active just isn't an option—that's why food becomes such an important part of the day. This can turn into a chronic problem: even when the illness is less active and you can be more active, there's a chance that you picked up some bad eating habits that are hard to break.

In this chapter, I'm going to help you learn how to eat better to move toward a healthier, leaner body weight. I firmly believe that achieving a healthy, lean body weight is even more important for people with chronic illness than it is for people without chronic illness. For example, a person with arthritis in the lower extremities has an easier time getting around and will have less pain if she is on the leaner side. People who rely on a wheelchair, crutches or a walker also have an easier time getting around if they are lighter in weight. Yet another reason why people with chronic illness should watch their weight: it helps prevent heart disease. This is important, because some people with chronic illness are more likely to get heart disease, either because they cannot be physically active or because they take certain medications that tend to predispose them to heart disease—and sometimes for both reasons.

Identify Problem Eating Patterns

Because it happens so surreptitiously, many people who eat for comfort don't realize that food has become their therapist. If you're faced with a weight problem, the first step to solve the problem is to identify what's causing it. And the best way to do that is to keep a food diary. In fact, weight loss experts says that tracking eating, and exercise, habits is one of the most important secrets to successfully taking weight off; in addition, people who shed excess weight and keep it off say that logging food and activity was their single most important strategy.

Start a food diary today, writing down:

➤ The time you ate.

➤ What you ate, including quantity (make sure to identify all condiments and sauces; ditto for sugar and cream in coffee).

➤ Who you ate with.

➤ The degree of hunger you had when you ate: were you hungry, or just eating to fill time or because the food was there?

➤ What emotions you had (if any) when you ate.

Your food log will help you identify the eating habits getting you into trouble. Maybe you didn't even realize, for example, how much food you ate after dinner as you watched television. Or, if you work outside the home, perhaps you didn't acknowledge that you were eating fast food nearly every day for lunch, complete with fries and a soft drink. If you're at home all day, perhaps you're skipping real meals, but nibbling every hour.

After analyzing your food log, target one unhealthy habit to change. For example, you might decide to start with breakfast. Perhaps you discovered that you skip breakfast, but then forage through the kitchen in the late morning for anything at all. Your solution might be to eat a good breakfast every day. Research shows, incidentally, that people who eat a good breakfast burn more calories throughout the day (because they give their bodies a jump start, so to speak). Breakfast eaters reap another important advantage: they can concentrate better, and therefore perform better at school and work.

Do Not Tackle Everything at Once

Let's say that your eating diary identified several habits you'd like to change. No matter how excited you are to get started on the path of a leaner version of you, just remember to tackle one or two issues at a time. Trying to wipe the slate clean and start over all at once will no doubt overwhelm you and frustrate you, eventually causing you to forget the whole process and revert to old ways.

For example, if you currently drink whole milk and want to switch to skim, don't make the switch cold turkey. Instead, cut down to 2%, then 1% and then skim. If you currently use regular cream cheese on morning bagels, first try the low-fat version and then (maybe) the no-fat version. Remember, it's far better to eat the low-fat version than it is to hate the no-fat version and then go back to eating the full-fat one.

Small changes that lead to the big changes are as simple as drinking a large glass of water between meals, or switching snacks from chips to fruit. These baby-step changes work best in the long run to slim you down and keep you that way.

Avoid Feeling Deprived

Most people who have tried to shed unwanted pounds have tried the crash dieting routine—you know, swearing off anything that resembles a calorie. While this may work to lose a pound or even a couple of pounds, it often backfires and leads to weight gain over the long run. After cutting back on food so drastically, your body rebels. So ravenous, you end up eating lots more food after this semistarvation state—some people would call this bingeing.

Other people don't cut back so drastically on calories, but they do strip their eating plan of interesting food. You know this routine, too: fill up on carrots, lettuce, broiled chicken and lots of other diet foods. But this, too, leads to deprivation, which eventually leads most people to go off the deep end and binge on the tastes and flavors of which they've deprived themselves.

Rather than cutting back on calories and tastes so drastically, strike a middle ground. In other words, bridge the gap between the so-called diet and nondiet plates, creating an eating plan that satisfies your taste buds, delights your eye and builds good health. Make sure this middle ground includes foods that you absolutely love—in some cases, just in smaller quantities. Do you love, for example, regular salad dressing, and despise the low-fat and non-fat versions? No problem, just use less. Maybe you enjoy a chocolate chip cookie and a glass of milk in the afternoon. Just limit yourself to one cookie, savoring every morsel. Lots of times, people end up "eating around" what they really wanted. In other words, trying to avoid the chocolate chip cookie (which usually ended up as three or four), a person eats carrots, celery and then an apple. Still not satisfied, that person frequently ends up eating the cookies, anyway and is even further behind in her weight-loss efforts than she would have been had she eaten just one cookie to begin with.

Redesign Your Dinner Plate

Most Americans need to redesign their dinner plates—as well as their breakfast and lunch plates. Traditionally, most Americans have planned meals around meat, often filling half of the dinner plate with a meat portion. A quarter of the dinner plate often has a baked potato, rice or pasta, usually topped with margarine, butter or sour cream. The other quarter of the plate may have a dinner roll or bread, and perhaps a sprinkling of vegetables. As a result of this eating style, Americans eat some 839 billion fat calories each year, or 34 to 36 percent of their calories as fat—much more than what's healthy. Official dietary goals urge us to limit fat calories to just 30 percent; many nutrition experts believe we should limit fat even more, stopping at 15 to 25 percent of calories.

But redesigning your plate to create the right fuel mix automatically slashes fat grams and calories to a healthier level. The first thing to modify is the meat portion, filling no more than 25 percent of the plate. As I said earlier, limit meat, fish or poultry to just two- to three-ounce portions, which is about the size of a deck of playing cards. While you're trying to lose weight, fill a generous half of the plate with vegetables (without added fat) and one quarter with whole grain foods, such as brown rice, bulghur, barley or a small baked potato with the skin. When you're achieved a healthy body weight and want to maintain your weight, play with the vegetable and grain proportions, sometimes allotting one-half to whole grains and one-fourth to vegetables. Not only will these proportions give you more nutrients for fewer calories, but they will also give you more fiber, which will help you feel full for a longer time.

Give Food Intense Flavor

A great way to enjoy smaller portions of food is to give them intense flavor. Bored with grilled chicken breasts? Instead, simmer them in an interesting flavor enhancer; try the recipes on pages 304 and 306. Similarly, are you tired of steamed broccoli and raw baby carrots? Pump up the flavors of these foods too, trying the recipes on pages 368, 387, and 394.

Plan Healthy Snacks

Let's face it: we all get hungry between meals. And some people feel better when they eat three small meals and two or three small snacks daily. But don't leave snack choices to chance. Instead, plan ahead with healthy items: low-fat yogurt, a whole grain bagel, low-fat cottage cheese, skim milk and a small cookie, or your favorite raw vegetables with low-fat or nonfat dip. Remember that you're using snacks to replenish your fuel tank—and you can't afford the consequences of putting poor-quality fuel into your tank (see below about overall dietary quality).

Stop the Body Bashing

No one knows better than I the frustration of not being able to exercise because of ill health, compounded by high-dose medication and the appearance changes it causes. But body bashing—beating up on yourself psychologically—because you don't like the way you look will get you nowhere. In fact, it will probably do more harm than good.

Here's why. If you're continually beating yourself up, telling yourself how bad you look, how can you take care of yourself? Repeated body bashing leads you to believe that you aren't worth taking care of—and that makes it hard to do all that you can do to look your best and be healthy.

Instead, focus on the positive. Don't equate your worth with your weight—they're just not connected. In other words, don't give the bathroom scale magical powers. After all, do you judge your friends by how much they weigh? Just as you do with your friends, look beyond the physical and see the good in yourself. And then you can start taking care of yourself. No doubt you'll have an easier time controlling what you eat and achieving the best body you can under the circumstances. In short, love yourself enough to begin living today.

Look Your Best

Maybe you have already gained a few extra pounds. Do you try to disguise the weight with slenderizing black or the baggy look? Starting today, update your closet with stylish, colorful clothes you love, replacing some of the boring black and baggy with lively, fresh clothes.

Ask for Help

One of my dearest friends presented me with at least a pound of my favorite chocolate every time I had a flare-up. I usually wasn't interested in the chocolate until I started to feel better—when my appetite was voracious from the increased dose of steroid medication I was taking. I know she brought the chocolate out of love, but I had to ask her to stop.

Ask your family and friends to help you in whatever way you need help to lose weight. Maybe someone doesn't bring you chocolate, but perhaps your spouse likes to go out to eat frequently, which wreaks havoc with trying to eat leaner. For some people, just asking someone else to do the grocery shopping is the help needed to resist temptation. Ask for that help.

Letting people who care about you know that you're trying to do something about the excess weight can be a help in another important way: perhaps they can help bolster your resolve when the going gets tough.

Weigh Yourself Just Often Enough

Remember the advice I gave about not giving the scale magical powers? That still holds, but I don't want you to ignore the scale altogether. An occasional journey to the scale does have value.

Weighing yourself occasionally lets you know if the small changes you're making are helping you achieve a leaner weight. While advice varies widely about how often to weigh, once a week seems to work best. You'll not be frustrated by the daily fluctuations in weight, and yet be able to see a trend. Waiting two weeks, however, might let you rationalize away less desirable habits—"Oh, I'll just skip exercising for a few days because I'm tired, and it's not making that much difference, anyway." Some people avoid the scale for a couple of weeks running when they know they've been ignoring their goals for portion control.

Learn the Difference Between Appetite and Hunger

When was the last time you felt that rumble in your tummy that signals real hunger? Many people who have some pounds to shed have forgotten what that feels like. True hunger is a sign that your fuel tank is approaching empty and needs fuel. Appetite, on the other hand, is the head's part of wanting to eat something—just a desire that stems from the psyche and not the stomach or fuel tank level. No doubt you've been in a situation—in a restaurant or at the family holiday table—when you were absolutely stuffed. Then, the dessert appeared on the scene and you somehow found room for it. You weren't hungry for the dessert, but your appetite went into overdrive because the dessert was so irresistible.

Sure, everyone needs a healthy appetite to live—without the desire to eat, some people would grow too thin and frail (see below). But because food takes on so many roles in our society and is often the focal point of events, appetite often goes into overdrive.

To achieve and maintain a healthier, leaner body weight, you have to teach your body to know the difference between hunger and appetite. When you think about it, this is an easy way to cut calories. Because your body really didn't want the calories anyway, it won't miss them. The first step is understanding when you're truly hungry.

If you think you're hungry between meals, or even at the end of a meal, don't give in to the temptation to eat right away. Instead, set a small timer for ten minutes. At the end of ten minutes, ask yourself if you're still hungry. In many cases, that ten-minute lag is enough to distinguish the desire to eat from true hunger. If you decide that you are still hungry, set the timer for an additional ten minutes. This will knock out another significant percentage of eating episodes. If you decide after the second ten minutes that you are hungry, split your normal portion in half and see if that satisfies you—my guess is that it will.

Fighting the Weight-Loss Trend

Losing weight as a result of having chronic disease can also be a tremendous problem. Some people lose their appetite because they are chronically in pain, others because of the medications they take. And still others go through stages of depression because of their illness, also losing the desire to eat.

Not eating enough and losing too much weight puts people with chronic illness at a real disadvantage to fight their disease. Excessive weight loss can lead to more weakness and fatigue. Most importantly, the body lacks enough fuel to engage in battle with the disease.

Whether you are trying to improve your own dietary intake or that of a family or friend you are caring for, here are some ideas that will help.

1. Make every calorie count. To quench thirst, avoid water. Instead, opt for a drink with calories and nutrients. Try, for example, plain milk, milk with instant breakfast mixed in (although people tire of this quickly, so don't overdo it) or peach, pear and apricot nectars, which are loaded with nutrients as well as calories. On the other hand, try not to load up on empty calorie beverages such as soda pop and lemonade. And try not to drink too much liquid before a meal, as it can kill your appetite.

2. Try small amounts of food more frequently. Many people with a poor appetite have trouble facing a big breakfast or a big any meal, for that matter. For example, start off with one slice of toast, but dress it up with good nutrition. Instead of butter or margarine, try peanut butter. The calories are about the same, but the peanut butter has loads more protein and nutrients. To add a few extra calories, add some jam or jelly. Later in the morning, try a glass of milk, or perhaps a banana. It's a lot easier to divvy up a breakfast meal into two smaller parts than to face the mass quantity.

3. Try to find alternatives to broth-based soups. While these soups are often favorites of people with poor appetites, they are virtually calorie-free. At the same time, though, they quickly fill up the stomach. Instead, try cream-based soups. Try the recipes for

thicker, higher-calorie and nutrition-loaded soups on pages 366–68. You'll note that one of the recipes for tomato soup sneaks in some cheese, which is full of the protein that people with poor appetites often are missing. If you're using canned cream soups, be sure to make them with milk instead of water to boost calories and protein.

4. Ask the doctor if any of the medications suppress appetite. If so, probe to find out if the medication can be taken at a different time of the day when it may not interfere with appetite so much.

5. If possible, take medications after eating. Sometimes, medications taken on an empty stomach can cause nausea, thereby preventing you from eating. By taking them after a meal, you can avoid this problem. Note that some vitamin/mineral supplements, especially iron, can also upset the stomach, taking away appetite. *Caution:* some medications must be taken on an empty stomach to be effective, so ask to make sure it's okay.

6. Try not to load up on fluids close to mealtime. While a cup of hot tea might make you feel better, drinking it before lunch or dinner may take away whatever appetite you did have. Try to avoid fluids for at least an hour before meals.

7. Think about nutrients as well as calories when you're choosing food. While you may have been advised to add butter, margarine or oil to food to beef up the calories, try not to overdo these fat-only calorie tricks. Other ideas to use to beef up calories and yet add nutrients include:

➤ Add low-fat cream cheese to mashed potatoes: I use low-fat because it has a decent protein content, and isn't just fat calories. See the recipe on page 394. This is a modification of an old family favorite recipe, and my family will only eat them this way. Note that while I didn't include skim milk powder in this recipe, you could certainly add a little to boost the protein even more.

➤ Get a yogurt strainer and turn yogurt into yogurt cheese. You can do this with any flavor, and it's a great way to concentrate calories, protein, calcium and riboflavin. See the recipes on pages 395–96 in which I've used yogurt cheese in gelatin dishes.

➤ Mash vegetables such as carrots, squash and sweet potatoes with low-fat cream cheese and milk, again beefing up nutrients and protein.

➤ Make hot cereals with milk and even a little extra skim milk powder to improve protein and calorie content. See the recipes on pages 248–49.

➤ Cook rice in milk, either for a breakfast food (see the recipe on page 248) or a dinner food. You'll just have to cook it a little slower, and avoid the instant varieties. Everyone will love the fuller tasting rice this cooking method produces.

➤ Use evaporated skimmed milk as much as possible. Because it's made of milk that has been dehydrated, you'll again get more calories, protein and nutrients in much less volume. While its slightly stronger taste might come through in some foods, causing you or the person you're trying to feed to reject them, it is perfectly acceptable in many foods. Give it a trial in hot cereals and to mix up creamed soups. Some people even like it in coffee and tea.

Overall Diet Quality

In trying to shed excess pounds or gain a few back, don't be content to just count calories. Instead, think about overall diet quality—that's the ticket to achieving the nutrition advantage to fight your illness.

How many times have you heard the advice "Eat a balanced diet"? Like most people, I bet you turn a deaf ear to this age-old advice. Perhaps more helpful advice would be "Eat a diverse diet."

"While there has always been good reason to eat a varied diet, there are now intriguing new reasons to emphasize this age-old advice," says nutrition researcher Ashima K. Kant, Ph.D., R.D., an associate professor in the department of family nutrition and exercise sciences at Queens College at the City University of New York. "Our research found that people who eat the least diverse diets have an increased risk of heart disease and cancer."

What is dietary diversity? There are two levels of dietary diversity. The first has to do with how many different food groups are represented by the foods eaten on any given day. There's even a scoring system, with five maximum points possible. A person earns a point for each food group from which he or she eats; the food groups are fruits, vegetables, grains, meats and dairy. (Although fats are a food group, a person does not have to include foods from this group in order to have a healthy diet.)

Americans don't score too well when it comes to dietary diversity. The National Health and Nutrition Examination Survey, a large and commonly cited nutrition survey, revealed disconcerting details about American dietary diversity: some one quarter of Americans eat foods from just three or fewer food groups. "Just one-third of Americans eat from all five food groups," says Kant. Fruit is the most common food group missing in action—about 46 percent of Americans eat no fruit—followed by dairy foods and then vegetables (the other two food groups, which are least likely to be missing in the American diet, are meat and grains).

"The theory behind urging people to include food from each of the five food groups is that it will help them harvest a wider variety of nutrients," says Dr. Kant, who explains that nutrients travel in groups. Fruits, for example, tend to be an excellent source of vitamin C, while dairy foods are the chief source of calcium and vitamin D. "In practice, we're beginning to prove the theory correct."

Kant's research, in fact, has shown a direct relationships with certain nutrient intakes and the number of different food groups from which a person eats. On average, people who eat foods from two or fewer food groups daily come up short on several nutrients; they come up short by the following percentages:

Riboflavin, 42%

Thiamin, 52%

Vitamin B$_6$, 61%

Vitamin C, 68%

Calcium, 65%

While people who eat from four of the five groups are in better shape nutritionally speaking than people who eat from just two, they are still, on average, 16 percent short on thiamine, 30 percent deficient in vitamin B_6 and 15 percent deficient in calcium.

But the significance goes beyond just getting too little of certain nutrients. "The research, in fact, strongly suggests that food plays a far more significant role than just preventing nutrient deficiencies and supporting growth and development," says Regina G. Ziegler, Ph.D., M.P.H., senior investigator at the nutritional epidemiology branch of the National Cancer Institute, and coauthor of the dietary diversity and chronic disease studies. Indeed, both Kant and Ziegler point out that an increasing number of studies hint at a whole new role for nutrients in disease prevention.

They are quick to point out, though, it is not nutrients in isolation, as they are in supplements, but nutrients harvested from real food. Studies of the ability of individual nutrients to prevent cancer, in fact, have been strikingly disappointing. "This study of dietary diversity dovetails with hundreds of others showing that diets high in fruits and vegetables prevent cancer and heart disease," says Dr. Ziegler, and, in a just released study, high blood pressure.

Why Dietary Diversity Rather Than Nutrients?

"There's so much about food that we just haven't discovered yet," says Susan Ahlstrom Henderson, M.S., R.D., health research associate in the Human Nutrition Program at the University of Michigan, who points out that we're just beginning to realize the potential importance of phytochemicals in food, for example. (Phytochemicals are the nonnutrient substances of foods thought to help fight chronic disease, including cancer and heart disease; see pages 5–6.) "No doubt there are other substances in food that are critical to health that we just haven't discovered. Eating a wide variety of foods—especially fruits, vegetables and grains—ensures not only that we get essential nutrients, but also these nonnutrient substances."

A Second Order of Diversity

It may be just as important to achieve a second order of diversity, says Dr. Ziegler. "Just as it seems wise to choose foods from all five food groups, it may be just as critical to choose a wide variety of foods within food groups—especially within the fruit, vegetable and grain food groups." The reasons are at least twofold: first, adding in different selections from the different food groups lends a different complement of nutrients. Even more diverse is the complement of phytochemicals for different foods within each food group. An orange, for example, has a different set of nutrients and phytochemicals than a bowl of strawberries—although both are a great source of vitamin C.

Let's take a look at two healthy days of eating, and demonstrate how different they are nutritionally—and see the importance of achieving diversity within food groups.

Menu A

Breakfast

   1 white bagel with margarine and jelly
   8 ounces of skim milk

Lunch

   1 ham sandwich on white bread with
      1 tablespoon mayonnaise
   1 can of soda
   1 apple

Dinner

   2 cups of spaghetti with pasta sauce
   2 cups of green beans
   2 slices Italian bread
   2 teaspoons margarine

Evening Snack

   1 apple

Menu B

Breakfast

   1 whole wheat bagel with peanut butter
      and jelly
   8 ounces of skim milk

Lunch

   1 ham sandwich on whole wheat bread
      with romaine lettuce leaves, tomato
      and 1 teaspoon mayonnaise
   1 apple
   8 strawberries
   8 ounces skim milk

Dinner

   1 cup of spaghetti noodles with meat
      pasta sauce
   1 cup of green beans
   ½ cup broccoli
   1 cup canned apricots
   1 slice Italian bread
   1 teaspoon margarine

Evening Snack

   2 fig bars

By most definitions, Menu A represents a very healthy diet: it includes at least one food from each of the five food groups mentioned above, and even includes six servings of fruits and vegetables. It also contains a healthy calorie, protein and fat level (about 1,625 calories with 15 percent of calories as fat), and even plenty of fiber (about 23 grams). As indicated by the bar graph, though, the meal plan comes up quite short on ten essential nutrients.

Diversifying the fruits, vegetables, grains and meats, though, rounds out the nutrients considerably in Menu B. Here's a summary of the most important ingredients added to Menu B and how the diversity brought the nutrients up so remarkably:

➤   The menu still contains just seven servings of fruits and vegetables, but in seven different forms rather than just the two in Menu A.

➤   Although there was plenty of protein in Menu A from the lunchtime ham sandwich, Menu B added two additional types of protein in the form of ground beef for the spaghetti and peanut butter at breakfast, cutting down on some of the ham and pasta.

➤   Menu B also diversified the grain components, substituting a whole wheat bagel for the white one, whole wheat bread for the white bread at lunch and fig bars for some of the Italian bread at dinner.

Menu A: Less Dietary Diversity

Serving Size:	58.20 oz-wt
Serves:	1.00
Water:	76%

% comparison to: US Female (25—50 years) — Bar Graph

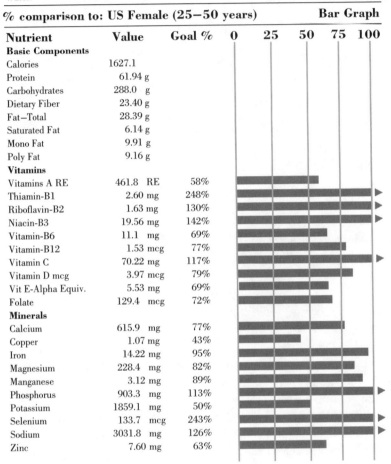

Nutrient	Value	Goal %
Basic Components		
Calories	1627.1	
Protein	61.94 g	
Carbohydrates	288.0 g	
Dietary Fiber	23.40 g	
Fat—Total	28.39 g	
Saturated Fat	6.14 g	
Mono Fat	9.91 g	
Poly Fat	9.16 g	
Vitamins		
Vitamins A RE	461.8 RE	58%
Thiamin-B1	2.60 mg	248%
Riboflavin-B2	1.63 mg	130%
Niacin-B3	19.56 mg	142%
Vitamin-B6	11.1 mg	69%
Vitamin-B12	1.53 mcg	77%
Vitamin C	70.22 mg	117%
Vitamin D mcg	3.97 mcg	79%
Vit E-Alpha Equiv.	5.53 mg	69%
Folate	129.4 mcg	72%
Minerals		
Calcium	615.9 mg	77%
Copper	1.07 mg	43%
Iron	14.22 mg	95%
Magnesium	228.4 mg	82%
Manganese	3.12 mg	89%
Phosphorus	903.3 mg	113%
Potassium	1859.1 mg	50%
Selenium	133.7 mcg	243%
Sodium	3031.8 mg	126%
Zinc	7.60 mg	63%

Menu B: More Dietary Diversity

Serving Size:	66.79 oz-wt
Serves:	1.00
Water:	76%

% comparison to: US Female (25–50 years)

Bar Graph

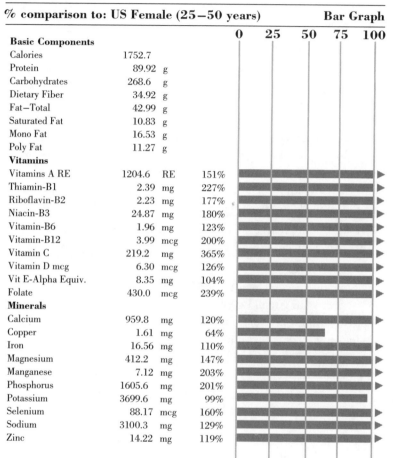

Basic Components			
Calories	1752.7		
Protein	89.92	g	
Carbohydrates	268.6	g	
Dietary Fiber	34.92	g	
Fat–Total	42.99	g	
Saturated Fat	10.83	g	
Mono Fat	16.53	g	
Poly Fat	11.27	g	
Vitamins			
Vitamins A RE	1204.6	RE	151%
Thiamin-B1	2.39	mg	227%
Riboflavin-B2	2.23	mg	177%
Niacin-B3	24.87	mg	180%
Vitamin-B6	1.96	mg	123%
Vitamin-B12	3.99	mcg	200%
Vitamin C	219.2	mg	365%
Vitamin D mcg	6.30	mcg	126%
Vit E-Alpha Equiv.	8.35	mg	104%
Folate	430.0	mcg	239%
Minerals			
Calcium	959.8	mg	120%
Copper	1.61	mg	64%
Iron	16.56	mg	110%
Magnesium	412.2	mg	147%
Manganese	7.12	mg	203%
Phosphorus	1605.6	mg	201%
Potassium	3699.6	mg	99%
Selenium	88.17	mcg	160%
Sodium	3100.3	mg	129%
Zinc	14.22	mg	119%

➤ In addition, Menu B cut down on the empty calorie fat (margarine and mayonnaise), which allowed for adding fat in the form of peanut butter and red meat, adding lots of nutrients.

Here's how to put diversity in the average American eating plan, without creating much more work in the kitchen:

➤ Try to get at least five servings of fruits and vegetables daily (counting each serving as one-half cup or a piece of fruit), but make them at least five different ones. In achieving variety, consider getting different colors and textures—for example, dark green leafy vegetables (such as spinach), red fruit (strawberries), orange vegetables (carrots), stalk vegetables (broccoli) and fruits with pits (apricots, peaches). For example, instead of tossing a whole bag of apples into your grocery cart, throw in two or three of five different types of fruit—two peaches, two pears, two apples and two bananas. Same with vegetables: rather than opting for a huge bag of carrots, buy five different ready-to-eat vegetables. Another easy way is to buy the frozen vegetable medleys; they add diversity with no extra work. Just be sure to skip the ones with sauces.

➤ Get six to eleven servings of grains daily, but mix them up. Instead of all white breads and pastas, try whole grain breads and bagels, rice, bulghur, barley, rye bread and quinoa.

➤ Have little bits of two or three different types of protein food—aiming for some animal protein (pork, beef, chicken) and vegetable protein (peanut butter, lentils). You'll get more diversity in having a little bit of pork for dinner and a little chicken on your lunchtime salad than just loading up on chicken at lunch.

➤ In addition, Menu B cut down on the empty-calorie fat (margarine and mayonnaise), which allowed for adding fat in the form of peanut butter and red meat, adding lots of nutrients.

An Extra Advantage: 8
Using Nutrition to Heal from Surgery and Injuries

In addition to the daily stress imposed on your body by your illness, you might face additional physical stress if you need surgery or suffer a major wound. But there are nutritional maneuvers you can take to recover optimally and more quickly from surgery or major injuries. Good nutrition can speed healing and also help you avoid the infections that can occur and delay healing.

As you're about to learn, certain nutrients play a more critical role than others in healing. Getting at least the Recommended Dietary Allowance (RDA, or DRI, that new term you'll be seeing more of) for these nutrients—and more in some cases—is necessary for about two to six weeks following surgery. But all nutrients are important in healing, which means that someone undergoing and recovering from surgery should be well nourished overall to ensure optimal healing.

Push Protein, Do Not Skimp on Calories

The body's complex strategy to heal wounds is amazing. It creates new blood vessels to replace those severed during surgery; makes new tissue and repairs injured tissue to close the wound; and produces more of certain white blood cells—fibroblasts and lymphocytes in particular—to help clean the wound. But not one of these healing steps can take place if the diet is short on protein, as adequate protein is required for each of these steps. Not eating enough protein, in fact, prolongs the healing process. Skimping on protein also decreases resistance to infection, one of the most common complications of surgery. Wounds that become infected take much longer to heal.

Although there are no official recommendations, boost protein to around sixty to eighty grams of protein following surgery or a major injury.

It's not enough, though, to get adequate protein. If you don't eat enough calories, the body can't use the protein as protein—instead, the body burns it for energy. Wound healing is a very energy-consuming process—and when calorie intake is low, the body searches for adequate fuel to burn. How do you know if calorie intake is too low? If you're losing weight after surgery, then you are not consuming enough calories—and that's a sign that you may be burning for fuel some of the protein your body needs for healing and to resist infections. Aim to maintain your weight until healing is complete.

Protein in Commonly Consumed Foods	*One 8-ounce glass nonfat milk = 8 g protein* *3 ounces cooked meat or fish = 26 g* *1 cup low-fat cottage cheese = 31 g*	*1 egg = 7 g* *2 tablespoons peanut butter = 8 g* *1 cup cooked lentils (or other beans) = 18 g* *1 ounce cheese = 7 g* *6 ounces tofu = 14 g*

Nutrients That Speed Healing

Vitamin A

Vitamin A boosts production of fibroblast, a type of white blood cell that is necessary to help fight infections. That's probably why it was dubbed the "anti-infective vitamin." It is also an essential ingredient in forming new cells to close and strengthen wounds.

And, if you take cortisone, vitamin A may be especially important in helping you heal properly and quickly after surgery. Cortisone interferes with the normal healing process by preventing collagen, one of the proteins that helps seal wounds, from "cross-linking," or weaving together to close the wound. While the RDA for vitamin A is 5,000 IU for men and 4,000 IU for women, people on cortisone medications may benefit from as much as 20,000 IU three times per day, beginning one week before surgery, and continuing for about two to three weeks after surgery. Don't continue to take vitamin A doses in excess of the RDA beyond three to four weeks, as such high doses quickly become toxic to the liver. Because it's fat soluble, the body stores excess vitamin A, which quickly becomes toxic. Also, always consult with your physician before doing this.

Foods rich in vitamin A include sweet potatoes, carrots, evaporated skim milk, apricot nectar, liver, part skim ricotta cheese, cantaloupe, tomatoes, squash and spinach.

Vitamin C

Vitamin C helps speed healing by encouraging the body's production of wound-closing cells; it also boosts white cell population, critical infection-fighting cells. There are no official recommendations for how much vitamin C to get after surgery, but I encourage people to get at least 100 milligrams, and getting 200 to 300 milligrams may be advantageous. But don't go overboard, as consuming too much can be dangerous. For one, taking megadoses changes the body's expectations. As a result, if a person cuts back to smaller doses (even though these smaller doses meet the RDA), she can experience deficiency signs, including prolonged wound healing.

Foods rich in vitamin C include orange juice, tomatoes, kiwis, papaya, strawberries, spinach, sweet potatoes and cantaloupe.

B Vitamins

At least three B vitamins help prevent wound infections, thereby speeding healing: pyridoxine (B_6), thiamin and riboflavin. These vitamins also help the body use protein and calories more efficiently.

Foods rich in pyridoxine include chicken, fish, pork, eggs, liver, oats, soybeans (and tofu) and bananas. Foods rich in thiamin include liver, unrefined whole grains, legumes (dried peas and beans) and brewer's yeast. Foods rich in riboflavin include meat, fish, poultry, eggs, dairy products, broccoli, asparagus, turnip greens and spinach.

Minerals

Several minerals also speed wound healing, including magnesium, iron, copper and zinc. While they all play many roles that help wounds to heal, they all are necessary in making the protein that builds new cells to close wounds. Iron and copper carry oxygen to the wound, another essential ingredient in wound healing.

Foods rich in magnesium include unprocessed whole grains, legumes, nuts and seeds, avocados and bananas. Foods rich in iron include lean meats, legumes, whole grains, nuts and seeds and green leafy vegetables. Foods rich in copper include shellfish, legumes, liver, whole grains, nuts and seeds. Foods rich in zinc include seafood, meats, whole grains and legumes.

Essential Fatty Acids

With all the talk of low-fat diets, some people go overboard to avoid dietary fat. But some fat is always necessary. And, during healing, essential fatty acids are especially critical.

Getting at least 25 grams of fat daily ensures an adequate intake of essential fatty acids for wound healing, as well as the needs of every day life.

*3 ounces chicken breast = 3 g
3 ounces lean roast beef = 5 g
3 ounces grilled salmon = 7 g
1 cup low-fat cottage cheese = 4.5 g
1 cup low-fat yogurt = 3.5 g
1 tablespoon margarine = 11.5 g
1 tablespoon olive oil = 13.5 g*

**How Much
Fat Is in
Ordinary
Foods?**

Essential fatty acids, fat the body cannot make, are critical ingredients in making cell membranes of newly forming cells in healing tissue; they also boost the immune system to help prevent infections. Most people eat a minimum of 25 grams of fat daily (and generally, around 40 to 60 grams); even the 25 grams is enough to supply necessary amounts of essential fatty acids.

Go Easy on Vitamin E

This fat-soluble vitamin illustrates well that too much of a good thing can be bad. While vitamin E is necessary for normal fat metabolism, critical in wound healing, too much slows healing by interfering with new cell production. Many people may benefit from vitamin E supplements to fight heart disease and possibly delay the onset of serious symptoms of Alzheimer's Disease. However, cut back on these supplements for one week before surgery and two to six weeks following surgery.

Do Not Smoke

Because smoking delays wound healing and also increases the risk of suffering complications from anesthesia, stop smoking before surgery. Surgeons say smokers have two to three times as many complications after surgery than nonsmokers. And substituting nicotine chewing gum isn't the answer, as nicotine is the main ingredient in cigarettes that delays wound healing.

Vitamin E and Aloe Vera: Do They Work?

Vitamin E creams. Although many people break open vitamin E capsules and rub the content into scars, there's no evidence that this has any benefit.

Aloe. If you've ever broken off an aloe leaf and rubbed the thick liquid into a minor burn, you know well that it seems to work well to relieve both pain and redness. Indeed, says burn researcher John P. Heggers, Ph.D., professor of surgery in the division of plastic and reconstructive surgery at the University of Texas Medical Branch and Shriner's Burn Institute in Galveston, Texas. "Research has proven that aloe helps ensure a rich blood supply to wounds, which is so necessary to healing," he says. It's been shown to work on many types of wounds, insect bites, rashes and itching. Ask your surgeon, though, if you can apply it to your surgical incision.

Nutritional Supplements

9

Millions of Americans take nutritional supplements. Some people take them "just to be sure" that they get all their nutrients. Other people take them to prevent cancer, failing eyesight and aging and to find more energy. And many people with chronic illness take nutritional supplements to cure or at least improve their condition.

Should anyone take supplements? Nutrition experts unanimously recommend that everyone get his or her nutrients from food instead of from pills (chapter 1). But certain people may benefit from a supplement. These include people with chronic disease, especially if they have a poor appetite or don't eat well for any other reason. In addition, some medications (see chapter 10) can affect nutrient metabolism, which means that people taking those medications might benefit from taking supplements. And people who frequently restrict calories, especially to 1,200 or less, heavy smokers and drinkers, and some elderly might also benefit from a supplement.

In each case, though, experts recommend a supplement containing no more than 100 percent of the Recommended Dietary Allowance (RDA). If you step beyond that, you're wandering into doses considered to be drugs and you need to be under a doctor's care.

When Supplements Get You into Trouble

About 10 percent of Americans take what are called solo nutrients, or pills containing just one nutrient or perhaps a specialized combination of nutrients. Typical of solo supplement aficionados, many often pop a few extra pills just to be sure, usually with no idea that ingredients overlap from pill to pill, nor that supplement manufacturers can put any dose into one pill. Often the dose is many, many times the RDA. Vitamin B_6, for example, is available as 500-milligram and 1,000-milligram tablets, although the RDA is a fraction of that: 2 milligrams for men and 1.6 milligrams for women.

Most solo supplement users do not win the health benefits for which they wager big bucks. All told, Americans spend at least $3 billion yearly on nutritional supplements.

Depending on the amounts they take, some *appear* to escape unharmed. Others suffer serious or potentially serious harm. And because the science of nutrition is not fully charted, some suffer consequences that experts have not yet linked to excess vitamin/mineral intake. No doubt negative effects of vitamin/mineral excess go unnoticed because we just don't know what to look for. Indeed, experts don't know the effects of being well nourished in one nutrient but not in others. Nutrients are meant to work in delicate balance with each other, not as free agents. Nor do experts always know the downside of taking doses ten, a hundred or a thousand times the RDA. They *do* know that very large doses are considered pharmacological—they act like drugs instead of nutrients.

Megatrouble

The following supplements, taken alone and/or in large quantities, are listed with their potentially negative consequences; the list is by no means complete.

➤ VITAMIN C: Nine of ten Americans take vitamin C supplements at widely varying doses up to thousands of milligrams. Fifteen hundred milligrams, a common "anticold" dose, interferes with copper absorption, leading to copper deficiency. Two thousand milligrams can cause diarrhea, nausea, abdominal cramps, headache, fatigue and hot flashes. Regular megadoses may create vitamin C dependency; dropping down to normal intakes induces "withdrawal," manifested as rebound scurvy or vitamin C deficiency—bleeding gums, malingering wounds, and skin problems. While some vitamin C functions as an antioxidant, an excess functions as a prooxidant, or actually causes the cellular damage it is supposed to stop; the higher the dose, the more likely it will function negatively.

Select populations are at special risk from vitamin C excess. For the 12 percent of Americans with a genetic defect causing excess iron absorption, extra vitamin C spells disaster. Because it enhances iron absorption, the extra C accelerates the speed with which they suffer negative consequences of iron overload, including heart attack. The red blood cells of people with sickle cell anemia who take excess vitamin C clump abnormally, exacerbating their condition. In iron-deficient people, megadoses of vitamin C destroy significant amounts of vitamin B_{12}.

➤ IRON: In select people, too much iron leads to iron overload, which can precipitate diabetes, liver disease, heart disorders; it also reduces zinc absorption.

➤ ZINC: The annals of medical history report the case of a fifty-seven-year-old man diagnosed with severe anemia and preleukemia; physicians later discovered he had for two years taken thirty times the RDA for zinc. Two months after he stopped the supplements, his blood tests normalized. The zinc had interfered with copper absorption, a mineral that prevents the anemia he had. While just twenty-five milligrams daily interferes with copper absorption, 150 milligrams per day causes overt copper deficiency, depresses immune function and reduces HDL, or good cholesterol. Getting so much more than the RDA is easy: some zinc supplements pack in eighty milligrams per tablet.

➤ FOLIC ACID: There's now conclusive evidence that boosting daily folic acid intake to 400 micrograms prevents neural tube defects in developing fetuses and very convincing evidence that it helps prevent heart disease. Because the average American intake is just 200 micrograms, many experts recommend a supplement. But supplementing even moderately can mean disaster for people who are vitamin B_{12} deficient: the folate corrects the blood abnormalities but not the underlying problem. Consequently, the associated nerve damage progresses silently, possibly to paralysis. Vitamin B_{12} deficiency becomes more common with age, as the body gradually loses its ability to split B_{12} from food and to absorb it.

➤ VITAMIN B_6: Even twenty-five milligrams daily can cause nerve damage; megadoses of 200 milligrams and up—those recommended for improving memory—cause more severe neurotoxicity and multiple sclerosis–like symptoms.

➤ NIACIN: In large doses, niacin becomes a drug capable of lowering too-high cholesterol levels in some people. The dose often used, one hundred milligrams, can cause itching, flushing and blurred vision. Taking the sustained release variety eliminates these discomforts. It doesn't, however, prevent liver damage that can occur with such large doses, allowing the damage to progress silently. Extra niacin may also strain the pathway by which it is shuttled through the body (its metabolic pathway), which could interfere with folate metabolism and send the body into deficiency even when folate intake is adequate. The message: large doses of niacin to lower cholesterol should only be taken under a physician's supervision.

➤ VITAMIN A: Hearing about a prescription drug containing vitamin A for acne, individuals in health food stores recommend the actual vitamin for healthier skin, not understanding the difference. Thinking they're saving money, many consumers buy big doses of vitamin A, and they're getting into huge trouble. Vitamin A is available as 10,000 IU tablets, and people are popping three to four, hoping for younger-looking skin.

Ironically, the very population that commonly takes more may need less: preliminary evidence suggests the aging body needs less vitamin A. Whatever the age, though, too much vitamin A toxicity is very dangerous. While 25,000 IU is toxic to most people—causing headache, hair loss, cracked lips, dry and itchy skin, liver enlargement, bone and joint pain—doses as low as 6,000 IU ingested chronically harm a select few. Discontinuing excess vitamin A generally reverses the symptoms, but in some cases permanent liver, bone and vision damage results. You can literally kill yourself with excess vitamin A and selenium, and it doesn't take a bushel to do it—one bottle is enough.

➤ SELENIUM: In another landmark case, thirteen people ingested toxic levels of selenium unwittingly—the supplement they took contained more than 180 times the amount stated on the label. As a result, they ingested from 27 to 2,387 milligrams of selenium daily. Even lower amounts cause diarrhea, hair and nail loss; it may even promote cancer. This example illustrates well the problem with some supplements: they are not always labeled fully or correctly.

➤ CHROMIUM: While experts don't know the long-term consequences of taking amounts over the recommended dosage, they know it can cause diarrhea, nausea and vomiting in the short run.

➤ VITAMIN E: While many experts say that doses up to 1,000 IU are safe, such doses can cause flulike symptoms—muscle weakness, fatigue, nausea and diarrhea—in some people. They may also impair immune function and disable white blood cells.

Extra vitamin E spells deeper trouble for some individuals. Because it prevents blood from clotting (how it's thought to help fight heart disease), it potentially causes bleeding problems, including hemorrhagic stroke, especially among those who take anticoagulants. People who take aspirin, vitamin E and garlic together may be at significant risk. No one knows how they work together, or magnify the effects of each other.

➤ BETA-CAROTENE: A 1994 Finnish study found that large doses of beta-carotene, taken as pills, failed to prevent lung cancer among smokers; beta-carotene users, in fact, had *higher* lung cancer rates. Some experts interpreted this to mean that beta-carotene had no effect, but others took this at face value, believing that beta-carotene taken as an isolated supplement may promote cancer. Similarly, a 1991 study suggested that beta-carotene increased cervical cancer risk. True, beta-carotene is a great substance, but get it from food, not supplements.

Medications and Nutrition

10

Fortunately, medical science has developed medications that make living with chronic illness much easier. Many medications, in fact, control symptoms and allow some people with a particular disease to live fairly normal lives. Other medications significantly alleviate pain and/or symptoms and help people return to a more active lifestyle.

Often, though, medications have undesirable side effects. This doesn't mean that you should avoid the drug, just that you should learn to manage your lifestyle to reduce, as much as possible, the chance of suffering these side effects.

In this chapter, we'll review how certain medications can affect nutritional status, or interfere with what happens to nutrients inside the body. Some medications reduce the amount of a particular nutrient that is absorbed; others increase the rate at which the nutrient is excreted from the body. And still others interact with the nutrient in yet other ways. Sometimes, certain foods interact with the medication to decrease its absorption, or, on the flip side, to increase its potency. In addition, some medications increase the chance of retaining excess fluid or are abrasive to the lining of the stomach.

Medications are listed alphabetically. Because so many of these medications are used in the treatment of several illnesses, I have not included any information about what diseases each is used for. Also, I have included at the end of the chapter information on foods high in the nutrients mentioned in this chapter. For example, if a medication causes potassium to be lost from the body, you'll find a chart on foods high in potassium.

While information on glucocorticosteroid medications is included in this chapter, please refer to chapter 11 for more details.

Acetaminophen   *Brand name(s)*: **Tylenol**
Interacting food(s) or nutrient(s): High-carbohydrate meal
Interaction : Slows absorption of acetaminophen
Solution: Take on an empty stomach

Advil: *See* **Ibuprofen**

Aspirin

Interacting food(s) or nutrient(s): Protein

Interaction: High doses of aspirin may interfere with breakdown of protein in the body

Solution: Maintain good protein intake; increases foods high in calcium and potassium to prevent muscle weakness

Aristocort: *See* **Triamcinolone**

Azulfidine: *See* **Sulfasalazine**

Betamethasone   *Brand name(s)*: **Celestone**

Interacting food(s) or nutrient(s): Caffeine

Interaction: Contributes to ulcer development

Solution: Avoid caffeine

Interacting food(s) or nutrient(s): High-sodium foods

Interaction: Increases fluid retention

Solution: Limit sodium intake

Interacting food(s) or nutrient(s): Potassium

Interaction: Medication may cause potassium to be lost from the body

Solution: Increase intake of potassium-rich foods

Interacting food(s) or nutrient(s): Protein

Interaction: High doses may interfere with breakdown of protein in the body

Solution: Maintain good protein intake

Bronkodyl: *See* **Theophylline**

Bumetanude   *Brand name(s)*: **Bumex**

Interacting food(s) or nutrient(s): Licorice

Interaction: Speeds potassium elimination, possibly quite rapidly and with dangerous consequences

Solution: Avoid licorice

Bumex: *See* **Bumetanude**

Celestone: *See* **Betamethasone**

Ciprofloxacin   *Brand name(s)*: **Cipro**

Interacting food(s) or nutrient(s): Caffeine-containing foods

Interaction: Greater than expected nervousness, insomnia, anxiety, tachycardia (rapid heart rate)

Solution: Avoid caffeine

Interacting food(s) or nutrient(s): Dairy products

Interaction: Calcium in dairy foods decreases drug absorption

Solution: Take medication on empty stomach

Coumadin: *See* **Warfarin**

Deltasone: *See* **Prednisone**

Dilantin: *See* **Phenytoin**

Dopar: *See* **Levodopa**

Eldepryl: *See* **Selegiline**

Etretinate   *Brand name(s)*: **Tegison**

Interacting food(s) or nutrient(s): Fatty foods

Interaction: High-fat foods enhance absorption of drug, but etretinate can cause increased triglyceride levels (triglyceride is one measure of the amount of fat in the bloodstream)

Solution: Take the drug with a food containing fat, but otherwise follow a low-fat diet (consume no more than 20 to 25 percent of calories as fat)

Interacting food(s) or nutrient(s): Milk
Interaction: Milk increases absorption of drug, allows smaller doses
Solution: Always take medication with milk

Feldene: *See* **Piroxicam**

Florinef: *See* **Fludrocortisone**

Fludrocortisone   *Brand name(s)*: **Florinef**
Interacting food(s) or nutrient(s): Caffeine
Interaction: Contributes to ulcer development
Solution: Avoid caffeine
Interacting food(s) or nutrient(s): High-sodium foods
Interaction: Increases fluid retention
Solution: Limit sodium intake
Interacting food(s) or nutrient(s): Potassium
Interaction: Medication may cause potassium to be lost from the body
Solution: Increase intake of potassium-rich foods
Interacting food(s) or nutrient(s): Protein
Interaction: High doses may interfere with breakdown of protein in the body
Solution: Maintain good protein intake

Fluphenazine   *Brand name(s)*: **Prolixin**
Interacting food(s) or nutrient(s): Beverages with caffeine (coffee, cola, tea) or apple juice
Interaction: Inactivates the medication
Solution: Avoid these substances. To dilute the liquid concentrate, use milk, noncola sodas, orange juice

Furosemide   *Brand name(s)*: **Lasix**
Interacting food(s) or nutrient(s): Licorice
Interaction: Speeds potassium elimination, possibly quite rapidly and with dangerous consequences
Solution: Avoid licorice
Interacting food(s) or nutrient(s): Potassium
Interaction: May cause potassium levels to fall too low
Solution: Increase intake of potassium-rich foods

Haldol: *See* **Haloperidol**

Haloperidol   *Brand name(s)*: **Haldol**
Interacting food(s) or nutrient(s): Coffee, tea (when drug is in the form of a liquid concentrate)
Interaction: Precipitate forms (the drug combines with an ingredient in coffee or tea to form a solid material, and then settles to the bottom of the glass)
Solution: Dilute liquid dose in water or milk instead of coffee or tea

Hydrocholorothiazide   *Brand name(s)*: **Oretic, Hydrodiuril**
Interacting food(s) or nutrient(s): Sodium (salt)
Interaction: High sodium intake causes excess potassium loss, possibly causing electrolyte disturbances
Solution: Decrease sodium intake
Interacting food(s) or nutrient(s): Potassium
Interaction: May cause potassium depletion
Solution: Increase intake of potassium-rich foods in diet
Interacting food(s) or nutrient(s): Licorice
Interaction: Can cause electrolyte imbalance
Solution: Avoid licorice

Hydrocortisone   *Brand name(s)*: **Solucortef**

Interacting food(s) or nutrient(s): Caffeine
Interaction: Contributes to ulcer development
Solution: Avoid caffeine
Interacting food(s) or nutrient(s): High-sodium foods
Interaction: Increases fluid retention
Solution: Limit sodium intake
Interacting food(s) or nutrient(s): Potassium
Interaction: Medication may cause potassium to be lost from the body
Solution: Increase intake of potassium-rich foods
Interacting food(s) or nutrient(s): Protein
Interaction: High doses may interfere with breakdown of protein in the body
Solution: Maintain good protein intake

Hydrodiuril: *See* **Hydrocholorothiazide**

Ibuprofen   *Brand name(s)*: **Advil, Motrin**

Problem: Can be irritating to the stomach
Solution: Take with food

Indocin: *See* **Indomethacin**

Indomethacin   *Brand name(s)*: **Indocin**

Problem: Can be irritating to the stomach
Solution: Take with food

Kenacort: *See* **Triamcinolone**

Larodopa: *See* **Levodopa**

Lasix: *See* **Furosemide**

Levodopa   *Brand name(s)*: **Larodopa, Sinemet, Dopar**

Interacting food(s) or nutrient(s): Foods very high in pyridoxine (vitamin B_6), including avocado,
    bacon, beans, beef liver, dry skim milk, oatmeal, pork, peas, sweet potato, tuna
Interaction: Pyridoxine decreases the action of this medication
Solution: Check with physician to determine how much of these foods may be eaten
Interacting food(s) or nutrient(s): High-protein foods
Interaction: Decrease absorption
Solution: Take on empty stomach or with low-protein snack (such as fruit)

MTX: *See* **Methotrexate**

Meticorten: *See* **Prednisone**

Methotrexate   *Brand name(s)*: **Mexate, MTX, Rheumatrex**

Interacting food(s) or nutrient(s): Folate (also called folic acid, which is one of the B vitamins)
Interaction: May interfere with folate metabolism and other nutrients
Solution: Increase intake of folate rich foods
Interacting food(s) or nutrient(s): Milk
Interaction: Delays drug absorption
Solution: Take on empty stomach

Mexate: *See* **Methotrexate**

Minocin: *See* **Minocycline**

Minocycline   *Brand name(s)*: **Minocin**

Interacting food(s) or nutrient(s): Dairy products, iron supplements
Interaction: Decreases absorption of drug
Solution: Take on an empty stomach

Motrin: *See* **Ibuprofen**

Oretic: *See* **Hydrochlorothiazide**

Penicillin G   *Brand name(s):* **Pentids, Pfizerpen**
  Interacting food(s) or nutrient(s): Coffee, citrus fruits, tomatoes, fruit juices
  Interaction: Destruction of drug in stomach
  Solution: Take on empty stomach

Pentids: *See* **Penicillin G**

Pfizerpen: *See* **Penicillin G**

Phenytoin   *Brand name(s):* **Dilantin**
  Interacting food(s) or nutrient(s): Charcoal-broiled meats
  Interaction: Decreases phenytoin blood levels
  Solution: Avoid charcoal-broiled meats
  Interacting food(s) or nutrient(s): Folate (or folic acid, which is one of the B vitamins)
  Interaction: May impair folate absorption
  Solution: Increase intake of folate-rich foods
  Interacting food(s) or nutrient(s): Pyridoxine (vitamin B_6)
  Interaction: May induce pyridoxine deficiency
  Solution: Increase intake of vitamin B_6-rich foods
  Interacting food(s) or nutrient(s): Vitamin D
  Interacting nutrient: May deplete vitamin D
  Solution: Maintain good calcium and vitamin D intake

Piroxicam   *Brand name(s):* **Feldene**
  Problem: Can be irritating to the stomach
  Solution: Take with food

Prednisone   *Brand name(s):* **Deltasone, meticorten**
  Interacting food(s) or nutrient(s): Caffeine
  Interaction: Contributes to ulcer development
  Solution: Avoid caffeine
  Interacting food(s) or nutrient(s): High-sodium foods
  Interaction: Increases fluid retention
  Solution: Limit sodium intake
  Interacting food(s) or nutrient(s): Potassium
  Interaction: Medication may cause potassium to be lost from the body
  Solution: Increase intake of potassium-rich foods
  Interacting food(s) or nutrient(s): Protein
  Interaction: High doses may interfere with breakdown of protein in the body
  Solution: Maintain good protein intake

Prolixin: *See* **Fluphenazine**

Rheumatrex: *See* **Methotrexate**

Selegiline   *Brand name(s):* **Eldepryl**
  Interacting food(s) or nutrient(s): High doses of aged and fermented foods, which contain a substance
    called tyramine
  Interaction: Tyramine-containing foods may cause blood pressure to rise quickly to an abnormally
    high level (called hypertensive crisis) if dose of the food is high.
  Solution: In most people, it takes an exceptionally high dose of tyramine-containing foods to
    cause this reaction. Discuss with your doctor what is appropriate for your dose of medication
    and your dietary habits.

Sinemet: *See* **Levodopa**

SloBid: *See* **Theophylline**

Slo-Phyllin: See Theophylline

Sulfasalazine   *Brand name(s)*: **Azulfidine**

   Interacting food(s) or nutrient(s): Folate (also called folic acid, one of the B vitamins)

   Interaction: Impairs ability to use food as source of folate

   Solution: Increase intake of folate-rich foods

Tegison: *See* **Etretinate**

Theo-24: *See* **Theophylline**

TheoDur: *See* **Theophylline**

Theophylline   *Brand name(s)*: **TheoDur, Theo-24, Slo-Phyllin, SloBid, Bronkodyl, Uniphyl**

   Interacting food(s) or nutrient(s): Caffeine-containing foods, including coffee, tea, chocolate, colas

   Interaction: Additive stimulant effect

   Solution: Avoid caffeine-containing foods

   Interacting food(s) or nutrient(s): Low-carbohydrate, high-protein diet

   Interaction: Increases the amount of theophylline the body eliminates without using, which means not as much drug is available to the body

   Solution: Balance protein/carbohydrates daily

   Interacting food(s) or nutrient(s): Charcoal-broiled meats

   Interaction: Increases theophylline elimination

   Solution: Avoid charcoal-broiled meats

Triamcinolone   *Brand name(s)*: **Aristocort, Kenacort**

   Interacting food(s) or nutrient(s): Caffeine

   Interaction: Contributes to ulcer development

   Solution: Avoid caffeine and caffeine containing food such as chocolate

   Interacting food(s) or nutrient(s): High-sodium foods

   Interaction: Increases fluid retention

   Solution: Limit sodium intake

   Interacting food(s) or nutrient(s): Potassium

   Interaction: Medication may cause potassium to be lost from the body

   Solution: Increase intake of potassium-rich foods

   Interacting food(s) or nutrient(s): Protein

   Interaction: High doses may interfere with breakdown of protein in the body

   Solution: Maintain good protein intake

Tylenol: *See* **acetaminophen**

Uniphyl: *See* **theophylline**

Warfarin   *Brand name(s)*: **Coumadin**

   Interacting food(s) or nutrient(s): Foods high in vitamin K, including green leafy vegetables, beef liver, broccoli, cauliflower, Brussels sprouts, asparagus, vegetable oil, egg yolk

   Interaction: Can increase the chances of abnormal bleeding

   Solution: Please note that this is generally only a problem if intake of these foods changes, such as during the summer time when people tend to eat more green leafy vegetables. Discuss with your physician the necessity of limiting these foods, depending on your dose; better yet, discuss with your physician how to have a consistent intake of these foods.

How to Limit Sodium

If you take medications that cause you to retain fluid, limit sodium to around 2,000 milligrams daily. To limit sodium, try the following suggestions:

➤ Concentrate on eating loads of fresh fruits and vegetables, as they are almost void of sodium. Frozen vegetables are also nearly sodium-free and are also nutritionally very strong; they're a great alternative if you can't include fresh ones. Do avoid canned vegetables, as they are high in salt.

➤ Cut down on salt in recipes you prepare at home; for example, don't add salt to cooking water when you prepare pasta, potatoes or vegetables. You can cut the amount of salt in most cookie and cake recipes without compromising quality; I generally cut it in half.

➤ Before you buy canned, frozen and packaged foods, read labels carefully. Check the amount of sodium per serving, avoiding foods that have more than 700 milligrams per serving. Yes, this is high, so limit use of convenience foods. Note that most canned soups are overwhelmingly high, so look for alternatives. There are some excellent and very easy soup recipes in this book, even if you say you can't cook.

➤ Use luncheon meats only rarely. While the sodium per ounce seems to fit into your eating plan, note that most people use more than one ounce, driving sodium intake up too high.

➤ Put away the salt shaker, finding alternatives to spice up food. For example, lemon juice, balsamic vinegar and herbs are no-sodium, healthy alternatives.

Here are just a few examples of high-sodium foods and the amount of sodium they contain per serving size indicated:

CANNED SOUPS

Regular canned soups: 800–1,200 mg per cup
Healthy Choice or Special Request soups: 400–500 mg per cup

FAST FOODS

Breakfast sandwich: 700–2,000 mg
Sandwich: 500–1,400 mg
Fried chicken: 300–800 mg per piece

CONVENIENCE FOODS

Luncheon meat: 300–500 mg per ounce
Lite luncheon meat: 200–400 mg per ounce
Snack foods (chips, etc.): 200–600 mg per ounce
Light frozen dinners: 300–1,000 mg per meal

How to Boost Potassium

Try to get around 3,500 milligrams of potassium daily (but always check with your doctor first to make sure it is safe for you and your medical condition)

FOODS WITH 300–400 MG POTASSIUM
½ cup prune juice
¾ cup vegetable juice cocktail (reduced-sodium variety)
½ cup broiled lentils
½ cup steamed spinach
3½ ounces baked flounder or sole

FOODS WITH 400–500 MG POTASSIUM
1 cup skim milk
1 medium banana
1 cup cantaloupe pieces
½ cup baked winter squash
3½ ounces cooked beef tenderloin
3 ounces cooked red snapper

FOODS WITH 500–600 MG POTASSIUM
8 ounces low-fat yogurt
10 dates

FOODS WITH MORE THAN 700 MG POTASSIUM
10 dried apricots
10 dried figs
10 dried prunes
1 medium baked potato with skin

How to Boost Vitamin B_6 (Pyridoxine)

The RDA for vitamin B_6 is 1.6 mg for women and 2 mg for men. Try to get at least this amount, especially if you take medications that interfere with the body's ability to use this vitamin. If you do take a supplement, don't overdo it. Too much B_6 can cause irreversible nerve damage.

3 ounces cooked pork loin = 0.32 mg
3 ounces cooked chicken breast = 0.48 mg
3 ounces cooked beef = 0.32 mg
8 ounces nonfat milk = 0.10 mg
1 cup cooked black beans = 0.12 mg
¼ cup wheat germ = 0.28 mg
½ cup cooked spinach = 0.14 mg

How to Boost Folate (Folic Acid)

If you take medications that break down folate, boost intake. Aim for about 400 to 600 micrograms daily. Note that if you take a supplement, and if you take too much of the supplement, you can mask signs of a vitamin B_{12} deficiency. This can be quite dangerous, as B_{12} deficiency leads to irreversible nerve damage.

1 cup cooked black beans = 256 mcg
¼ cup wheat germ = 99 mcg
½ cup cooked spinach = 102 mcg
8 ounces fresh orange juice = 69 mcg
2 cups chopped romaine lettuce = 152 mcg

Nutritional Concerns   11
of the Glucocorticoid (Steroid) User

When glucocorticoids (also called steroids) were introduced in the 1950s, they were widely hailed as a wonder drug. People with arthritis who took them could move again, and often with little or no pain. Those with asthma could breathe again, and people with lupus and multiple sclerosis finally had some relief from their symptoms.

As more and more people started using this type of medication, however, they found it brought with it some not so wonderful side effects. Some of the most noticeable are water retention, a moonface and an increased appetite. Of more serious consequence are the effects cortisone has on nutritional stores and metabolism. Let's take a look.

Increased Protein Needs

Steroids bind with proteins in the body, sometimes causing loss of protein needed to repair tissues, fight infections and maintain muscle mass. Fortunately, most Americans eat considerably more protein than needed for optimal health, enough even to offset the steroid-induced losses. But steroid users with a poor appetite or poor dietary habits, however, can become protein deficient. To be on the safe side, plan generous servings of protein-rich foods daily, paying attention to include some at each meal. (*Caution*: patients with kidney disease should check with their physician about how much protein is safe for them.)

GOOD SOURCES OF PROTEIN
One 8-ounce glass nonfat milk = 8 g
3 ounces cooked meat or fish = 26 g
1 cup low-fat cottage cheese = 31 g
1 egg = 7g
2 tablespoons peanut butter = 8 g
1 cup cooked lentils (or other beans) = 18 g
1 ounce cheese = 7 g
½ package (4.5 ounces) tofu = 9 g

Balancing Sodium and Potassium

Steroid users must watch sodium intake carefully. Sodium, or salt, causes fluid retention, which can lead to significant weight gain and undesirable appearance changes; it can also raise blood pressure. This is compounded by another side effect of steroids: it interferes with the body's fluid-balancing hormones, causing fluid retention both with and without excess sodium, but the problem is definitely much worse with sodium (see page 75).

While steroids cause the body to latch onto too much sodium, they tend to drain the body's potassium stores. This can cause muscle weakness, and it can also interfere with the normal rhythm of the heart if really excessive amounts of potassium are lost. For most people who take steroids, it is a good idea to boost potassium intake to around 3,500 milligrams per day; see page 76. (*Caution*: if you have kidney disease, check with your physician about a safe level of potassium intake for your condition.)

Plan for Healthy, Strong Bones

A devastating consequence of long-term steroid use is osteoporosis, or brittle bones. Taking steroids every day for just six months can result in rapid bone loss, which can lead to osteoporosis and then fractures, some of which can be life-changing. Osteoporosis and fractures can greatly reduce mobility, which can be particularly serious in someone who has a chronic illness that already restricts mobility. Steroids not only interfere with the body's ability to absorb calcium, but they also cause the body to excrete higher than normal amounts of calcium in the urine. The effects of this calcium shortage are intensified by another undesirable effect of steroids: changes in the way the body uses vitamin D, which helps the body absorb and use calcium. It's sort of like the key that allows calcium into the body where it is needed; without it, all the calcium in the world could not prevent osteoporosis.

There is now evidence that substantially increasing calcium and vitamin D intake can help stop and reverse corticosteroid-induced bone loss. In one study, researchers studied 130 patients with rheumatoid arthritis who took steroids. Some of the patients (mostly women) received 1,000 milligrams per day of calcium, in the form of calcium carbonate, along with 500 IU of vitamin D. Another group of patients received a placebo, or pills that looked and tasted like the vitamin D/calcium supplements but were just sugar pills. Bone density was measured both before and after the study, and researchers found that the women taking the real thing (the vitamin D and calcium) had greater bone density of the spine and the femoral bone.

The American College of Rheumatology recommends patients using steroids get 1,500 milligrams of calcium daily, either from food or supplements, or some combination of the two. Many doctors also recommend 800 IU of vitamin D daily. Unfortunately, a study published in the *British Medical Journal* in 1996 found that very few steroid users take calcium and vitamin D. In their study of 303 patients taking continuous oral steroids for three or more months, just seven patients were receiving calcium and only six were receiving calcium plus vitamin D. Take responsibility to raise the issue with your physician—you'll be in charge of your bone strength and of your independence in the future.

Other ways to help preserve bone mass include:

➤ Quit smoking.

➤ Limit alcohol to one drink daily.

➤ Do at least thirty minutes of weight-bearing exercise daily.

➤ Postmenopausal women should discuss estrogen therapy with their physician.

Get Enough Zinc

Although information is limited, there is some evidence that long-term steroid use may cause low zinc levels. Try to get the Recommended Dietary Allowance (RDA) for zinc, which is fifteen milligrams for men and twelve milligrams for women. The following foods are good sources of zinc: meat, liver, eggs, seafood (especially oysters) and whole grains (but the zinc in whole grains may be partially "bound up" and therefore unavailable to the body). Don't go overboard, as doses just slightly more than the RDA can cause problems.

Control Hyperlipidemia

Steroids can cause hyperlipidemia, or high levels of blood fats. This increase in blood fats is similar to that seen in people with poorly controlled diabetes: a moderate rise in cholesterol, but a significant increase in blood triglycerides. The long-term consequences of hyperlipidemia are a much greater chance of developing artery-clogging heart disease.

While this hyperlipidemia may be unavoidable with certain doses, one can at least minimize other contributions to undesirable blood fats by maintaining a desirable weight and limiting saturated fats, cholesterol and concentrated sweets. (See chapter 3 for information on how to prevent heart disease.)

Steroids and Blood Sugar Problems

Steroids may interfere with carbohydrate metabolism or the body's ability to break down and use sugar and other starches. The higher the dose of steroids, the more serious this problem. Some people who take steroids actually become diabetic, especially those with an inherent or latent tendency to have blood sugar problems. This includes people with a history of diabetes in their family, and people who are overweight. Some individuals can solve the problem by following a special diet, but others need oral medication or even insulin.

Maintaining a lean weight is crucial to reducing the chances of becoming diabetic. Let's review the blood sugar problems that can arise with steroid use.

More Than One Type of Sugar

Most people think of table sugar when they hear the word *sugar*. What's puzzling, though, is hearing that foods like peas and rice have sugar, too. The confusion results from using the term *sugar* in place of the more accurate word, *carbohydrate*. One reason that carbohydrates are often called sugars is that all carbohydrate-containing foods—fruits, vegetables, grains and legumes—are composed of one or more types of sugar units hooked together.

Understanding two additional terms will help you plan sweets into your eating plan healthfully: *simple* and *complex carbohydrates*. Sweets are simple carbohydrates; whole grains are complex carbohydrates. Complex carbohydrates contain lots of sugar units hooked together, while simple carbohydrates commonly consist of just a few sugar units.

But there's another critical difference between complex and simple carbohydrates. Complex carbohydrates aren't the most complex just in terms of the individual sugars forming them, but also because they are complex nutrition packages. Wrapped into their elaborate packages are lots of vitamins, minerals and fiber. Eating more complex than simple carbohydrates means harvesting more nutrients—and that translates into a healthier you.

The Larger Picture

How often should the average diabetic include a sweet treat? There are two factors to consider, the most important of which has nothing to do with being diabetic. Everyone should evaluate how sweets fit into a healthy diet. If you have treats every day in place of healthier, complex carbohydrates, you'll come up short nutritionally; because they are generally higher in calories, you'll also be more likely to gain weight. And if you add them to a nutrient-rich diet, you may gain weight. Realistically and healthfully, most people should plan in no more than two or three desserts weekly.

Exercise to Improve Blood Sugars

The benefits of exercising frequently are no secret: it helps control weight, reduce heart disease risk and relieve stress. For people with diabetes, there is an additional and compelling reason to exercise regularly: it helps control blood sugars.

Exercise helps lower blood sugars in several ways. Most importantly, exercise changes the manner in which the body uses insulin by:

➜ SENSITIZING THE BODY. Making the body more sensitive to insulin means that exercise helps the same amount of insulin lower blood sugar more significantly.

➜ CONTROLLING WEIGHT. For diabetics, maintaining a healthy weight is critically important, as being overweight makes blood sugar control more difficult.

➜ REDUCING STRESS. Research has proven that diabetics under less stress have an easier time controlling blood sugar readings.

GETTING STARTED The first step you should take to make exercise a regular part of your diabetes care plan is to consult with your health care providers about what's best for you. Your medical team will make sure you're ready to exercise and then help you design an individualized exercise plan by:

➤ Evaluating your current blood sugar control, and determining if you'll need changes to your insulin dose and/or food intake to accommodate the type of exercise you choose.

➤ Determining how healthy your heart is. If you haven't been a regular exerciser, it's important to know if you have heart trouble, which could make it dangerous for you to exercise. For other previously inactive people, these tests help prescribe the safest form of exercise.

➤ Considering your other medical condition. Many times, a physical therapist can be a tremendous help in devising the safest exercise plan for you.

If you've had diabetes for a while, here are some other concerns to have as you devise an exercise program:

➤ Examine your feet for sores and/or signs of nerve damage. Because diabetics often experience slow wound healing, they shouldn't engage in exercise that can irritate already existing sores on their feet. Patients who have diabetes-associated nerve damage (neuropathy) in their feet are less able to feel when blisters or sores are developing on their feet. These people may be advised to avoid running, choosing instead walking, cycling or swimming.

➤ Have your eyes examined for signs of retinopathy, a common complication of people who have diabetes. People with this condition must avoid activities that require rapid head movements, heavy lifting or straining.

Managing the Steroid Appetite

One of the most frustrating side effects of steroids is a voracious appetite.

If you've been on steroids for any length of time, you probably know the feeling. You have likely fought the urge to put away a package of cookies chased with a quart of milk. You may have found yourself in front of the opened refrigerator, praying for the strength to close the door before you polish off the leftover pizza and meat loaf, and part of tonight's dinner as well. You've likely endured the frustration of feeling hungry after appetizers, dinner and dessert. Don't despair: you *can* fight the steroid appetite.

Why Appetite Goes into Overdrive

The insatiable hunger experienced by people on steroids is real, not psychological in nature. Here's how that happens. Steroids suppresses the normal activity of two of the body's hormone-producing glands, the hypothalamus and the pituitary. Consequently, the body's delicate hormone balance is upset. Among many other things, a proper hormone balance is necessary to regulate appetite. Steroids, then, take away the ability to control food intake by taking away the appetite signal.

As a result, the idea of eating until you are satisfied, which works well for most people, goes right out the window when steroids comes into the picture. Because your body can no longer provide internal signals to control appetite, you have to take the initiative of controlling what you eat through careful menu planning.

Preventing weight gain while on any substantial dose of steroids is critically important for all the obvious reasons and at least one more: it's nearly impossible to lose weight while taking these higher doses. If you take steroids, no longer can you allow yourself to give in to a few temptations today because you'll crash diet tomorrow to drop the extra three to five pounds. Unfortunately, each extra pound adds up, and you'll soon be looking at many excess pounds you can't shed.

Don't wait until the scales start to tip unfavorably. Planning ahead for the increased appetite that goes with taking steroids will keep you in control. Here are some ideas:

1. PLAN AHEAD. Plan your meals before you eat, preferably on a full stomach when you're better able to think about food rationally. Planning a few days of menus in advance not only ensures variety, but also makes shopping easier. If you aren't sure where to start, you may find it helpful to consult a registered dietitian. He or she can help you determine how many calories you need to consume for your size and your unique physical condition.

2. PORTION CONTROL. This is just as important as choosing the appropriate foods. An example will help explain. Let's say you've consulted with a registered dietitian and have learned that at dinner, you should have a 3-ounce meat or fish portion; 2 servings of a starch (where a serving is ½ cup or 1 slice of bread) and 8 ounces of skim milk. So, for Wednesday night, you've planned a healthy dinner of 3 ounces of grilled salmon, 1 cup of rice, 1 cup of broccoli and 8 ounces of skim milk. But, in a hurry, you didn't bother with the food scale or measuring cups, and you just guessed on portion sizes. Just eyeballing portions, you served up a 7-ounce portion of salmon, 1½ cups of rice and 12 ounces of milk—and a couple of hundred extra calories for that meal alone. Consuming just 300 extra calories each day leads to a pound of weight gain every 12 days, based on the fact that to gain a pound, you have to eat 3,500 extra calories over and above those needed to maintain weight.

   Use the food measuring tools regularly in the beginning to help you learn servings sizes, and you'll be more confident to "eyeball" them. Then, just use them on occasion—once a week or so—to make sure you're still on target. Remember, you can overeat even on food that's "good for you" such as lean beef and chicken. This is especially true when you are taking steroids and your appetite is out of whack.

3. DO NOT SKIP MEALS. Eat regularly, preferably three small meals and three nutritious snacks daily. Skipping meals may leave you insatiably hungry and less able to stick to your meal plan when you finally eat. The three small snacks, preferably of fruits, raw vegetables or plain popcorn, help satisfy that never-ending urge to nibble.

4. AVOID TEMPTATION. Don't tempt yourself by keeping high-calorie treats around your house or office. Rid your surroundings of all those things you have trouble passing up under normal circumstances—cookies, cakes, chips, and so on—and replace them with acceptable munchies. Keep a container of chopped raw vegetables in the refrigerator to grab when you're about to chew through your fingernails. Clearing kitchen counters of bread baskets, cookie jars and fruit bowls also removes temptation. By the same token, try filling your plate from the stove rather than serving from the table where you may be tempted to have seconds.

5. RETHINK COMFORT FOODS. Remember, too, that steroids can have a psychological effect, sometimes leaving you a little down in the dumps. It is common for people who are feeling down to turn to comfort foods, usually fat-laden choices like macaroni and cheese or french fries. You can bypass these disastrous moments by simply not stocking up on your favorite comfort foods. Again, only have available what you can safely afford to eat. Try some of the flavorful herbal teas for these difficult moments.

6. DO NOT GROCERY SHOP. Grocery shopping while on any significant dose of steroids is like placing a kid in a candy store and telling him he can only look. Even though you go armed with a list of healthy foods, it's the snack and sweet aisles that will beckon you. Send your spouse, teenager or a good friend if you can't go shopping without coming out a candy bar or two heavier.

Ensuring Safe Food 　　12

While preventing foodborne infections—often called food poisoning—is important for everyone, it is especially important for people who take medications that suppress the immune system—immunosuppressed people. Some of these medications are steroids, methotrexate, cyclophosphamide and other antimetabolites. In addition, people who are weakened by a chronic medical condition need to be more attentive to food safety.

Although healthier people can sometimes get away with eating a raw egg (although this is never recommended), or tasting cookie dough containing raw eggs (again, not recommended), or even eat leftovers that aren't heated through properly, immunosuppressed people and those weakened by chronic disease cannot. In this chapter, we'll look at how you can avoid foodborne infections.

Purchasing Food: Safety Guidelines

1. Check the "sell by" and "use by" dates—and pay attention to them.
2. Don't purchase food if the safety seal is broken.
3. If you reach into the freezer case and find something is defrosted, don't purchase it.
4. When purchasing raw meat and poultry, place them in plastic bags available in the produce section. Meat packages often leak, and the juice can contaminate fresh foods in your cart, such as fruits and vegetables.
5. Purchase dairy foods last in the grocery store even though you often encounter them first in the grocery store.
6. Don't run other errands after grocery shopping. Refrigerate food within thirty minutes to an hour after purchase.

Storing Food Safely

1. Don't pack the refrigerate tightly. Leave enough room for air to circulate around food so that it can cool down properly. This is especially true for leftovers put in the refrigerator warm.

2. Check refrigerator temperature from time to time. The optimal refrigerator temperature is 35° to 40°F and 0°F in the freezer.

3. Clean the refrigerator regularly. A vinegar solution not only freshens the refrigerator, but also helps kill bacteria.

4. Refrigerate leftovers promptly. It is an old wives' tale that you should bring cooked foods to room temperature before refrigerating them. Similarly, just putting plastic wrap or foil wrap on food and then allowing it to cool at room temperature provides absolutely no protection against food contamination. Divide large portions into smaller ones so they cool down quickly. For example, package up several containers of leftover chili rather than placing the whole pot in the refrigerator. Similarly, cut the meat from a turkey, transferring it to several shallow containers rather than refrigerating the whole carcass.

5. If perishable food has been out on a buffet for more than two hours, discard it. This would include meats, sauces, dips, casseroles. Leftover veggies, fruits, cheeses, breads and desserts generally don't have to be discarded.

Egg Safety

1. Don't eat any foods that contain raw or improperly cooked eggs, including eggnogs (pasteurized ones are okay) and egg-based sauces like hollandaise sauce.

2. Cook all eggs properly. Scrambled eggs should be cooked past the runny stage. Better to avoid sunny-side-up eggs and flip them briefly (over easy). Make sure the white is thoroughly cooked with no runny spots. When using eggs in meringue-topped pies, bake the pies for at least fifteen minutes at 350°.

Meat, Poultry and Fish Safety

1. Defrost foods in the refrigerator rather than on the kitchen counter at room temperature. Take out frozen meat a day or two before you plan on using it, transferring it to the refrigerator.

2. Cook meat directly from the refrigerator—don't bring it to room temperature first. Bacteria can multiple rapidly at room temperature, and cooking might not destroy it.

3. Marinate meat in the refrigerator. Also, limit marinating time, not exceeding the recommended storage for fresh meat or poultry. That is, marinate red meat for no longer than three to five days, poultry for no more than one to two days. Discard marinating liquid, as any organisms that might have been in the meat can contaminate the marinating liquid.

4. When roasting or baking a whole chicken or turkey, place a cooking rack in the bottom of the pan—this allows hot air to circulate under the bird, and ensures more thorough cooking.

5. Do not partially cook or brown foods and then plan on cooking them later. This can only encourage bacterial growth. If you need to cook food early in the day, cook it all the way, refrigerate promptly and then reheat thoroughly at meal time.

6. If something smells wrong, then it's probably not safe. You shouldn't detect any odor from meat, fish or poultry when you unwrap it. If you do, it might not be safe. Fish, for example, should never smell fishy.

7. If meat or fish feels slimy, discard it. Washing off the slime doesn't get rid of the bacteria that are inside.

8. Cook all ground beef to well done (past the pink stage, even in the center). A type of bacteria called *E. coli 0157:H7* is often found on the surface of beef. Cooking destroys this surface bacteria on cuts of beef, even if you don't cook them to well done. However, beef with this bacteria that is ground into hamburger meat becomes contaminated throughout. The only way to kill it is to cook the hamburger to the well-done stage.

9. Wash (preferably in the dishwasher) all utensils and cutting boards used with use raw meat and poultry. Don't reuse these utensils to prepare other foods, such as fruit and produce.

10. When cooking outside on the grill, take the raw meat out on one platter and then place that platter in the dishwasher (or wash it). Bring in the meat using a clean platter.

11. Avoid raw fish, especially raw shellfish.

12. Purchase shellfish only from safe waters and cook it properly.

13. If meat or poultry juice spills on to the counter, don't reuse the sponge or cloth with which you mopped it up. Place the cloth in the dirty laundry, and the sponge into the dishwasher. Better yet, use paper towels.

Produce Safety

1. Wash all produce with lots of clean, drinkable water. Include on this list melons and other fruits and vegetables that you peel before eating. Cutting into melons, for example, can transfer bacteria on the rind into the interior.

2. Use one cutting board for produce and one for meat—or at least wash the board in a dishwasher or in the sink with lots of hot, soapy water.

3. If you have your own garden, don't use manure to fertilize. It may contain dangerous organisms that you cannot wash off properly.

Reheating Leftovers Safely

1. Eat all leftovers within three to four days.

2. Reheat all food to 160°F, or to steaming hot. Be aware that the microwave can leave pockets of cold or inadequately warmed food. Stir food at least once if using the microwave, and make sure it, too, is piping hot.

3. Discard any leftovers that have any degree of off-odor—no matter how slight. Never skim off the molded portion of anything and use the food underneath (not even of jellies and jams)—discard the whole container. (You can however, safely cut off the moldy portion of cheese—just include a quarter-inch margin.)

4. Reheat sauces and gravies to a rolling boil for at least one minute before serving.

Miscellaneous

1. Wash hands thoroughly with hot water and soap before cooking and eating. While this is always important, pay special attention to this detail if you touch animals. Consider carrying baby wipes in your car or purse for days when you eat out—or wash your hands in the rest room after ordering to be on the safe side.

2. Purchase only pasteurized milk and juice. Homemade apple cider, for example, can contain dangerous organisms. Raw milk isn't safe for anyone.

3. Wash (in the washing machine) and dry (in a hot dryer) your kitchen cloths and towels. If you use a sponge, wash it daily in the dishwasher.
   Remember: When in doubt, throw it out!

For more information

For more information on safe food handling practices, call the United States Department of Agriculture Meat and Poultry Hotline at 800/535-4555.

HIV/AIDS

To say that good nutrition is important to HIV-positive people is an understatement. Staying well nourished "is the single greatest enhancement of the immune system" after medications used to treat HIV, says Martin Delaney, founding director of a San Francisco–based Project Inform, an organization that advocates for experimental drug trials and seeks to educate potential participants. Indeed, agrees Paul Skolnik, M.D., assistant professor of medicine at Tufts University School of Medicine and director of the HIV Laboratory at New England Medical Center, "Nutritional interventions, combined with potent antiviral drugs, may lead to optimal treatment outcomes."

Good nutrition is key to fighting the HIV infection and preventing it from progressing to full-blown AIDS. It's also critical to steering clear of the opportunistic infections that are a real problem for HIV-positive patients. Experts, in fact, say that the most cost-effective approach in treating HIV/AIDS is to prevent malnutrition.

In this chapter, we'll review the key nutrition goals for every patient who is HIV positive. They include:

→ Preventing progressive wasting: contrary to what many people think, progressive wasting is not an invariable consequence of AIDS.

→ Eating to preserve not only body weight, but also lean body mass.

→ Making every calorie count: eat nutrient-dense foods.

→ Concentrating on taking in the optimal amount of all nutrients, and understanding the special role that certain nutrients play in battling HIV/AIDS.

→ Accommodating taste changes and mouth sores.

→ Dealing with lactose intolerance.

→ Eating when nausea and diarrhea make it difficult.

→ Paying careful attention to safe food handling practices.

→ Using safe water.

→ Trying to get enough fruits and vegetables to boost your intake of phytochemicals.

Preventing Progressive Wasting and Preserving Lean Body Mass

Keeping weight on is a challenge for the person who is HIV positive. The disease process itself puts the body's metabolic machinery into overdrive, demanding more calories, protein and nutrients than normal. Even before symptoms arise in HIV-positive people, calorie needs are increased. In addition, both the infection and the medications used to treat it can significantly diminish appetite, as can such diverse problems as depression and constipation. And even when appetite does pick up, mouth sores (and mouth infections) as well as swallowing difficulties make it difficult to eat.

But weight loss is not an inevitable consequence of HIV/AIDS. As difficult as it can be, it is essential to take charge of keeping weight on: doing so can slow the course of the infection. HIV experts have documented a close relationship between weight loss and mortality—the more weight lost, the greater the chance of mortality. Indeed, most deaths from AIDS are due to starvation. The time of death in AIDS patients has been linked to weight loss, commonly occurring when body weight falls below 66 percent of ideal weight.

Be aware of the factors that cause wasting: opportunistic infections, fever, diarrhea (from infections and medications), nausea, and altered metabolism. Work with your health care provider to find solutions to these problems—and to keep weight on.

As you take charge of keeping weight on, you have to think about one very important factor: preserving lean body mass. *In fact, HIV/AIDS experts say that the amount of lean body mass is a more accurate predictor of survival than T-cell counts.*

The body is composed of two basic types of tissues: lean body mass and fat mass, as well as bone and water. Keeping the optimal amount of lean body mass, which is basically muscle, is important to fighting the HIV infection. Often, when people with HIV/AIDS lose weight, they lose more lean body mass than fat mass—this is especially true when they are already thin. In fact, when a thin person does not take in enough calories, the body turns to any available energy source. When there is no more fat to burn, the body turns to lean tissue. Because the muscles are on the bottom of the totem pole when it comes to figuring out what is most essential for the body to function, they get burned for fuel first.

If protein intake is low—even if calories are sufficient—the body will gradually turn to the vital organs, breaking them down to harvest the protein that is needed to drive the thousands upon millions of chemical reactions that run the body's machinery.

To make matters worse, people more commonly regain fat mass than lean body mass. When an individual goes through several cycles of weight loss and weight gain, the body composition can gradually change to too little lean body mass and too much fat mass—though the person is still quite thin. Even if a person is at a good weight, he might not be healthy if lean body mass is too low.

In any case, gaining back lost weight is no easy task. If you lose 10 pounds, for example, you'd have to eat 35,000 extra calories to gain it back (1 pound is worth 3,500 calories). That would take 140 cans of Ensure—3 cans daily for nearly 50 days—in addition to your regular food intake. Although it's work to keep weight on. It's a much easier proposition than putting it back on.

Boost Calories and Protein

While there are no official recommendations for how much protein to eat each day, it seems prudent to try to get 50 percent to 100 percent more than people without HIV need. Translation: instead of needing 50 grams to 60 grams per day, try to eat 75 grams to 100 grams. During the times that you're fighting a secondary infection, try to get the higher amount—the protein can be a big help in winning the battle.

Getting this much protein isn't as hard as it seems—most people in America eat far more protein than they actually need. The charts at the end of this chapter list high-protein foods and the amount of protein they contain. The menus following them are designed to supply 100 grams of protein daily. Because high-protein foods tend to be more expensive, I've included some of the best protein buys—foods that pack in a lot of protein per penny spent.

HIV-positive people without symptoms should eat 17 or 18 calories for every pound they weigh. For example, someone who weighs 160 pounds should eat about 2,800 calories. Those who have full-blown AIDS need more calories—19 or 20 calories per pound. Often, though, you are the best judge of how many calories you need. If you're losing weight, then you're not getting enough calories. The menus at the end of this chapter target a caloric intake of around 2,500 calories. If you're not keeping weight on at this caloric level, or if you need to gain weight, boost calories with foods from the chart of calorie/nutrient dense foods.

Making Calories Count: Eating Nutrient-Dense Foods

When you're trying to gain or keep weight on, it's tempting to turn to such calorie-loaded foods as candy bars, potato chips and soda pop. But don't be tempted—do yourself a favor and think about making every calorie count. Choose calories that aren't just calories, but carry with them loads of the nutrients that your body demands to fight the HIV infection, as well as secondary infections. In other words, avoid empty-calorie foods.

Think of the calories you consume as medicine to fight the infection and to preserve lean body mass. If you fill up on potato chips and pop, which are indeed loaded with calories, you won't have room left for the protein- and nutrient-rich foods that your body really needs.

Here's a good way to think about nutrient density. If you plant a garden in nutrient-poor soil, the plants will grow if you give them enough water. But they might be pale in color, more of a yellow-green instead of a healthier, deeper green color and spindly—tall with relatively fewer leaves than you'd expect. In addition, they might not produce as many vegetables as they would under better conditions. If you plant them in better soil or fertilize them, the plants should look dramatically better and also produce more vegetables. Think of your body as the plant, and calories as the water. Also think of your immune system as the color of the garden plants and the amount of produce they bear. If you feed your body enough calories but not enough protein and nutrients, it will keep going, but your immune system will be as weak and spindly as those plants that got water but not enough nutrients. Feeding your immune system with both enough calories and nutrients, it will be more robust and stronger to fight the infection.

So, when you're thirsty, choose a glass of high-calorie fruit juice, fruit nectar or milk. (See the section, page 97, on dealing with lactose intolerance if that is a problem for you.) You'll be loading up on not only calories, but also nutrients. And, if getting enough protein is a problem for you, the milk can help you take a giant step toward taking in an optimal amount.

When you reach for a snack, skip the chips and cookies and instead grab a peanut butter and jelly sandwich—loaded with calories, but also rich in protein and several nutrients. Or grab a fruited yogurt—higher in calories than plain yogurt, but again bursting with good nutrition, including the protein that is so essential to preserving lean body mass. Yogurt, by the way, might be a help in replenishing the good bacteria in the intestinal tract that can be diminished when you must take antibiotics. Refer to the charts at the end of this chapter for other high calorie snacks that are also nutrient dense.

Optimizing Nutrients

In choosing nutrient-dense foods, you'll be making great strides toward taking in all essential nutrients. Indeed, a wide range of nutrients is necessary to make the immune system strong—as well as just to live. The following list of nutrients are known to be essential for a healthy immune system, along with the foods containing the richest amounts:

- ➤ PROTEIN: Milk, cheese, meat, legumes (such as lentils).

- ➤ ZINC: Good sources include seafood, meats, whole grains, legumes.

- ➤ IRON: Red meat (the best source), fish, poultry, legumes, nuts and seeds, whole grains.

- ➤ MANGANESE: Rice cakes, brown rice, whole wheat bread, oatmeal, wheat germ, tea.

- ➤ COPPER: Legumes, meats, seafood, shellfish, whole grains, nuts and seeds.

- ➤ MAGNESIUM: Foods that are a good source of protein are generally a good source of magnesium; in addition, whole grains, legumes, nuts and seeds, green vegetables, avocados, bananas are good sources.

- ➤ SELENIUM: Protein-rich foods are also a good source of selenium; whole grains are also a good source. One of the richest sources is Brazil nuts.

- ➤ VITAMIN B_6: Chicken, fish, pork, eggs, liver, whole grains, legumes, avocados, bananas.

- ➤ RIBOFLAVIN: Meat, poultry, fish, eggs, and dairy products.

- ➤ FOLIC ACID: Dark green leafy vegetables, such as romaine lettuce and spinach; orange juice.

- ➤ VITAMIN B_{12}: This vitamin is found only in foods of animal origin, including meats, seafood, dairy products and eggs.

- ➤ THIAMIN: Whole grains, legumes, seeds, pork and brewer's yeast.

➤ VITAMIN C: Citrus fruits, tomatoes, broccoli, cantaloupe, berries, cabbage, asparagus, green and red sweet peppers.

➤ VITAMIN A: Sweet potatoes, carrots, evaporated skim milk, apricot nectar, liver, part skim ricotta cheese, cantaloupe, tomatoes, squash, spinach.

➤ VITAMIN E: Asparagus, beet greens, broccoli, cabbage, mustard greens, soybeans, spinach, tomatoes, hams, almonds, peanut butter, sunflower seeds, blueberries, papaya, quinoa, wheat germ, tuna steak, salmon, sole, shrimp.

As you can see, the list of nutrients that build a healthy immune system is long! While it's not good to concentrate on getting one nutrient to the exclusion of others, it makes sense to mention two nutrients that are a little more difficult to get, or at least keep in the body, when you have HIV/AIDS. In addition, researchers have shown that staying well nourished in one of these nutrients can be a big help in preventing bacterial infections and another checks the progression of HIV into full-blown AIDS. Let's take a look at zinc and vitamin B_{12}.

Zinc

HIV/AIDS researchers from the San Francisco General Hospital have shown that HIV-positive people who are deficient in zinc are far more likely to get systemic bacterial infections. These same researchers found that 29 percent of hospitalized patients had very low blood levels of zinc and another 21 percent had just borderline blood levels.

Unlike other essential minerals, the body does not store any significant amount of zinc. In addition, zinc deficiency occurs rapidly during periods of weight loss, when large amounts of zinc are lost in the urine. Moreover, chronic diarrhea causes big zinc losses, further compounding the problem.

Try to include plenty of zinc-rich foods, aiming to get the Recommended Dietary Allowance (RDA) of fifteen milligrams if you're a man and twelve milligrams if you're a woman, or just a little more. Don't overdose, though, with high dosed supplements. Too much can cause gastrointestinal irritation and vomiting; it can also lower blood levels of copper, which in turn shrinks red blood cells and also impairs immunity.

Foods High in Zinc

Food★	Zinc (mg) amount per serving
Dry-roasted peanuts, ¼ cup	1.2
Oil roasted peanuts, ¼ cup	2.4
Pumpkin seeds, roasted kernel portion only, ¼ cup	4.2
Sesame seeds, dried kernels only, ¼ cup	3.8
Canned mackerel, ½ can	1.8
Canned pink salmon, ½ can	2.1
Ground beef, 3 ounces cooked	4.5
Chicken, 3 ounces cooked	2.4
Instant Breakfast, 1 envelope	3.0
Dry milk powder, ½ cup	1.0
Yogurt, 1 cup	2.0
Clams, 1 cup canned	4.4

Food	Zinc (mg) amount per serving
Pork, 3 ounces cooked	1.5 to 2.0**
Oysters, 3.5 ounces cooked	182
Split peas, 1 cup cooked	2.0
Refried beans, 1 cup canned	3.5
Canned pork and beans, 1 cup	2.6 to 4.8
Canned vegetarian baked beans, 1 cup	3.6

All of these high-zinc foods are also excellent sources of protein!
**Depending on cut.*

Vitamin B_{12}

Studying 300 HIV-positive men, researchers at Johns Hopkins University found that those who had good amounts of vitamin B_{12} in their blood remain AIDS-free several years longer than HIV-positive people with low B_{12} blood levels. This study found that the B_{12}-adequate people did not progress to full-blown AIDS for 8 years, compared to just 4 years for people with low concentrations of B_{12}. Researchers took into account CD 4 levels, age, and use of HIV-fighting drugs, which did not differ between groups.

The problem for HIV-positive patients generally isn't getting enough B_{12}. In the Johns Hopkins study, for example, just 2 of the 300 men fell short of the RDA for B_{12}, which is 2 mcg (for both men and women). Rather, people with HIV have trouble hanging on to the B_{12} they do take in, for at least two reasons. In order to absorb B_{12}, the body has to produce enough stomach acid. For some reason, this acid production falls off in HIV-positive people, even before they develop full-blown AIDS. As a result, a greater than usual amount of the B_{12} just passes through the body unabsorbed. This is compounded by diarrhea, which washes out more of the B_{12}.

Pay attention to getting the RDA for vitamin B_{12} (2 mcg for men and women), plus a little extra. There aren't yet any official recommendations for how much extra B_{12} you should get to keep up blood levels. In some cases, you may need to work with your health care providers to determine if you'll need to get B_{12} in another form, such as through injections.

Foods High in B_{12}

Food	B_{12} (mcg) amount per serving*
Milk, whole, 2%, 1% or skim, 1 cup	1
Skim milk powder, ½ cup	1.35
Yogurt, 1 cup	1.3
Shrimp, 3.5 ounces cooked	1.5
Sole, 3.5 ounces cooked	2
Salmon, ½ can of pink salmon	10
Clams, 1 cup canned	158
Ground beef, 3 ounces cooked	2
Chicken, 3 ounces cooked	0.3
Braunschweiger, 2 ounces	11.5
Cottage cheese, 1 cup	1.5

Vitamin B_{12} is found only in foods of animal origin—that's why vegetarians who exclude dairy products cannot possibly get enough. They need to turn to a supplement.

Taste Changes and Mouth Sores

Sometimes, taste acuity goes down in people with HIV, because of either medications, mouth sores or infections. When taste acuity goes down, food tastes more bland, or tastes different than it usually does. Lacking its normal taste, food then becomes less appealing, which leads to undereating and undernourishment. In addition, mouth sores can make eating painful.

You'll have to experiment with what works best for you, but here are some suggestions that typically work:

➤ Choose foods that smell good to you: smell is an important part of taste.

➤ Go for your favorite foods, even if you eat them repeatedly.

➤ Sometimes heavily spiced food makes up for your diminished sense of taste. Choose your favorite spice, whatever it is—oregano, parsley, basil, chili and so on. If you have sores in your mouth, you might want to avoid spicy foods with a bite, such as hot chilis, salsa and the like.

➤ Practice impeccable hygiene: brushing your teeth frequently and even using mouthwash helps kill the normal bacteria in the mouth that can also alter your taste sensation.

➤ When mouth sores are troublesome, go for cool, soothing foods that are smooth in consistency. Good, high-nutrition foods that fit this ticket include yogurt, custard (try the recipes on pages 399–402, which give you both more variety and more nutrition than regular custard), cream soups, ice cream, rice pudding, scrambled eggs or mashed potatoes. Try mashing potatoes with ricotta cheese or low-fat cream cheese, which is higher in protein and nutrients than regular cream cheese. Avoid orange juice and other acidic foods, which can burn the mouth.

Lactose Intolerance

Lactose is the technical term for milk sugar; to digest lactose, the intestine must produce an enzyme called lactase. While infants of all races make plenty of lactase, people of some races produce less and less of the enzyme after the first year of life. Just 10 percent to 15 percent of adults of northern and western European ancestry have lactose malabsorption, but 90 percent of Asian Americans do. In addition, taking antibiotics for any length of time can temporarily affect the intestine and decrease its ability to make the enzyme lactase; similarly, chronic diarrhea can diminish lactase production. Both of these problems occur in HIV/AIDS patients, leading to temporary bouts of lactose intolerance.

While for a long time people used to think that lactose intolerance is an all-or-nothing phenomenon, there is now good evidence that lactose-intolerant people can indeed handle some milk. According to researchers at the Minneapolis Veterans Affairs Medical Center and the University of Minnesota, people with even severe lactose intolerance can drink two cups of milk per day without suffering symptoms. The caveat: divide the milk into two portions and drink it with meals.

In the study, nineteen people with documented lactose intolerance drank one cup of either lactose-reduced milk or regular milk twice daily. They reported no greater incidence of lactose intolerance symptoms after consuming regular milk than after lactose-reduced milk.

While people with lactose intolerance may not be able to stomach a pint of milk straight up—suffering bloating, gas and/or diarrhea—most can enjoy half a pint when it's "diluted" by breakfast, and another half pint several hours later diluted by dinner. Having smaller portions and consuming milk with meals slows the rate at which lactose hits the intestine, thereby improving lactose tolerance.

If dividing milk into smaller portions doesn't work for you, there are other solutions. Try yogurt, which has less lactose than milk and so is often tolerated by lactose-intolerant people. You can buy lactose-reduced milk in the dairy section of most grocery stores; because the milk sugar is already "digested," lactose-reduced milk does taste a little sweeter than other milk. Or, you can purchase pills that contain a version of the lactase enzyme (available from most drugstores without a prescription) made by the body; taking these pills before consuming dairy products solves the problem for most people.

It is worth the extra effort to either purchase lactose-reduced milk or take pills with the lactase enzyme. Milk and other dairy products are a great source of protein and calories for people with poor appetites (milk is also a good source of vitamin B_{12}). In addition, milk, custards, yogurts and cottages cheese are nonirritating and even soothing to people with mouth sores. They're also easy foods to consume when energy is low and you don't feel like cooking or even like chewing.

Nausea and Diarrhea

It seems like the times when you most need good nutrition—when the virus becomes more active and/or you acquire a secondary infection—that you have the most trouble with nausea and diarrhea. Just being sicker can cause these problems, but they're often compounded by the medications. These problems make eating difficult if not seemingly impossible.

To work around nausea, try the following suggestions:

➤ Try getting a little fresh air or a short walk just before eating; you might even try eating outside in the fresh air.

➤ Eat in a well-ventilated room to avoid being bothered by smells.

➤ Eat very small meals, but frequently.

➤ Try drier foods, such as bread and crackers.

➤ Turn to cold foods; because they have less smell, you often tolerate them better.

➤ Have someone else do the cooking. Sometimes, just being around food uses up your tolerance for it. Save that tolerance for eating.

➤ Practice good oral hygiene. A fresh-tasting mouth helps diminish that nauseous feeling.

➤ Believe it or not, sniff a fresh cut lemon.

To get good nutrition when you have diarrhea, work with your health care provider first to figure out what is causing the diarrhea—that is essential to treating it properly. In addition, the cause will determine how you should eat. If the diarrhea is caused by lactose intolerance, see the section above. You can help prevent diarrhea by preventing coming down with foodborne infections (see the section below). In addition, staying well nourished helps keep the intestinal tract strong and healthy to properly break down food and absorb the nutrients in food rather than passing them through unabsorbed. Finally, if antibiotics are causing diarrhea, try eating yogurt with active cultures daily—this can be a big help for many people.

Below are foods that people with diarrhea seem to tolerate better. You may have to experiment to determine the best choices for you:

- Rice

- Potatoes, prepared without added fat

- Bananas

- Rice cakes (they're low in calories, so don't fill up on them)

- Apple juice (make sure it is pasteurized)

- Tea; find the type that works best for you, perhaps plain or chamomile

- Chicken, without the skin and prepared without added fat

- Creamed soups, such as the ones on pages 366–68, or even canned cream soup

Avoid fatty foods, as they tend to be the most difficult to digest and break down when you have diarrhea.

Safe Food Handling Practices

Most people don't think too much about foodborne infection, commonly called food poisoning, but it is a real concern for people with HIV. Because the immune system isn't as strong, it is less able to tolerate even the low levels of bacteria that generally don't trouble people without HIV. Refer to the chapter on safe food handling practices for more detailed information.

Using Safe Water

In addition to food, you should be concerned about what type of water you use for preparing food, drinking and brushing your teeth. While you need to be concerned about any organism that can contaminate water, one particular of organism poses a problem. While people without HIV can tolerate certain levels of the organism without difficulty, HIV-positive people cannot. Unfortunately, chlorination doesn't get rid of this particular organism, called *Cryptosporidium*. While not all water contains this organism, people with HIV need to be concerned about it.

The safest water for people with HIV is either sterile water, which you can purchase in a pharmacy, or tap water that is boiled and then cooled. The latter, however, just isn't practical for most people. Many people use tap water, as long as it comes from a municipal water supply (there is less chance that well water will be safe for people with HIV). Call your municipal water company and ask if your tap water comes largely from surface water supplies or deep wells. While water originating from deep wells in the earth is only rarely contaminated with Cryptosporidium, approximately 85 percent of surface water is. If you find that your tap water originates largely from surface water, you may want to boil and then cool it, use safe bottled water (see below) or sterile water, or install an appropriate type of filter (see below). Whatever choice you make, make sure you use it exclusively, not just for drinking. For example, use it to make ice cubes, reconstitute drink powders and concentrates, wash produce and brush your teeth.

Bottled Water

Some people wonder if bottle water is safer than tap water. It just depends. Be aware that just by virtue of being bottled, water isn't necessarily safer or purer. Many bottled waters, in fact, are made from tap water. Neither is spring water or spring water necessarily safe. The only bottled water that is treated sufficiently to prevent Cryptosporidium is water that undergoes a specific type of filtering (not even all filtered water is safe). The water has to be filtered through a filter with pores the size of one micron or less.

But there is another issue with bottled water. While certain brands of bottled water may be filtered appropriately to get rid of Cryptosporidium, they can still pose another problem. Bottled waters, if stored too long, can lose their ability to keep other bacteria in check. In addition, if you purchase large bottles of water and drink out of them for a couple of days (especially if they are unrefrigerated, although even if they are refrigerated from time to time), they can develop too-high levels of bacteria that can cause problems. So, if you choose a brand of bottled water that is supposed to be treated properly to get rid of Cryptosporidium, make sure it isn't past the expiration date stamped on the bottle. Also, purchase smaller bottles that you'll consume in a short period of time (on the same day), or throw out any remaining water at the end of the day.

If you use bottled water at home dispensed from a large bottle placed upside down on a dispensing system (this type is generally delivered to the home), make sure that you clean the system on a regular basis. At least once per month, flush the system with a weak bleach solution, and then rinse very thoroughly. Otherwise, the moist environment becomes a perfect breeding ground for all sorts of organisms.

Sparkling waters are generally one of the safer choices as they are more acidic and provide a less-favorable environment for bacteria.

Water Filters

There are water filters—and then there are water filters. What's critical to know is that many filters are actually an excellent environment for growing bacteria, causing more problems than they prevent.

Most countertop filters, either those you pour tap water into or just place on your faucet, simply cannot produce safe enough water for the HIV patient, nor for anyone who is immunosuppressed. Instead, you'll need a more sophisticated unit that installs under the sink. When choosing a filter, insist that it meets the following criteria:

➤ It should filter to one micron or less.

➤ It should be a Class no. 1 filtration system with a National Sanitation Foundation certification "NSF Standard 53 Cyst Removal" designation (call the National Sanitation Foundation at 800/673-8010 for a list of acceptable filters and purchase locations).

If you do use an appropriate filtering system, learn how often you need to replace the filter to make it function properly. Some filters have a special feature that doesn't allow you to use it when the filter can no longer function properly to cleanse water optimally.

Boost Phytochemical Intake

This is the most speculative advice of any given in this chapter. But because it can't hurt you, and is a great way to work toward being well nourished overall, it is probably worth doing. Although it sounds very complicated, phytochemicals are simply plant chemicals—*phyto* is the Greek word for plant. Nutrition experts believe that phytochemicals take nutrition science to the next level. Phytochemicals have many functions in plants. Their most visibly obvious function, though, is to give fruits and vegetables their rainbow range of brilliant colors. Although they've been in food for millions of years, we're just now discovering what they are, how intriguing they are *and* how powerful they are. Phytochemicals are classified as nonnutrient constituents of foods because they have no calories and aren't essential for the body to function normally (unlike essential vitamins and minerals). Although we don't need them to function normally, we probably do need them for good health.

Food scientists first became aware of phytochemicals in the 1950s and '60s. From then until very recently, they knew that phytochemicals protected plants against disease, pests and the insults of handling. But then food scientists and pharmacologists (experts in drugs and biologically active substances) discovered that phytochemicals can also protect humans from disease. Now, there is rapidly accumulating evidence that phytochemicals can play a role in preventing cancer, heart disease, and infections.

There are literally thousands of phytochemicals, many yet to be discovered. Now, there is some preliminary evidence that at least certain ones might help squelch HIV.

Turmeric is a wonderfully interesting spice used commonly in Indian food. It contain a specific phytochemical (among others) called curcumin, which shows promise in fighting heart disease, cancer and even infectious diseases. Very preliminary research suggests that curcumin may keep the AIDS virus from reproducing itself. The evidence goes beyond the test tube and the laboratory: in clinical studies, AIDS patients given curcumin showed improvement in blood tests that reveal how active the' virus is in the body, CD-4 and CD-8 levels.

Use this spicy spice in curry mixtures, chutneys, lamb, winter squash, rice and couscous. While curcumin is the only phytochemical identified so far that may play a role in battling HIV, there are thousands of others in fruits, vegetables and grains that offer loads of health benefits. Those in garlic, apples and onions, for example, may help fight infections. When your digestive system permits it, make it a point to include lots of different colors of fruits and vegetables, which ensures that you'll get lots of different phytochemicals from nature's wonderful bounty (just make sure to wash all produce thoroughly). But even if there isn't, the other substances in these foods contain so many wonderful things that you should make it a point to include them in your eating plan regularly.

Remember, though, that you should add this to your other treatment plan: continue to take prescribed medications and eat to achieve good nutrition overall. No one substance is the magic bullet that will eradicate HIV.

A Note About Fat and Cholesterol

Taking in enough calories is difficult, if not impossible, if you try to keep fat intake low. Certainly, we all hear about the importance of reducing dietary fat and dietary cholesterol to reduce cancer and heart disease risks. But for the HIV-positive person, keeping weight on takes higher priority. And that takes more calories than most people can consume eating a low-fat diet. Also, note that many people who are HIV-positive have low blood cholesterol readings, anyway.

Menus
HIV/AIDS

These menus are loaded with the fabulous nutrition that will give you the nutrition advantage in fighting your illness. The calories are high, around 2,500 per day. In addition, each day contains at least 100 percent of the RDA for all nutrients (with a few minor exceptions, but generally, another day makes up for one day that may lag by 2 percent or 3 percent in reaching 100 percent)—most often, each day provides greater than 125 percent of the RDA, and for some nutrients much more.

The recipes included are very simple. In addition, you'll notice that I've used leftovers; as long as you're going to the trouble of cooking up a recipe, you might as well use it for more than one night. Also, don't hesitate to freeze a serving or two for another night down the road.

You'll notice that there is a lot of milk on these menus: it's an inexpensive source of protein and vitamin B_{12}. Finally, I've tried to use less-expensive foods, so that eating healthy won't break your budget.

Part 1: Seven Days of Menus Incorporating All the Guidelines

DAY ONE

Breakfast
Breakfast Bulghur (page 246)
1 cup 2% milk

Morning Snack
1 cup orange juice

Lunch
Kielbasa Corn Chowder (page 377)
1 cup 2% milk
1 orange

Snack
¼ cup peanuts

Dinner
Cheeseburger: 3-ounce well-cooked
lean hamburger patty and 1 slice
American cheese (4 ounces before
cooking) on whole grain bun with
2 large romaine lettuce leaves
1 cup steamed broccoli (frozen is fine)
1 cup 2% milk

Evening Snack
2 fig bars

2335 calories, 105 g protein, 42 g fiber, 70 g fat
RDA: 240% for vitamin B$_{12}$; 111% for zinc; 466% for vitamin C

DAY TWO

Breakfast
2 poached eggs
2 slices whole wheat toast
1 tablespoon margarine
1 tablespoon jam
1 cup 2% milk

Morning Snack
1 apple
1 cup orange juice

Lunch
Grilled cheese sandwich: 3 slices
American cheese, 2 slices whole
wheat bread, 1 tablespoon margarine
2 carrots

Afternoon Snack
1 cup fruited yogurt

Dinner
Dinner Pancakes (page 256)
1 cup 2% milk
1 cup frozen green peas, steamed in
microwave

Evening Snack
2 oatmeal raisin cookies

2565 calories, 111 g protein, 29 g fiber, 101 g fat
RDA: 290% for vitamin B$_{12}$; 96% for zinc; 246% for vitamin C

DAY THREE

Breakfast
Eggs Goldenrod (page 252)
1 cup 2% milk

Morning Snack
1 banana
1 cup apricot nectar

Lunch
Lentil and Brown Rice Chili (page 374)
1 cup 2% milk

Afternoon Snack
1 orange
¼ cup peanuts

Dinner

   5 ounces roasted chicken (skin removed)

   1 large baked potato

   1 tablespoon margarine

   1 cup frozen carrot slices, steamed in microwave

   1 cup 2% milk

2294 calories, 126 g protein, 37 g fiber, 72 g fat

RDA: 192% for vitamin B$_{12}$; 98% for zinc; 406% for vitamin C

DAY FOUR

Breakfast

   Oatmeal: Mix ½ cup oats with 1 cup 2% milk; cook slowly or microwave on low; plus 2 tablespoons raisins and 1 tablespoon brown sugar

   1 cup orange juice

Morning Snack

   ¼ cup roasted sunflower seeds

Lunch

   3-Bean Pasta Salad (page 272)

   1 cup 2% milk

   1 banana

Afternoon Snack

   1 apple

Dinner

   Chicken Noodle Casserole (use leftover roast chicken from previous day and recipe, page 281, but divide into four servings, instead of six, and enjoy one)

   1 cup frozen broccoli pieces, steamed with 1 tablespoon margarine

   1 cup 2% milk

2527 calories, 106 g protein, 37 g fiber, 80 g fat

RDA: 168% for vitamin B$_{12}$; 88% for zinc; 417% for vitamin C

DAY FIVE

Breakfast

   2 poached eggs

   2 slices whole wheat toast

   1 tablespoon margarine

   1 tablespoon jam

   1 cup 2% milk

Morning Snack

   1 cup peach nectar

Lunch

   Brown Rice and Lentil Chili (leftover from day three)

   1 banana

   1 cup 2% milk

Afternoon Snack

   2 chocolate chip cookies

   1 cup 2% milk

Dinner

   Favorite Tuna Pasta Salad (page 275)

   1 cup 2% milk

   1 cup grapes

Evening Snack

   1 cup low-fat fruited yogurt

   ¼ cup peanuts

2619 calories, 130 g protein, 25 g fiber, 88 g fat

RDA: 448% for vitamin B$_{12}$; 130% for zinc; 277% for vitamin C

DAY SIX

Breakfast
Eggs for Brunch (page 252)
1 cup 2% milk
1 orange

Morning Snack
1 banana

Lunch
Tuna sandwich: 6 ounce can tuna,
2 slices whole wheat bread, 2 thick
tomato slices, 2 romaine lettuce leaves,
2 tablespoons mayonnaise
1 cup 2% milk

Afternoon Snack
Trail mix: ¼ cup sunflower seeds,
2 tablespoons raisins, 2 tablespoons
chocolate chips

Dinner
Chicken Noodle Casserole
(leftover from day 4)
1 cup steamed broccoli
1 tablespoon margarine
1 cup 2% milk

2526 calories, 151 g protein, 29 g fiber, 93 g fat
RDA: 432% for vitamin B$_{12}$; 104% for zinc; 446% for vitamin C

DAY SEVEN

Breakfast
Eggs Goldenrod (leftover from
day three)
1 cup 2% milk

Morning Snack
1 orange

Lunch
Kielbasa Corn Chowder
(leftover from day one)
1 cup 2% milk
1 whole wheat bagel
1 apple

Afternoon Snack
2 cups grapes

Dinner
5 ounces pot roast★
1 potato
2 carrots
½ onion
1 cup 2% milk
★Roast carrots, onion and potato with pot roast.

Evening Snack
Trail mix: 2 tablespoons sunflower seeds,
2 tablespoons raisins, 2 tablespoons
chocolate chips

2436 calories, 147 g protein, 32 g fiber, 68 g fat
RDA: 365% for vitamin B$_{12}$; 117% for zinc; 288% for vitamin C

Part 2: Seven Days of Menus for People with Mouth Sores

These menus use several recipes from the back of this book. Please note, though, that you should use some higher calorie ingredients than what they call for. These ingredients are marked by as asterisk on that particular menu item. There's a caveat, though: most of these higher calorie ingredients are also higher in fat. If you're having a problem with diarrhea, you may not be able to tolerate this extra fat; in those cases, try the lower fat version. Also note that while these foods are arranged in three meals and three snacks, you should feel free to eat them as you are able.

DAY ONE

Breakfast
Creamy Scrambled Eggs (page 250)
1 cup apricot nectar

Morning Snack
Raspberry Cream Gelatin (page 397)

Lunch
Chicken Noodle Casserole
(page 281)
1 cup peach nectar

2711 calories, 128 g protein, 18 g fiber, 73 g fat

Afternoon Snack
1 banana

Dinner
6 ounces broiled salmon
2 cups brown rice: simmer 1 cup raw
rice slowly in 1 cup whole milk, to
boost protein, nutrients and calories

Evening Snack
1 cup ice cream

DAY TWO

Breakfast
Creamy Oatmeal★ (page 249)
1 cup pear nectar

★Change skim milk to whole milk; change
skim milk powder to whole milk powder.

Morning Snack
Pumpkin Custard★ (page 400)
★Change evaporated skim milk to evapo-
rated whole milk

Lunch
1 banana milk shake: 1 cup vanilla ice
cream, 1 banana, ¼ cup whole milk,
1 packet vanilla Instant Breakfast

3000 calories, 98 g protein, 20 g fiber, 85 g fat

Afternoon Snack
1 cup apricot nectar

Dinner
Fettucine Alfredo★ (page 279)
1 cup peach nectar

★Change nonfat cream cheese to regular
cream cheese; change nonfat milk to whole
milk.

Breakfast
    Cream of wheat★
    1 cup apricot nectar
    ★Make with whole milk instead of water; for example, 1 instant packet with 1 cup whole milk.

Morning Snack
    Creamy Gelatin (page 395)

Lunch
    Cream of Broccoli Soup★ (page 368)
    ½ peanut butter and jelly sandwich: 2 tablespoons peanut butter, 1 slice soft white bread, 1 tablespoon jam

2645 calories, 116 g protein, 16 g fiber, 86 g fat

    1 cup peach nectar
    ★Change nonfat milk to whole milk and increase cheese to 8 ounces.

Afternoon Snack
    1 cup fruited yogurt

Dinner
    Chicken Noodle Casserole (leftover from day one)
    1 cup pear nectar

Evening Snack
    1 cup ice cream

DAY FOUR

Breakfast
    Rice and raisins: simmer for about 45 minutes 1 cup brown rice and ¼ cup raisins in 2 cups whole milk, or until rice is tender; stir in sugar to taste after it has cooked

Morning Snack
    Raspberry Cream Gelatin (leftover from day one)

Lunch
    Potato Soup★ (page 367)
    1 cup peach nectar
    ★Change nonfat cream cheese to regular cream cheese

2682 calories, 75 g protein, 23 g fiber, 72 g fat

DAY FIVE

Breakfast
    Creamy Scrambled Eggs (page 250)
    1 cup pear nectar

Morning Snack
    Pumpkin Custard (leftover from day two)

Afternoon Snack
    1 banana milk shake: blend 1 cup ice cream, 1 banana, ¼ cup whole milk in blender

Dinner
    White Cheddar Macaroni and Cheese★ (page 278)
    The Best Mashed Potatoes (page 394)
    1 cup pear nectar
    ★Change nonfat milk to whole milk

Evening Snack
    1 cup apricot nectar

Lunch
    Cream of Broccoli Soup (leftover from day three)
    1 cup peach nectar

Afternoon Snack
   Strawberry-banana milk shake: 1 cup
      vanilla ice cream ¼ cup whole milk,
      1 packet strawberry Instant Breakfast,
      1 banana

2742 calories, 143 g protein, 16 g fiber, 94 g fat

DAY SIX

Breakfast
   Creamy Oatmeal★ (page 249)

   ★Change skim milk to whole milk; change
   skim milk powder to whole milk powder.

Morning Snack
   1 cup peach nectar

Lunch
   Chicken Noodle Casserole
      (leftover from day one)
   1 cup apricot nectar

2698 calories, 103 g protein, 23 g fiber, 100 g fat

Dinner
   4 ounces steamed sole
   1 cup brown rice
   1 cup apricot nectar

Evening Snack
   1 cup low-fat fruited yogurt

Afternoon Snack
   Peanut butter shake: 1 cup ice cream,
      ¼ cup peanut butter, ¼ cup whole milk

Dinner
   The Best Mashed Potatoes
      (leftover from day four)
   White Cheddar Macaroni and Cheese
      (leftover from day four)

Evening Snack
   1 cup pear nectar

References

Bacon, P. "Nutritional Care of the Patient with HIV/AIDS." *Nursing Standard* 11(12) (1996): 44–46.

Melchior, J.C., et al. "Efficacy of 2-Month Total Parenteral Nutrition in AIDS Patients: A Controlled Randomized Prospective Trial." *AIDS* 10 (1996): 379–84.

Selberg, O., et al. "Effect of Increased Protein Intake and Nutritional Status on Whole-Body Protein Metabolism of AIDS Patients with Weight Loss." *Metabolism* 44(9) (1995): 1,159–65.

Alzheimer's Disease 14

At least 2.5 million Americans have Alzheimer's disease, the most common form of dementia among the elderly. As people age, the chances of getting Alzheimer's disease increase dramatically. While the rate of Alzheimer's among people between the ages of sixty to sixty-five is just 0.1 percent, it rises to 47 percent by the age of eighty-five.

The mental and physical deterioration occurs gradually, with memory, thought and behavior problems becoming worse and worse. In the first stage, called the amnestic stage, people experience a mild memory deficit. In the second stage, called the dementia stage, a marked memory deficit is experienced. In the final stage, the vegetative stage, there is communication loss, incontinence of bladder and bowel and difficulty in caring for yourself, including difficulty in eating.

There is now evidence that people can use good nutrition to reduce their chances of ever getting Alzheimer's disease, as well as slowing the progression of the disease, and to improve quality of life after the disease advances.

Nutrition and Prevention

While there is no cure for Alzheimer's disease, there are some things that people can do, nutritionally speaking, to reduce their risk of getting Alzheimer's disease. A possible answer? Reduce the risk of stroke, which people can do with several nutrition maneuvers.

Researchers recently found that by reducing the risk of stroke, it seems possible to reduce the risk of getting Alzheimer's disease. This is because there is a connection between the brain's blood supply and dementia. When the blood supply remains good, the chances of getting dementia are much less. However, when the blood supply becomes interrupted, which it does after a stroke, the chance of dementia increases. Experts think that the interrupted blood supply caused by a stroke, which creates a reduced flow of oxygen to brain cells, might "tip the balance" in brain cells that have the early changes of Alzheimer's disease, making these changes more likely to cause the actual symptoms of dementia. In other words, while someone's brain cells, upon microscopic examination, as during an autopsy, may have shown the physical changes that are characteristic of Alzheimer's disease, that person may not necessarily show the symptoms of dementia that occur in Alzheimer's disease.

After being deprived of oxygen, though, these diseased cells somehow are more likely to spur symptoms of dementia.

We know this from research conducted on 102 Catholic nuns who were followed for several years during later life. The research team gave them a thorough neurological exam every year to detect changes in memory or mental acuity that would indicate Alzheimer's disease was present. In addition, the nuns agreed to donate their brains to research after their death. All nuns were between seventy-six and a hundred years of age when they died.

When researchers examined the brain tissue, they were looking for signs of Alzheimer's disease and signs of stroke. Even though people may not have been diagnosed as suffering a stroke, examining the brain tissue at death can reveal oxygen-deprived areas of the brain characteristics of little strokes. Similarly, brain tissue can show the changes indicating the presence of Alzheimer's disease, even though someone doesn't show signs of dementia while alive.

The researchers found that those nuns whose brains showed evidence of the tissue changes characteristic of both stroke and Alzheimer's disease were eleven times more likely to have had symptoms of dementia while alive than the nuns who had no evidence of stroke in their brains but who did have evidence that Alzheimer's disease had settled in their brain cells. On the other hand, women whose brains showed the tissue changes of Alzheimer's disease but not of stroke were much less likely to have demonstrated symptoms of Alzheimer's dementia while alive. Certainly more research is necessary, but there is no reason to wait to prevent stroke—even the little ones you don't realize occurred.

Eat to Prevent Stroke

In trying to prevent stroke—even the ministrokes that may not be recognized as stroke but that indeed deprive the brain of oxygen—you may be able to compensate for some of the early Alzheimer's damage to brain cells. You should:

➤ Eat for a lower blood pressure, which includes decreasing dietary sodium and boosting the intake of potassium, magnesium and calcium. See the charts on page 114 for foods high in these nutrients.

➤ Keep weight at a healthy, lean level. Staying on the lean side helps cut stroke risk in two ways. First, staying leaner helps keep blood pressure lower. Also, staying leaner cuts the chances that you'll develop diabetes, which is a powerful risk factor for having a stroke. If you have diabetes, work hard to keep blood sugar readings at the healthier readings your doctor suggests, which at least helps reduce the chance of suffering stroke.

➤ Limit alcohol intake. Having more than two drinks per day raises blood pressure, which of course increases the risk of stroke (for women, one drink per day may increase risk). In addition, binge drinking (even just one session of drinking too much) can lead to a stroke. One drink is defined as 12 ounces of regular beer, 5 ounces of wine, and 1.5 ounces of 90-proof distilled spirits.

➤ Decrease the chance that you'll develop atherosclerosis, or artery-clogging disease. This can lead to ischemic strokes, or strokes that cut off the oxygen supply to brain cells (the kind the nuns in the study suffered). You can decrease the chances of getting atherosclerosis by following a low-fat, low-saturated fat diet that is high in dietary fiber. Refer to chapter 3 on preventive health for more information on preventing atherosclerosis.

Vitamin E: The Nutrition Advantage

For years, neuroscientists suspected that vitamin E could help Alzheimer's patients. It made sense, after all, as they believed that free radicals play some role in the brain cell destruction leading to Alzheimer's disease, and hoped that vitamin E, as the powerful antioxidant it is, could help arrest that damage. In support of their theory, an early, small trial comparing ten patients with Alzheimer's disease to twenty controls (people without Alzheimer's disease), found that Alzheimer's patients had significantly lower vitamin E blood levels than their disease-free counterparts.

Then, in April 1997, researchers reported that high doses of vitamin E may modestly slow the progression of Alzheimer's disease. Indeed, said the research team from Columbia University in New York reporting in the prestigious *New England Journal of Medicine,* vitamin E appears to work by absorbing the free radicals. The researchers also studied the effects of a drug used to treat Alzheimer's disease, selegiline, whose brand name is Eldepryl.

They studied 341 men and women with midstage disease not living in an institution but who needed help with routine tasks, dividing the patients into four groups. Patients in group one received 2,000 international units (IU) of vitamin E; group two, 10 milligrams of selegiline; group three, both 2,000 IU of vitamin E and 10 milligrams selegiline; and group four, a placebo, or sugar pill.

The research team then followed the Alzheimer's patients, checking on four major milestones that are important in assessing the progression of the disease: the inability to care for oneself, or perform "activities of daily living," including bathing, feeding oneself, dressing, and so on; admission to a nursing home; progression to severe dementia; or death. The researchers found that it took 230 days longer for people taking the vitamin E to reach one of these milestones; on average, 670 days versus 440 for people receiving the placebo, or dummy drug. It took 215 days longer for people who took the selegiline. The researchers were surprised to find that the people who took both the vitamin E and the selegiline actually did worse than both the vitamin E only and selegiline only groups—it took them just 145 days longer, or a total of 585 days.

This study provides good reason for Alzheimer's patients to take vitamin E in large doses; the 2,000 IU used in the study is more than 60 times the recommended intake of 30 IU daily. Always check with your physician first, though, to make sure this is safe for you. People who take anticoagulant medications (such as coumadin), for example, may significantly increase the chances that they could suffer dangerous bleeding complications by taking large doses of vitamin E.

There is currently no evidence that taking vitamin E if you don't have Alzheimer's disease will prevent the disease, although it just may be that the research hasn't yet been done. As you contemplate your decision, note that many heart disease experts believe that vitamin E, at doses between 100 to 400 IU, may help prevent heart disease. That may be reason enough to take it. Those doses appear to be safe, and may indeed give you the nutrition advantage in fighting off Alzheimer's disease and heart disease.

Nutrition and Caring for Alzheimer's Patients

As Alzheimer's progresses, patients gradually become unable to prepare meals and then even to feed themselves. But helping Alzheimer's patients stay well nourished and not grow too thin (both real problems for them) can improve their quality of life. For example, helping them avoid growing too thin and to get enough dietary calcium and vitamin D can help keep bones strong, which can reduce the chances of getting osteoporosis. In turn, this can reduce the chance of suffering fractures, which can make caring for Alzheimer's patients even more difficult.

Nutrition experts at the Hebrew Home for the Aged in Riverdale, New York, have received an award from the New York State Association of Homes and Services for their innovative nutrition programs that help to improve the nutritional well-being of Alzheimer's patients. With their nutrition program, dementia patients who were undernourished and underweight gained weight; in addition, they become less angry and agitated, apparently because they could feed themselves once again. Among their suggestions are:

➤ Prepare bite-sized portions of items such as fruits, vegetables, cheese and sandwiches that patients can pick up with their hands rather than with forks and spoons, as they may not understand how to use these eating utensils anymore. Another reason these finger foods work better is that people with dementia like to wander about and they can eat finger foods as they do.

➤ When serving soups, opt for thick, creamy soups in which all ingredients are evenly pureed rather than vegetable soup in which ingredients settle to the bottom. In addition, serve the thick, creamy soups in a mug rather than a bowl, so that people can drink the soup. See the recipes on pages 365–68.

➤ Make sure that someone with Alzheimer's is hungry when you feed him. This may mean feeding him outside of normal mealtimes. In addition, make sure you allow him plenty of time to eat and even to wander about as he eats.

Studies have also shown that people with Alzheimer's disease are more likely to come up short on protein than other people their age, usually because of poor dietary habits. This makes sense, given that cutting up and chewing meat, the most commonly used source of protein, becomes difficult for these people. Becoming protein deficient can make a person more susceptible to infection and also to feeling less energetic and therefore even less able to care for himself. Try to keep protein intake at around fifty to sixty grams (see page 79). To ensure a good protein intake for people with Alzheimer's, opt for easy-to-eat protein sources, such as:

➤ Scrambled eggs or hard-boiled eggs (the latter they can pick up on their own); don't worry about the cholesterol content of the eggs.

➤ Thick, creamy soups made with pureed white beans as the thickener, which greatly increases the protein content (see the recipes on pages 364–65).

➤ Finger-sized peanut butter and jelly sandwiches, which are easy to chew and easy to swallow.

➤ Try to offer milk as a beverage rather than an empty calorie beverage such as tea or coffee. You can try adding chocolate powder or chocolate syrup to it to make it more interesting.

➤ If you're serving gelatin, make it with cottage cheese or yogurt to increase the protein content (see the recipes on pages 395–99).

Also important to helping Alzheimer's patient stay well nourished is helping them maintain good oral health. Studies have shown that people with Alzheimer's disease generally produce less saliva, which can cause teeth to decay faster. This happens for two reasons: saliva is necessary to clean the teeth and it contains minerals that help keep the teeth hard and therefore more resistant to decay. Lacking enough saliva, the teeth become especially vulnerable to decay and loss. In addition, the gums can be affected, causing periodontal disease, which you'll recognize by red, swollen gums that bleed easily. This, too, can cause tooth loss: the more affected are the gums, the more likely is the gum line to shrink away from the teeth. When more of the tooth surface is exposed, it is more likely to decay. In addition, the bone holding the teeth in place (the jawbone) can become infected if it becomes exposed; this in turns causes teeth to loosen and fall out.

Lacking their own teeth, people have greater difficulty chewing and swallowing, making eating a nutritionally balanced diet very difficult. Help Alzheimer's patients keep their own teeth by:

➤ Having them rinse with water after each meal.

➤ Helping them brush their teeth at least twice daily. Researchers have shown that when someone helps people with Alzheimer's perform oral hygiene, they have less plaque and less gum disease.

➤ Ask the dentist about fluoride treatments that can make teeth more resistant to decay, helping the Alzheimer's patient keep his or her own teeth longer.

➤ Take the person you care for to regular dental checks.

➤ If saliva production becomes quite low, offer the person more frequent sips of water and/or ask the dentist about saliva replacement solutions.

Foods High in Potassium

Dried apricots
Dried figs, dried prunes
Baked potato with skin
Banana
Low-fat yogurt
Prune juice
*Red snapper (which is also a lean source of protein, another aid in helping
    to reduce dietary fat)*
Skim milk (the best choice of milk to reduce dietary fat)

Foods High in Magnesium

Baked potato with skin
Banana
Beets, broccoli, corn
Halibut (another lean source of protein)
Milk
*Oatmeal (make the oatmeal with milk instead of water to really boost magnesium,
    as well as calcium, protein and potassium intake)*

Foods High in Calcium

Calcium-fortified orange juice
Skim milk
Yogurt

Soft, High-Protein Foods

*Cooked meat or fish, 3 ounces/26 grams (fish is a wonderful, soft source of protein,
    easy to chew and swallow; when using chicken or beef, cut the meat into finger-
    sized portions, such as chicken strips, and serve that way)*
Low-fat cottage cheese, 1 cup/31 grams
Milk, 8 grams
Scrambled egg, 7 grams

Menus

ALZHEIMER'S DISEASE

The menus are intended for people with moderate to severe Alzheimer's disease. They use finger foods and foods that are more calorically and nutrient-dense—or foods that pack in more calories and nutrients. In addition, you'll note that some of the same recipes (from the back of this book) appear on more than one menu; that way, you can use leftovers to cut down on the amount of cooking you, as caretaker, must do.

The menus are high in calcium, which helps keep your loved one's bones strong, to prevent the osteoporosis that can make caring for them a little more difficult. You'll also note that nectar is listed as a beverage fairly frequently—that's because it's higher in calories and nutrients than juices. Finally, this is the only set of menus for which I use 2% milk. Again, it's to get in more calories in less food—it makes the fat (and saturated fat) higher than in other menus. While both are still within recommended limits, the saturated fat tends to be a little higher than I recommend. While the menus are given as three meals and often two or three snacks, don't hesitate to divide up the food differently throughout the day, to accommodate special appetites.

DAY ONE

Breakfast
Creamy Scrambled Eggs (page 250)
½ cup apricot nectar

Morning Snack
Creamy Strawberry-Banana Gelatin
(page 396)

Lunch
Peanut butter and jelly sandwich:
3 tablespoons peanut butter, 1 tablespoon jam, 2 slices whole wheat bread
(cut into bite-sized pieces)
1 cup 2% milk
1 banana

Afternoon Snack
6 brown sugar baby carrots, cooked
until tender, cooled (cook in just
enough water to cover and 2 tablespoons brown sugar; make more and
use again during the week)

Dinner
Everyone's Favorite Chicken and Rice
Casserole (page 302)
1 cup frozen green peas, steamed, and
then slightly cooled, as a finger food

1834 calories, 104 g protein, 20 g fiber, 64 g fat (20 g saturated fat), 871 mg calcium, 2461 mg sodium

DAY TWO

Breakfast
2 Oat Muffins (page 259)
1 tablespoon margarine
1 cup 2% milk

Morning Snack
1 pear, cored and cut into bite-sized
pieces

Lunch
Grilled cheese sandwich: 2 ounces
cheese, 2 slices whole wheat bread,
2 teaspoons margarine
1 cup 2% milk

Afternoon Snack
4 fig bars

Dinner
Dinner Pancakes (page 256), with
1 tablespoon margarine, rolled as a
finger food (make up the whole
batch, and you'll use again during the
week; also, you can freeze the extras)
1 peach, cut up into bite-sized pieces

Evening Snack
1 cup apricot nectar

1857 calories, 65 g protein, 22 g fiber, 71 g fat (30 g saturated fat), 1237 mg calcium, 1619 mg sodium

DAY THREE

Breakfast
3 French toast sticks★
1 cup 2% milk
★Buy in the freezer section.

Morning Snack
1 banana

Lunch
3 cheese sticks
8 crackers
1 cup nectar
4 frozen broccoli spears, steamed
(as finger food)

Afternoon Snack
1 apple, cored and sliced

Dinner
2 roasted chicken legs (as finger food)
1 baked sweet potato, peeled, sliced and
slightly cooled, as finger food
1 pear, cored and sliced
1 cup 2% milk

Evening Snack
Bread Pudding (page 264)
1 cup nectar

1844 calories, 70 g protein, 23 g fiber, 51 g fat (15 g saturated fat), 970 mg calcium, 1218 mg sodium

DAY FOUR

Breakfast
1 frozen oat bran waffle, toasted
2 teaspoons margarine
1 cup 2% milk

Morning Snack
3 fig bars
½ cup nectar

Lunch
1 mug Cream of Broccoli Soup (page 368)
8 crackers

Afternoon Snack
Creamy Strawberry-Banana Gelatin
(leftover from day one)

Dinner
3 ounces tender pork roast, as bite-sized
pieces
1 baked potato with skin, halved, and
then sliced into bite-sized pieces (melt
1 tablespoon margarine onto halves
before slicing)
1 cup frozen cauliflower pieces, steamed,
and slightly cooled, as finger food
1 cup nectar

Evening Snack
1 cup ice cream

1946 calories, 83 g protein, 18 g fiber, 64 g fat (26 g saturated fat), 886 mg calcium, 1991 mg sodium

DAY FIVE

Breakfast
Bread Pudding (leftover from day three)
1 cup 2% milk

Morning Snack
1 banana

Lunch
8 crackers with peanut butter
1 cup 2% milk
6 brown sugar baby carrots
(leftover from day one)

Afternoon Snack
    1 peach, cut into quarters

Dinner
    Everyone's Favorite Chicken and Rice
        Casserole (leftover from day one)
    1 cup 2% milk

Evening Snack
    ½ cup dry Cheerios
    1 cup nectar

1761 calories, 83 g protein, 16 g fiber, 63 g fat (20 g saturated fat), 1181 mg calcium, 2010 mg sodium

Day Six

Breakfast
    2 Oat Muffins (leftover from day two)
    1 cup 2% milk

Morning Snack
    1 cup nectar

Lunch
    Grilled cheese sandwich: 2 ounces
        cheese, 2 slices whole wheat bread,
        2 teaspoons margarine
    1 cup frozen green peas, steamed and
        slightly cooled, as finger food

Afternoon Snack
    1 pear, cored and sliced

Dinner
    3 frozen fish sticks
    1 baked sweet potato, peeled and sliced,
        as finger food
    1 cup green beans, steamed, as finger
        food
    1 cup 2% milk

Evening Snack
    2 oatmeal cookies

1815 calories, 73 g protein, 30 g fiber, 60 g fat (28 g saturated fat), 1342 mg calcium, 1892 mg sodium

Day Seven

Breakfast
    Creamy Scrambled Eggs (page 250)
    1 cup nectar

Morning Snack
    1 pear, cored and sliced

Lunch
    Turkey sandwich: 3 ounces turkey
        breast, 2 slices whole wheat bread,
        1 tablespoon mayonnaise

    1 cup 2% milk
    1 cup steamed green beans, as finger
        food

Afternoon Snack
    Bread Pudding (leftover from day three)

Dinner
    Dinner Pancakes (leftover from day two)
        with 1 tablespoon margarine, rolled as
        finger food
    1 cup 2% milk

1779 calories, 101 g protein, 19 g fiber, 63 g fat (20 g saturated fat), 1317 mg calcium, 1665 mg sodium

References

Bansun, Hans, et al. "Cobalamin Levels Are Not Reduced in Alzheimer's Disease: Results from a Population-Based Study." *Journal of the American Geriatric Society* 42(2) (1994): 132–36.

Clibbens, R. "Eating, Ethics and Alzheimer's." *Nursing Times* 92(50) (1996): 29–30.

Gomes-Trolin, C., et al. "Influence of Vitamin B_{12} on Brain Methionine Adenosyltransferase Activity in Senile Dementia of the Alzheimer's Type." *Journal of Neural Transmission* (General Section.) 103(7) (1996): 861–72.

Joosten, E., et al. "Is Metabolic Evidence for Vitamin B_{12} and Folate Deficiency More Frequent in Elderly Patients with Alzheimer's Disease?" *Journal of Gerontology* 52(2) (1997): M76–79.

Sano, M., et al. "Rationale and Design of a Multicenter Study of Selegiline and Alpha-Tocopherol in the Treatment of Alzheimer Disease Using Novel Clinical Outcomes." Alzheimer's Disease Cooperative Study. *Alzheimer's Disease and Associated Disorders* 10(3) (1996): 132–40.

———. "A Controlled Trial of Selegiline, Alpha-Tocopherol, or Both As Treatment for Alzheimer's Disease." The Alzheimer's Disease Cooperative Study. *New England Journal of Medicine* 336(17) (1997): 1,216–22.

Schiaffino-Purvis, Ellen. "Protein-Energy Malnutrition in Alzheimer's Disease." *Journal of Environmental Pathology, Toxicology, and Oncology* 10(4–5) (1990): 193–97.

Serra, J.A., et al. "Copper-Zinc Superoxide Dismutase Activity in Red Blood Cells in Probable Alzheimer's Patients and Their First-Degree Relatives." *Journal of Neurological Science* 122(2) (1994): 179–88.

Ship, J.A. "Oral Health of Patients with Alzheimer's Disease." *Journal of the American Dental Association* 123 (1992): 53–58.

Sopher, B.L., et al. "Neurodegenerative Mechanisms in Alzheimer Disease. A Role for Oxidative Damage in Amyloid Beta Protein Precursor-Mediated Cell Death." *Molecular and Chemical Neuropathology* 29(2–3) (1996): 153–68.

Spindler, A.A., et al. "Nutritional Status of Patients with Alzheimer's Disease: A 1-Year Study." *Journal of the American Dietetic Association* 96(10) (1996): 1,013–18.

Teunisse, S., et al. "Dementia and Subnormal Levels of Vitamin B_{12}: Effects of Replacement Therapy on Dementia." *Journal of Neurology* 243(7) (1996): 522–29.

Wolf-Klein, G.P. et al. "Energy Requirements in Alzheimer's Disease Patients." *Nutrition* 11(3) (1995): 264–68.

Yi, E.S., et al. "Alzheimer's Disease and Nursing: New Scientific and Clinical Insights." *Nursing Clinics of North America* 29 (1994): 85–99.

Asthma

15

Some asthma sufferers say that breathing during an asthma attack is like trying to breathe through a straw stuffed with cotton.

The mother of a child with asthma described the condition this way: "It's as if a powerful vacuum is trying to suck his chest through his back, forming a big cavity. He's rapidly gasping and still not getting enough air; his skin is white as parchment, his lips blue. Every ounce of energy he has is invested in breathing."

To appreciate what happens during an asthma attack, you have to understand the normal breathing process. When you breathe, air first enters the nose where it is filtered, warmed and humidified. It next travels through the trachea, or windpipe to the lungs. Inside each lung, there is a main stem, called the bronchus, which is analogous to the main stalk of a bunch of grapes. The tiny "stems" running off the stalk are the bronchioles. Finally, the bronchioles lead to little air sacs, called alveoli, that look like clusters of grapes. It is in the alveoli that air exchange takes place and fresh oxygen is exchanged for carbon dioxide (the waste product produced in the process of breathing) in the blood to be carried to all the body tissues.

During an asthma attack, several things happen inside the lungs. Inflammation of the airway tissue, the most common feature of asthma, is triggered by any one of a number of factors (such as respiratory infection, allergic reaction, vigorous exercise, cold air, smoke and other air pollution). Bronchospasm, which is a tightening or squeezing of the muscles wrapped around the airways, narrows the airways, making it even more difficult for air to move in and out. Some asthmatics also produce excessive, thick mucus, which further obstructs the airway. The increased mucus stimulates coughing as the body attempts to clear the airways. The classic sign of an asthma attack, wheezing, occurs as the air tries to pass in and out of these vise-gripped airways.

Ultimately, asthmatics in an attack trap "used" air in the narrowed airways of their lungs and are unable to take in enough fresh air because there simply is no room. Although inhaling is a problem, exhaling stale air is even more challenging.

Asthma attacks range from mild to severe and life-threatening. Some begin slowly and develop over the course of several days; others strike abruptly. Fortunately, mild episodes are the norm, and even when severe episodes occur, airway obstruction is usually fully reversible, either spontaneously or as a result of treatment.

The Nutrition Advantage

There are several things with regard to nutrition that asthma patients can do to be their healthiest:

➤ Boost dietary intake of foods high in antioxidant nutrients, especially vitamins E and C. (As I'll emphasize later, harvest these nutrients from food, not supplements.)

➤ Boost dietary intake of magnesium, an essential mineral.

➤ Eat to increase resistance to infection, especially respiratory infections.

➤ If you take steroid medications, compensate nutritionally.

➤ If you take theophylline medications, compensate nutritionally and to maximize their benefits.

➤ Accommodate food allergies.

While never proven, there is one additional dietary maneuver that may prove of some benefit to asthma patients:

➤ Reel in a couple of fish twice a week to boost intake of omega-3 fatty acids.

Boost Intake of Dietary Antioxidants

Of all vitamins, vitamin E boasts the longest and most diverse list of potential benefits, from reducing the risk of heart disease and adult-onset diabetes to improving exercise performance. Banking on profiting at least once, consumers pop ten or even a hundred times the Recommended Dietary Allowance (RDA); others squeeze the glistening gel onto skin, hoping to erase scars and wrinkles. Consumer demand is so great, increasing 10 percent yearly for the past five years as the list of health claims increases, that health food shelves are turning up empty. Is there any evidence that vitamin E can help ameliorate the symptoms of asthma, as you may have read?

Vitamin E was named tocopherol from the Greek *tos* for "childbirth" and *phero* meaning "to bring forth" after scientists discovered in 1922 that it prevented fetal death in animals; thirty to forty years later researchers found that humans literally cannot live without it. It's not one, but several compounds, tocopherols and tocotrienols, varying widely in their "active" vitamin E content. Alpha-tocopherol is both the most biologically active and the most widely distributed in nature.

Vitamin E deficiency is rare, occurring only in premature infants and people who do not absorb fat normally; adult deficiencies take five to ten years to develop. The recommended dietary allowance (RDA), the amount necessary to prevent the deficiency signs of anemia, fragile red blood cells and neurological abnormalities, is 15 IU for men (10 mg alpha-TE) and 12 IU for women (8 milligrams alpha-TE). That's in sharp contrast to amounts proposed for vitamin E's other touted benefits: 100 to 800 IU.

Why the colossal discrepancy? "As we probe vitamin E-disease relationships, we have to start somewhere, essentially guessing at potentially helpful doses," explains Jeffrey Blumberg, M.D., professor of nutrition at Tufts University. In contrast, assigning recommended allowances for essential nutrients is relatively easy and more exacting: they search for the dose that prevents deficiencies (adding a generous pinch of safety). Researchers withdrew vitamin C, for example, until gums started to bleed and then added it back until bleeding disappeared.

But quantifying a nutrient's role in disease prevention is more challenging, and researchers are treading unfamiliar territory. The line demarcating the start of a chronic disease process isn't as crisp as the one defining the beginning of an acute nutrient deficiency. For example, if a nutrient purportedly guards against cancer, we cannot measure exactly how much arrests cancer, as we don't fully understand cancer's genesis. The same is true for its role in stopping or at least relieving asthma.

The new focus on vitamin E is its role as the body's key chain-breaking antioxidant, or scavenger of cell-damaging free radicals. By neutralizing these stray, high-energy particles that otherwise ricochet wildly, scarring and punching holes in cells, vitamin E could theoretically prevent many chronic diseases. Now, research is beginning to bridge the theoretical and the possible.

Studying nearly 78,000 women from the Nurses Health Study for ten years, Harvard researchers found that women who consumed the most vitamin E from foods (an average of 8.9 milligrams), but not supplements, were 25 percent less likely to develop asthma compared to women who consumed the least (3.2 milligrams on average). As an antioxidant, vitamin E could theoretically reduce asthma risk by minimizing free radical induced inflammation in the respiratory tract. In addition, it might boost prostaglandin production, which checks natural chemicals that initiate asthma.

Pulmonologist Scott T. Weiss, M.D., of the Channing Laboratory at Brigham and Women's Hospital notes that this is the first suggestion that vitamin E might play a protective role and that evidence is even stronger for vitamin C. "Bear in mind that benefits were for relatively small amounts gotten from food—there is no evidence that high doses of vitamin E from supplements offer any additional benefit."

Vitamin E aficionados who carefully follow new studies might be puzzled to read that food intakes of just tens of units seem to confer the same benefit as hundreds of units of supplemental vitamin E. "But when studies associate vitamin E benefits with higher food intake, the vitamin E might simply be a marker for a healthier diet that as a whole confers the benefit," says Charles Hennekens, chief of preventive medicine at Brigham and Women's Hospital. People who get vitamin E from food, for example, generally consume diets packed with other disease-fighting substances, such as fiber, folic acid and phytonutrients. It's not to say that vitamin E isn't important, just that it may take less vitamin E if several protective factors work together—yet more support for getting nutrients from food not supplements.

If you're thinking that getting vitamin E from foods is difficult—at least without taking in a lot of fat—you're correct. But you can do it by choosing carefully. Use the following table to plan a generous intake of vitamin E. The menus at the end of this chapter contain good amounts of vitamin E, too, so don't hesitate to rely on them.

Foods Rich in Vitamin E

It is possible to get at least 10 IU of vitamin E without eating a lot of high-fat foods. Use our table to boost your intake of vitamin E and yet follow a diet that meets the American Heart Association's guidelines for limiting fat, especially saturated fat. Another benefit: you'll also be reaping lots of other key nutrients that may help fight heart disease, cancer and keep you healthy in general. Remember the key: lots of fruits, vegetables and whole grains.

Food	Serving Size	IU Vitamin E Per Serving	Other Nutrients
Asparagus, steamed	1 cup	2.7	fiber, vitamin C, folate, iron, potassium
Beet greens, boiled	1 cup	3.0	fiber, beta-carotene, vitamin C, calcium, iron, potassium
Broccoli, boiled	1 cup	2.6	fiber, vitamin C, folate, calcium, iron, potassium
Cabbage, raw, shredded	1 cup	1.7	fiber, vitamin C
Cabbage, boiled	1 cup	3.7	fiber, vitamin C
Dandelion greens, boiled	1 cup	3.1	fiber, beta-carotene, calcium, iron, potassium, vitamin C
Mustard greens, boiled	1 cup	4.2	fiber, beta-carotene, vitamin C, folate, calcium, iron, potassium
Soybeans, boiled	1 cup	5.0	fiber, calcium, iron, folate, potassium
Spinach, boiled	1 cup	3.5	beta-carotene, folate, calcium, iron, potassium, vitamin C
Spinach, raw	1 cup	1.5	beta-carotene, folate, calcium, iron, potassium, vitamin C
Sweet potato	1 each	0.7	fiber, beta-carotene, vitamin C, potassium
Swiss chard, cooked	1 cup	1.8	fiber, beta-carotene, vitamin C, calcium iron, potassium
Tomato paste, canned	¼ cup	1.6	vitamin C, iron, potassium
Tomato, raw	1 medium	1.5	vitamin C, beta-carotene, potassium
Turnip green, boiled	1 cup	3.7	fiber, beta-carotene, vitamin C, folate, calcium, iron, potassium
Yam, white boiled	1 cup	9.2	fiber, vitamin C, potassium
Almonds, whole, toasted	1 ounce	10.2	fiber, calcium, iron
Filberts, dry or oil roasted	1 ounce	10.6	fiber, calcium, iron
Peanut butter	2 tablespoons	3.6	iron
Sunflower seed	1 tablespoon	6.7	iron
Blueberries	1 cup	2.2	fiber, vitamin C, potassium
Guava	1 each	1.5	fiber, vitamin C, potassium
Kiwi	1 each	1.3	vitamin C, fiber, potassium
Papaya	1 each	5.1	vitamin C, fiber, potassium
Prunes	10 each	1.7	fiber, vitamin C, potassium
Barley	1 cup	1.8	B vitamins, minerals, fiber
Quinoa, uncooked	½ cup	6.2	B vitamins, minerals, fiber
Wheat germ, toasted	2 tablespoons	4.2	B vitamins, minerals, fiber
Catfish, steamed	3 ounces	1.9	

Food	Serving Size	IU Vitamin E Per Serving	Other Nutrients
Crab, broiled, baked	3 ounces	2.1	
Halibut, baked or broiled	3 ounces	0.9	
Salmon, steamed	3 ounces	2.4	Omega-3 fatty acids
Shrimp, steamed	3 ounces	2.2	
Sole, poached	3 ounces	3.0	
Tuna steak, baked or broiled	3 ounces	2.5	
Chicken breast, skinless, baked	3 ounces	0.2	
Chicken thigh, skinless, baked	3 ounces	0.6	
Turkey meat, dark, baked	3 ounces	.8	
Canola oil	1 tablespoon	4.7	
Corn oil	1 tablespoon	4.3	
Olive oil	1 tablespoon	2.4	
Sunflower oil	1 tablespoon	12.2	

Vitamin C, another potent dietary antioxidant, has long been suspected to play a role in preventing asthma attacks or at least making them less severe. Probably the earliest association was made in 1803, when Reisseissen noted "convulsive" asthma in sailors with scurvy. Another historically important data in asthma–vitamin C history was in 1953, when Irish researchers reported five cases of asthma treated with vitamin C. Their work seemed to indicate that asthma attacks were more common in people with vitamin C deficiency. This research also found that people tend to "waste" more vitamin C in the urine during an asthma attack. Over the years, literally dozens of studies have examined the role of vitamin C in asthma. While not all have found a benefit of vitamin C, the evidence leans in favor of a benefit.

The RDA for vitamin C (for adults) is just sixty milligrams. Try, though, to take in at least 200 milligrams of vitamin C, but as food. Doing so greatly improves the quality of your diet in general. As you plan ways to increase vitamin E and vitamin C intake, use the table above, choosing foods high in both of these important antioxidant nutrients. Note another benefit: you'll also harvest lots of other antioxidant nutrients, such as carotenoids, which will be of great benefit to your general health.

Boost Intake of Magnesium

The role of magnesium in asthma continues to be researched. Current results, while hopeful, are still inconclusive, though. Animal research suggests the role that magnesium could play in relieving asthma: it appears to relax bronchial smooth muscle, which could help to dilate the airways that constrict in asthma. While further research is needed about magnesium's role in asthma, it is definitely worth making sure that you get enough magnesium from the food you eat. I want to emphasize that *there is no evidence that magnesium supplements over and above the RDA might in any way help prevent asthma attacks*. The point of mentioning this is simply to make you aware that the research may someday prove useful in treating this disease.

Foods high in magnesium include unprocessed whole grains, legumes, nuts and seeds, avocados and bananas. Each day's menu at the end of the chapter contains sufficient amounts of magnesium to help you meet the RDA, with a generous extra cushion.

Increase Resistance to Respiratory Infection

Respiratory infections, such as a cold or bronchitis, can irritate the lung tissue enough to bring on an asthma attack. Eat healthy to keep your immune system strong, and to give yourself the nutrition advantage in resisting infection. Among the nutrients that will help you fight off infections (and the foods rich in these nutrients) are:

- ➤ PROTEIN-RICH FOODS: Meat, fish, peanut butter, eggs, cheese, milk, legumes (split peas, lentils, black beans), poultry.

- ➤ VITAMIN A–RICH FOODS: Sweet potatoes, carrots, evaporated skim milk, apricot nectar, liver, part skim ricotta cheese, cantaloupe, tomatoes, squash, spinach.

- ➤ VITAMIN C–RICH FOODS: Orange juice, tomatoes, kiwis, papaya, strawberries, spinach, sweet potatoes, cantaloupe.

- ➤ AT LEAST THREE B VITAMINS: Pyridoxine (B_6), thiamin and riboflavin. Pyridoxine-rich foods: chicken, fish, pork, eggs, liver, oats, soybeans (and tofu), bananas. Thiamin-rich foods: liver, unrefined whole grains, legumes (dried peas and beans), brewer's yeast. Riboflavin-rich foods: meat, fish, poultry, eggs, dairy products, broccoli, asparagus, turnip greens, spinach.

- ➤ ZINC-RICH FOODS: Seafood, meats, whole grains, legumes.

If You Take Steroid Medications

Fortunately, new asthma medications have greatly reduced the need for steroid medications, such as prednisone, in treating asthma. When these drugs are necessary, though, they are literally a life-saver, so don't hesitate to take the drug when you need it. To minimize side effects of the drug, compensate nutritionally by doing the following:

- ➤ Get plenty of protein.

- ➤ Balance sodium and potassium.

- ➤ Plan for healthy, strong bones.

- ➤ Get enough zinc.

- ➤ Eat to prevent hyperlipidemia, or too-high levels of fats in the bloodstream—commonly known as hardening of the arteries or atherosclerosis.

- ➤ Watch out for blood sugar problems, such as diabetes, that can crop up when you take high doses of steroid medications.

- ➤ Watch out for the "steroid appetite," or your appetite kicked into high gear by this medication, and try not to gain weight while on the medication, a common problem among people who take steroid medications.

If You Take Theophylline Medications

Newer medications are also gradually replacing theophylline in many patients, but some people still do take this old standby. Theophylline has what is called a narrow therapeutic window, which means it works well only within a very small range of how much is in the blood. Too much can quickly become toxic, and too little won't work at all.

When you take theophylline, the doctor will perform blood tests to determine how much of the drug is necessary to give you that optimal blood level. But certain foods (and other drugs) can increase or decrease the rate at which the body absorbs and/or metabolizes the drug. That means that on days when you eat more of the foods that increase the rate at which the body absorbs the drug, the blood level will be higher than on days when you don't. Similarly, blood levels will be lower on days when you eat foods that cause the body to "waste" or excrete more of the drug.

The best advice is to eat a consistent amount of foods that in any way influence the amount of theophylline absorbed or the rate at which it is absorbed. Research has shown, for example, that diets higher in protein tend to speed up the rate at which theophylline is excreted from the body. The advice isn't to avoid protein, but to eat a consistent amount of protein daily. For example, you wouldn't want to eat a lot of carbohydrate foods one day—breads, salads and vegetables—and then the next day load up on protein, such as lots of steak. Instead, regularly include good quality protein foods, as I've done with the meal plans at the end of this chapter.

Research has also shown that people taking theophylline medications tend to have lower blood levels of one of the B vitamins, B_6 or pyridoxine, probably because the medication speeds up the rate at which the body excretes this water-soluble vitamin. Although there has been considerable research, there is no evidence that taking higher than recommended amounts of vitamin B_6 helps to improve asthma symptoms; you definitely want to make sure you get enough of this vitamin, however. Foods high in vitamin B_6 include chicken, fish, pork, eggs, liver, oats, soybeans (and tofu) and bananas. The menus at the end of this chapter have plenty of vitamin B_6. Note that loading up on a vitamin B_6 supplement can be dangerous: too high levels can cause irreversible damage to peripheral nerves, or those in the limbs. If you want to take a supplement for insurance, take it in the form of a one-a-day vitamin/mineral supplement that supplies no more than 100 percent of the RDA for essential nutrients.

Accommodate Food Allergies

Exposure to allergens can trigger an asthma attack. The most common allergy-producing substances in people with asthma are dust, pollens and other inhaled substances. Some people, though, are allergic to certain food components and/or additives.

It's very hard to prove that someone has a true allergy to food. Many times, people with asthma think they have a food allergy because it appears as though the symptoms of their asthma worsen after eating a certain food. While estimates vary, about 24 percent of adults with asthma believe themselves to have at least one food sensitivity. As many as 28 percent of parents of children with asthma report that their children are allergic to at least one food. Allergy testing, however, turns up quite different numbers: the confirmed incidence of adverse reactions to food is probably less than one percent in adults; about 1 to 2 percent in young children and 4 to 6 percent in infants. The most common allergy-producing foods are eggs and milk, with other common offenders including wheat, soy, peanuts, fish and shellfish. In addition, sulfites, a food preservative, can make asthma worse in people who are allergic to it. Fortunately, many infants and children gradually outgrow their food allergies.

The point of comparing the percentage of people who believe themselves allergic to food versus the number confirmed by testing is this: many people place themselves (or their children) on very restrictive diets, believing that this will make the asthma better or decrease the number of attacks. But this can lead to nutritionally inadequate diets. Before placing yourself (or your child) on a restrictive diet, always check with a doctor first to confirm your suspicion. Then, if you really do have a food allergy, work with a registered dietitian to make sure your diet is nutritionally adequate without the substance you're eliminating. For example, if you have a milk allergy, make sure you plan for ways to get enough vitamin D and calcium, two essential bone-building nutrients that milk is rich in.

Eat Fish Twice a Week

After noticing that heavy fish-eating Eskimos suffer less asthma, researchers have tried to prove that fish protects against this chronic lung condition. Theoretically, research suggests that the type of fat found in fish could help reduce the inflammation that causes asthma to flare up. Currently, though, research hasn't yet proved the association. Here's the scoop.

While the word *fat* almost always conjures up negative connotations, the fat in fish swims to a first place victory when it comes to doing good. Fish contain a special type of polyunsaturated fatty acids called omega-3s. You may have even read about two of these omega-3s that are especially abundant in fish, eicosapentaenoic acid and docosahexaenoic acid.

This special type of "body fat" helps fish adapt to the cold water in which they live; it's also thought to confer the health benefits fish eaters realize. Here's how. Omega-3s seem to keep the body's immune system from working overtime. Specifically, they put the brakes on the body's production of prostaglandins, leukotrienes and thromboxanes. While the body needs some of these chemicals to function normally, too-high concentrations can lead to inflammation associated with several conditions, including asthma.

When leukotrienes and prostaglandins rage out of control, they cause the airway tubes to clamp down, trapping air in the lungs. This leads to the wheezing and shortness of breath that asthma sufferers know all too well.

While evidence isn't yet conclusive that eating fish protects against asthma or even reduces asthma attacks, there is considerably more definitive evidence that fish may protect smokers from getting chronic lung inflammation. While quitting is still the best idea, this is good news for smokers.

Try to eat fish at least twice a week. Canned white tuna (albacore) is one of the most inexpensive and easy ways to increase omega-3 intake. Other excellent sources include salmon, mackerel, whitefish (except smoked); pickled Atlantic herring, European anchovies, rainbow trout, Atlantic sardines, Atlantic and Pacific oysters, swordfish, bluefin tuna and rainbow smelt. Try to cook these omega-3-rich fish at lower temperatures, such as in the microwave, which helps preserve the omega-3.

Menus

ASTHMA

The following menus incorporate all the nutritional guidelines recommended in this chapter:

→ They're high in vitamin C, with each packing in at least 200 milligrams of this great vitamin.

→ They're high in vitamin E, with each day having somewhere between seven and ten milligrams (10.5 to 15 IU).

→ They contain a couple of fish meals for the week.

→ The protein/carbohydrate ratio is consistent throughout the day.

→ They contain plenty of vitamin B_6.

→ They contain ample amounts of all nutrient necessary to boost the immune system to resist infections.

→ The calorie level is an excellent one to keep from gaining weight while on steroid medications. Some people, especially those who are more active, may have to boost calories a little. If you do so, always do it in the form of nutrient-dense foods, such as fruits, vegetables and whole grains.

DAY ONE

Breakfast
  2 slices whole wheat toast with 2 tablespoons peanut butter, 1 tablespoon jam
  1 cup skim milk

Morning Snack
  1 orange

Lunch
  Tuna sandwich: ½ can tuna (packed in water), 2 slices whole wheat bread, 2 leaves romaine lettuce, 2 slices tomato, 1 tablespoon low-fat mayonnaise

  1 apple
  1 cup skim milk

Afternoon Snack
  1 cup vegetable juice

Dinner
  One-Pot Chili (page 375)
  1 cup steamed broccoli
  1 cup skim milk

Evening Snack
  1 ounce almonds
  ½ cup skim milk

1763 calories, 106 g protein, 43 g fiber, 55 g fat (27% of calories from fat), 12 g saturated fat (6% of calories from saturated fat), 1540 mg calcium, 2567 mg sodium

Supplies more than 120% of the RDA for the following nutrients: vitamin A, thiamin, riboflavin, niacin, vitamin B_6, vitamin B_{12}, vitamin C, vitamin D, folate, magnesium, manganese, phosphorous, selenium and zinc.

DAY TWO

Breakfast
½ cup nonfat cottage cheese
1 whole wheat English muffin
1 tablespoon jam
1 cup skim milk

Morning Snack
½ cup low-fat fruited yogurt
1 kiwi

Lunch
Salad: 2 cups chopped romaine lettuce,
1 tomato (sliced), 1 cup garbanzo
beans (okay to use canned, just drain
and rinse to reduce sodium), 2 tablespoons low-fat dressing
1 ounce whole wheat pretzel sticks
1 cup vegetable or tomato juice

Dinner
Honey Glazed Carrots and Parsnips
with Chicken Thighs (page 298)
1 cup skim milk
1 tomato slice

Evening Snack
½ cup ice cream
1 cup sliced strawberries

1948 calories, 101 g protein, 43 g fiber, 34 g fat (16% of calories from fat), 11 g saturated fat (5% of calories from saturated fat), 1417 mg calcium, 2761 mg sodium

Supplies more than 120% of the RDA for the following nutrients: vitamin A, thiamin, riboflavin, niacin, vitamin B$_{12}$, vitamin C, folate, magnesium, manganese and selenium.

DAY THREE

Breakfast
Creamy Breakfast Barley with Bananas
and Dried Cranberries (page 247)
1 cup orange juice

Lunch
Peanut butter and jelly sandwich:
2 tablespoons peanut butter,
1 tablespoon jam, 2 slices whole
wheat bread
1 cup skim milk
1 orange
6 baby carrots

Afternoon Snack
2 fig bars
½ cup skim milk

Dinner
Lentil Vegetable Soup (page 371)
Salad: 2 cups romaine lettuce, ½ tomato
(chopped), 2 tablespoons dressing
1 cup skim milk

Evening Snack
1 cup fresh or frozen raspberries with
½ cup milk and a sprinkle of sugar if
you desire

1839 calories, 81 g protein, 58 g fiber, 35 g fat (16% of calories from fat), 7 g saturated fat (3% of calories from saturated fat), 1643 mg calcium, 1538 mg sodium

Supplies more than 120% of the RDA for the following nutrients: vitamin A, thiamin, riboflavin, niacin, vitamin B$_6$, vitamin B$_{12}$, vitamin D, vitamin E, folate, magnesium, manganese and selenium.

Breakfast
1 poached egg
2 slices whole wheat toast
1 teaspoon margarine
1 cup skim milk

Morning Snack
1 cup cantaloupe pieces
1 cup vegetable or tomato juice

Lunch
Favorite Tuna Pasta Salad (page 275)
5 whole grain rye crisps
1 cup skim milk

Afternoon Snack
1 chocolate chip cookie
½ cup skim milk
1 peach

Dinner
5 ounces grilled salmon
1 medium-sized sweet potato, baked
1 teaspoon margarine
1 cup steamed broccoli

Evening Snack
1 cup nonfat frozen yogurt

1756 calories, 121 g protein, 29 g fiber, 39 g fat (27% of calories from fat), 9 g saturated fat (6% of calories from saturated fat)

Supplies more than 120% of the RDA for the following nutrients: vitamin A, thiamin, riboflavin, niacin, vitamin B$_6$, vitamin B$_{12}$ (578%), vitamin C (507%), folate, magnesium, manganese and selenium.

Day Five

Breakfast
Oatmeal: Mix ½ cup oats with 1 cup
    skim milk. Microwave on high for
    2 minutes; stir and microwave for
    2 minutes more. Or combine in a
    heavy pot and simmer 7 minutes.
1 sliced banana
1 cup orange juice

Lunch
Turkey sandwich: 3 ounces lean turkey,
    1 slice American cheese, 2 slices
    whole wheat bread, 1 tablespoon
    light mayonnaise, romaine lettuce,
    2 slices tomato
1 orange
1 cup skim milk

Afternoon Snack
10 thin pretzel sticks
1 cup peach or apricot nectar

Dinner
Chicken and Zucchini Spaghetti
    (page 283)
1 peach
1 cup skim milk

Evening Snack
½ cup trail mix: 2 tablespoons sunflower
    seeds, 2 tablespoons peanuts, 4 table-
    spoons raisins

1942 calories, 108 g protein, 28 g fiber, 51 g fat (23% of calories from fat), 14 g saturated fat (6% of calories from saturated fat), 1309 mg calcium, 1914 mg sodium

Supplies more than 120% of the RDA for the following nutrients: vitamin A, thiamin, riboflavin, niacin, vitamin B$_6$, vitamin B$_{12}$, vitamin C, vitamin D, vitamin E, folate, magnesium and selenium.

DAY SIX

Breakfast

½ cup nonfat cottage cheese

1 whole wheat English muffin

1 tablespoon jam

1 cup skim milk

Morning Snack

1 peach

Lunch

Barley and Bacon Soup (page 370)

6 baby carrots

1 cup skim milk

Afternoon Snack

2 tablespoons sunflower seeds

½ cup skim milk

Dinner

Hamburger: 3 ounces very lean ground beef, 1 hamburger bun, 1 slice tomato (ketchup and mustard as desired)

Salad: 2 cups chopped romaine lettuce, 1 tomato (chopped), ¼ cup grated carrot, ½ red bell pepper (chopped), 2 tablespoons fat-free salad dressing

1 cup skim milk

Evening Snack

1 orange

1 cup vegetable or tomato juice

1917 calories, 123 g protein, 34 g fiber, 40 g fat (19% of calories from fat), 12 g saturated fat (6% of calories from saturated fat), 1942 mg calcium, 4124 mg sodium

Supplies more than 120% of the RDA for the following nutrients: vitamin A, thiamin, riboflavin, niacin, vitamin B_6, vitamin B_{12}, vitamin C (657%), vitamin D, vitamin E, folate, magnesium, manganese, selenium and zinc.

DAY SEVEN

Breakfast

1 poached egg

2 slices whole wheat toast

1 tablespoon jam

½ cup skim milk

Morning Snack

1 cup orange juice

Lunch

Cream of Broccoli Soup (page 368)

1 tomato, sliced, sprinkled with balsamic vinegar and basil (dried or fresh)

1 whole wheat bagel

2 teaspoons margarine

1 cup skim milk

Afternoon Snack

2 fig bars

½ cup skim milk

Dinner

5 ounces grilled tuna

1 baked potato

2 tablespoons nonfat sour cream

½ cup frozen peas and carrots, steamed in microwave

1 cup blueberries

Evening Snack

½ cup nonfat frozen yogurt

1 sliced banana

1882 calories, 115 g protein, 30 g fiber, 37 g fat (17% of calories from fat), 11 g saturated fat (5% of calories from saturated fat), 1290 mg calcium, 1804 mg sodium

Supplies more than 120% for the following nutrients: vitamin A, thiamin, riboflavin, niacin, vitamin B_6, vitamin B_{12} (965%), vitamin C, vitamin D, vitamin E, folate, magnesium, manganese and selenium.

References

Allergy and Asthma Network. "Mothers of Asthmatics." The MA Report. 11(9) (July 1996).

Asthma and Allergy Foundation of America. "What Is Asthma?" The Asthma and Allergy Advance.

Asthma and Allergy Foundation of America. "How to Reduce Exposure to Allergens: The Bedroom Is Your First Line of Defense."

Bielory, L., and R. Gandhi. "Asthma and Vitamin C." *Annals of Allergy* 73 (1994): 89–96.

Clark, N.M., and N.J. Starr-Schneidkraut. "Management of Asthma by Patients and Families." *American Journal of Respiratory Critical Care Medicine* 149 (1994): S54–66 (S67–8).

Dawson, K.P., et al. "Childhood Asthma: What Do Parents Add or Avoid in Their Children's Diets?" *New Zealand Medical Journal* 103 (1990): 239–40.

Gastaminza, G., et al. "Pickled Onion-Induced Asthma: A Model of Sulfite-Sensitive Asthma?" *Clinical and Experimental Allergy* 25(8) (1995): 698–701.

Greene, L.S. "Asthma and Oxidant Stress: Nutritional, Environmental, and Genetic Risk Factors." *Journal of American College of Nutrition* 14(4) (1995): 317–24.

Guill, M.F. "Management of Childhood Asthma: More Than Juggling Medication Doses." *Journal of the Medical Association of Georgia* 83(6) (1994): 358–63.

Hauptman, R.S. "Chronic Asthma Management. What to Do After the Diagnosis." *Canadian Family Physician* 40 (1994): 1313–16.

Henderson, W.R. "Role of Leukotrienes in Asthma." *Annals of Allergy* 72 (1994): 272–78.

Kaslow, J.E. "Double-Blind Trial of Pyridoxine (Vitamin B_6) in the Treatment of Steroid-Dependent Asthma." (letter to the editor). *Annals of Allergy* 71(5) (1993): 492.

Lezaun, A., et al. "Asthma and Contact Urticaria Caused by Rice in a Housewife." *Allergy* 49(2) (1994): 92–95.

Park, H.S., et al. "Occupational Asthma Caused by Two Herb Materials, Dioscorea Batatas and Pinellia Ternata." *Clinical and Experimental Allergy* 24(6) (1994): 575–81.

Sakai, K., et al. "Fatty Acid Compositions of Plasma Lipids in Atopic Dermatitis/Asthma Patients." *Arerugi* 43 (1994): 37–43.

Sur, S., et al. "Double-Blind Trial of Pyridoxine (Vitamin B_6) in the Treatment of Steroid-Dependent Asthma." *Annals of Allergy* 70 (1993): 147–52.

Troisi, R.J., et al. "A Prospective Study of Diet and Adult-Onset Asthma." *American Journal of Respiratory Care Medicine* 151(5) (1995): 1401–08.

Urbink, J.B., et al. "The Relationship Between Vitamin B_6 Metabolism, Asthma, and Theophylline Therapy." *Annals of New York Academy of Sciences* 585 (1990): 285–94.

Dry, J., and D. Vincent. "Effect of a Fish Oil Diet on Asthma: Results of a 1-Year Double-Blind Study." *International Archives of Allergy and Applied Immunology* 95 (1991): 156–57.

Arthritis

16

Nearly forty million Americans, or one in seven, have arthritis. Causing pain and swelling in the joints and connective tissue, arthritis is the number-one cause of limited movement in this country. There are more than a hundred different types of arthritis, but the three most common are fibromyalgia, osteoarthritis, and rheumatoid arthritis.

People who have fibromyalgia—about seven million to ten million in this country—experience widespread pain in muscles and attachments to the bone. In osteoarthritis, the cartilage covering the ends of bones in the joints deteriorates, causing pain and limiting movement as bone begins to rub against bone. This type of arthritis affects more than 15.8 million Americans, the great majority over the age of forty-five. Rheumatoid arthritis (RA) is an autoimmune disease, or one in which the immune system causes inflammation. In this case, it is a chronic inflammation of the lining of the joints, causing joints to deteriorate, a painful process that can greatly limit movement. The most serious and disabling type of arthritis, RA affects about 2.1 million Americans.

As you can see, each type of arthritis is due to a different type of disease process. Similarly, treatment varies considerably. That's also true when it comes to what you can do nutritionally to gain an advantage in feeling better and fighting your disease. In this section, we'll take a close look at how nutrition can help if you have fibromyalgia, osteoarthritis or rheumatoid arthritis. In addition, we'll take a look at some new evidence about diet and two other types of arthritis called Reiter's syndrome and reactive arthritis.

Fibromyalgia Syndrome

A little-understood disease, fibromyalgia strikes some seven million to ten million Americans; like other rheumatic diseases, it strikes a disproportionate number of women (about twenty women for every man). By some estimates, about 2 percent of all adults in the United States have this painful condition. While fibromyalgia occurs in people of all ages, it begins most commonly during the second and third decade of life.

Although doctors don't know what brings on fibromyalgia or by what mechanism it wreaks havoc in the body, fibromyalgia causes widespread body pain originating in the muscles. While some people feel as though the pain originates in the joints, true fibromyalgia doesn't. Sometimes, though, people with fibromyalgia have other conditions that can cause joint pain, including rheumatoid arthritis, osteoarthritis, Lyme disease, systemic lupus erythematosus or other conditions. In fact, about one-third of people with fibromyalgia have one of these other diseases.

Repetitive activities involving the muscles often results in the worst pain, but some patients experience pain even while they are resting. One patient described the pain this way: "Imagine how it would feel to fall out of a speeding car and bounce along the pavement"; another as an "aching all over" feeling, much like what those coming down with the flu describe. Fibromyalgia experts say that the pain often prevents people from exercising; this, in turn, creates a vicious cycle. Because not exercising leads to being out of shape, the fibromyalgia only grows worse. Other symptoms of fibromyalgia include low energy and not sleeping well.

At least one study has found that a portion of fibromyalgia patients have Sjögren's Syndrome. Among 72 patients with fibromyalgia, about 6.9 percent were diagnosed with probable Sjögren's Syndrome and another 11 percent with possible Sjögren's Syndrome. This condition, among other symptoms, can cause severe mouth dryness, which can interfere with achieving good nutrition.

The Nutrition Advantage

Finding therapies for fibromyalgia is difficult due to the lack of understanding of what causes the disease or what it does inside the body. Similarly, there is an incredible void of knowledge about how nutrition can help people with fibromyalgia. Let's review what is known, and also when to eat to maximize energy and good health.

Here are some ideas that will help all people with fibromyalgia:

➤ Eat to maximize energy and to fight the chronic disease process.

➤ Fuel before and refuel after exercising.

➤ Don't take certain medications on an empty stomach.

➤ If you have Sjögren's Syndrome in addition to fibromyalgia, see chapter 22 for more information on Sjögren's Syndrome and how to create a nutrition advantage.

And here are some nutritional issues that have been explored but not proven:

➤ Magnesium and malic acid supplements.

➤ Vitamin B_1 supplementation.

➤ Avoiding an overdose of vitamin A.

Eat to Maximize Energy and Fight Disease

According to Mary Anne Saathoff, R.N., B.S.N., executive director of The Fibromyalgia Alliance of America, many people with fibromyalgia have a short period during the day when they feel their best. Often, she says, this is between 11 A.M. and 3 P.M. You can use this window to your nutrition advantage: plan to prepare your biggest meal during this time, and, if it's convenient, eat it then, too.

Most people try to prepare the biggest, most elaborate meal of the day in the evening. But by the time evening rolls around, many people with fibromyalgia are too tired and sore to even think about cooking; sometimes, the discomfort level is so high that they aren't even interested in eating anything substantial. Take advantage of your peak time during the day and cook up a meal complete with vegetables, a grain and a good-quality protein. There are many one-pot meal recipes in this book that make even more elaborate meal preparation much easier and more accessible for people with limited mobility and/or low energy. If you do work outside the home during your peak period, be sure and bring along or order out a meal complete with fruits and vegetables.

What about those other times of the day? Even though mornings might be particularly difficult for you, try to bolster your body to fight the pain by getting enough calories and a good source of protein. Remember, fighting pain is hard, exhausting work. If all you can manage is milk with an instant breakfast powder, that's excellent. Custards, yogurt with fresh fruit and scrambled eggs are also great choices. Do avoid starting your day off with on an empty tank or with just coffee, as this quickly leads to fatigue for just about anyone—including people who do not have a chronic painful condition such as fibromyalgia. Be sure to read chapter 2, "Eat to Energize."

Fuel Before and After Exercising

Many people with fibromyalgia benefit greatly from an exercise program, an appropriately designed program that is not too strenuous and allows a day of rest in between exercise days. According to Jon Russell, M.D., associate professor of medicine and director of the University Clinical Research Center at the University of Texas Health Science Center in San Antonio, people with fibromyalgia should push themselves to the point of shortness of breath twice during each exercise period.

While replenishing the fuel that exercise burns from muscles is important for everyone, it may be even more important for fibromyalgia patients. Although the significance isn't yet totally understood, doctors do know that in people with fibromyalgia, the amount of energy in muscle cells (as well as in blood cells) is lower than normal. Officially speaking, they are low in a substance called adenosine triphosphate (ATP), which is the body's energy currency. Using a special scan called nuclear magnetic resonance spectroscopy, doctors have noticed that in people with fibromyalgia, exercising muscles use up abnormally large amounts of energy. While this may be because of the disease, it may also be because people with fibromyalgia tend to be deconditioned, or out of shape.

Here's how to restore energy in muscle cells and also to help muscle cells repair themselves after exercise:

➤ One hour *before* exercise, drink a cup of orange juice, skim milk, pear nectar or some other good quality, nutritious and low-fat beverage. Beverages with any amount of fat in them won't be digested and absorbed as rapidly, so you may not benefit from the energy they do contain soon enough to boost energy during your exercise session.

➤ Immediately after exercise, drink another cup of orange juice or other high-carbohydrate (and nutritious) beverage. This will help restore burned energy.

➤ About two to four hours after exercise, eat a nutritious meal with a good source of complex carbohydrate (grains such as pasta, whole wheat bread, barley, rice) and a good source of protein (lean meat, fish, lentils or other dried beans).

Do Not Medicate on an Empty Stomach

Many fibromyalgia patients find that nonsteroidal anti-inflammatory medications, such as ibuprofen and naproxen, help their condition (take them only under a doctor's care, though). Be sure to take these medications with food, as they can be quite irritating to the stomach—to the point where you have to stop taking them. See chapter 10 for information on medications you take and how they might affect nutritional status.

Magnesium and Malic Acid Supplements

These two substances occur naturally in the body, and both are known to be necessary to make adenosine triphosphate, the body's energy currency. Knowing this, some researchers speculated that giving supplements of magnesium and malic acid might help restore energy to low-energy muscle cells, and thereby relieve fibromyalgia symptoms.

One controlled trial was done to explore this possibility. Researchers from the University of Texas Health Science Center studied twenty-four patients with fibromyalgia. Some of the patients were given three tablets twice each day of a supplement containing 200 milligrams of malic acid and fifty milligrams of magnesium and others were given a placebo, a sugar pill that looked and tasted like the real thing. After four weeks, there was no clear evidence that that amount of the magnesium/malic acid supplement helped the fibromyalgia patients. However, after the four-week study period, some of the patients increased the dose to as much as six tablets twice day. Many of those who did reported significant reductions in the severity of all three primary pain/tenderness measures. These researchers suggest that higher doses are beneficial and recommend further studies to verify that premise

Always discuss potential therapies with a physician, including the possibility of taking this supplement. High dose magnesium, which is how the poststudy dose of magnesium would be regarded, can have several side effects, including diarrhea, nausea, vomiting, low blood pressure, breathing difficulties, coma and even heart attack. If a person did take the maximum dose taken by patients after the formal study (six tablets twice daily), the total dose of magnesium would be 600 milligrams. In contrast, the recommended dietary allowance is 350 milligrams for men and 280 milligrams for women.

Vitamin B₁ Supplementation

The theory behind supplementing this B vitamin (also called thiamin) also has to do with the idea that fibromyalgia patients do not have enough energy in their cells, possibly because they do not metabolize carbohydrates normally. Vitamin B_1 is necessary, among other functions, to unleash energy from carbohydrates. While this is true, there is no evidence that taking more than the recommended amount can work "overtime" to make up for the lack of energy that fibromyalgia patients (or anyone) experience.

While the recommended dietary allowance of vitamin B_1 is just 1.1 milligrams for women and 1.5 milligrams for men, some people recommend doses of 100 milligrams a day to as high as 500 milligrams a day for fibromyalgia patients. Note, however, that controlled trials have not been conducted. Also, taking such high doses of thiamin may be dangerous. For one, prolonged use of more than 250 milligrams per day of vitamin B_6 may cause irreversible nerve damage, loss of coordination, loss of sensation and extreme sensitivity to light.

Avoid Overdosing on Vitamin A

While the evidence is quite limited, there is some suggestion that an overdose of vitamin A may worsen fibromyalgia symptoms. In one study of nine patients who showed no improvement after the usual treatments for fibromyalgia, blood levels of vitamin A were substantially higher than normal. All of these patients had been taking supplemental vitamin A preparations. After discontinuing the excess vitamin A supplements, all patients improved to varying degrees.

Again, remember that this is only one study and so definitive conclusions cannot be made. It makes sense, though, that loading up on a vitamin to the point of abnormally raising blood levels could cause problems. As with all vitamins, take only the recommended amount. If you do take extra, take it only under the care of a physician as if it were a medication—at higher than suggested doses, it really is a medication.

Putting It All Together

I've devised seven days' worth of menus that accommodate all the dietary advice given above. Each day's menu has two calorie levels—1,500 if you need to lose weight and 1,800 calories if you wish to maintain your weight.

Menus

FIBROMYALGIA

The menus for fibromyalgia feature a very easy to prepare breakfast, a midmorning snack, a larger lunchtime menu (as energy is generally best between 11 A.M. and 3 P.M.), and a smaller dinner meal. Remember, do not begin your day on an empty tank, as you'll only feel worse very quickly. I've chosen some particularly easy menus from the recipe section. Note that I have used frozen vegetables in most of the menus to save energy; feel free to use fresh in place of any of them.

Part 1: Weight Maintenance—1800 calories

DAY ONE

Breakfast
  1 cup Fiber One cereal
  1 sliced banana
  1 cup nonfat milk

Morning Snack
  1 cup low-fat fruited yogurt

Lunch
  Turkey sandwich: 3 ounces turkey breast, 1 slice American cheese, 2 slices whole wheat bread, romaine lettuce, 2 thick slices tomato, 2 teaspoons mayonnaise

  1 cup frozen broccoli pieces, steamed with 1 tablespoon soft margarine
  1 apple
  1 cup skim milk

Dinner
  6 ounces salmon fillet, broiled
  1 cup frozen peas, microwaved
  1 medium baked sweet potato
  1 tablespoon soft margarine

Evening Snack
  ½ cup fresh or frozen raspberries

1860 calories, 112 g protein, 43 g fiber, 48 g total fat (13 g saturated fat), 1489 g calcium

DAY TWO

Breakfast
  1 whole wheat English muffin
  2 tablespoons peanut butter
  1 tablespoon jam
  1 cup skim milk

Morning Snack
  1 large pear

Lunch
  Salad★: 2 cups romaine lettuce; ¼ cup chopped green onion; 1 red bell pepper, chopped; 1 cup garbanzo beans (chickpeas); 1 tablespoon low-calorie French dressing
  1 whole wheat bagel

  1 tablespoon soft margarine

  ★You can purchase the salad makings from the grocery store salad bar already chopped up, with the exception of the garbanzo beans, which you can purchase in a can.

Dinner
  Grilled cheese sandwich: 2 ounces cheddar cheese, 2 slices whole wheat bread, 1 teaspoon soft margarine
  6 baby carrots
  1 orange
  1 cup skim milk

Evening Snack
  1 peach (or 2 canned peach halves)

1760 calories, 77 g protein, 40 g fiber, 60 g total fat (23 g saturated fat), 1471 mg calcium

DAY THREE

Breakfast

1 slice whole wheat toast with ½ cup
2% low-fat cottage cheese

1 cup orange juice

Morning Snack

½ cup fruited, low-fat yogurt

Lunch

Ham sandwich: 3 ounces lean ham,
1 slice American cheese, 2 slices whole

wheat bread, 2 romaine lettuce leaves,
2 teaspoons low-fat mayonnaise

1 cup skim milk

1 green bell pepper, sliced

1 orange

Dinner

1 serving Italian Chicken and Rice
(page 302)

2 apricots (or 4 canned apricot halves)

1785 calories, 115 g protein, 25 g fiber, 29 g total fat (11 g saturated fat), 1347 g calcium

DAY FOUR

Breakfast

Oatmeal: Mix ½ cup oats with 1 cup
skim milk. Microwave on high 2 minutes; stir and microwave for 2 minutes
more. Or combine in a heavy pot and
simmer 7 minutes.

1 banana

Morning Snack

3 fig bars

½ cup skim milk

Lunch

Peanut butter and jelly sandwich:
2 tablespoons peanut butter, 1 tablespoon jam, 2 slices whole wheat bread

1 cup skim milk

1 apple

Salad: 2 cups chopped romaine lettuce;
1 tomato, chopped; 2 tablespoons
low-fat French dressing

Dinner

1 serving Onion and Cheesy Tomato
Soup (page 366)

Ice water

Evening Snack

½ cup skim milk

DAY FIVE★

Breakfast

1 hard-boiled egg

½ whole wheat English muffin

2 teaspoons soft margarine

1 tablespoon jam

1 cup orange juice

Morning Snack

1 cup low-fat yogurt

Lunch

4 ounces roasted lean beef (such as eye
of round)

1 large baked potato

1 tablespoon margarine

1 cup frozen peas and carrots, steamed
in microwave

1 cup skim milk

1 peach (or 2 canned peach halves)

Dinner

Tuna sandwich: ½ can tuna (packed
in water) with 2 tablespoons light
mayonnaise, 2 slices whole wheat
bread, 2 romaine lettuce leaves

1 banana

Ice water

★This has a rather large lunch, intended for
a Saturday or Sunday.

1785 calories, 102 g protein, 24 g fiber, 45 g total fat (11 g saturated fat), 1000 mg calcium

DAY SIX

Breakfast

1 cup Fiber One cereal (or some other high-fiber cereal)

1 cup fresh or frozen raspberries

1 cup skim milk

Morning Snack

1 large banana

Lunch

Grilled cheese sandwich: 3 ounces low-fat American cheese, 2 slices whole wheat bread, 2 teaspoons margarine

1 cup grapes

1 cup frozen vegetable blend (such as broccoli, cauliflower, red peppers), steamed in microwave

1 cup skim milk

Dinner

3 ounces roasted chicken

1 medium sweet potato, baked with 2 tablespoons brown sugar, 1 tablespoon margarine

1 cup frozen green beans, steamed in microwave

1 cup skim milk

Evening Snack

1 cup vanilla ice cream

1856 calories, 96 g protein, 33 g fiber, 51 g total fat (19 g saturated fat), 1957 mg calcium

DAY SEVEN

Breakfast

Oatmeal: Mix ½ cup oats with 1 cup skim milk. Microwave on high 2 minutes; stir and microwave for 2 minutes more. Or combine in a heavy pot and simmer 7 minutes.

2 tablespoons raisins

Morning Snack

2 crackers

2 tablespoons peanut butter

½ cup skim milk

Lunch

Scrambled Eggs for Dinner (page 254)

1 whole wheat English muffin

1 tablespoon margarine

1 orange

Dinner

Turkey sandwich: 3 ounces lean turkey, 1 slice American cheese, 2 slices whole wheat bread, 1 tablespoon low-calorie mayonnaise

1 large banana

1843 calories, 104 g protein, 26 g fiber, 67 g total fat (19 g saturated fat), 1312 mg calcium

Part 2: Weight Loss—1500 Calories

DAY ONE

Breakfast
1 cup Fiber One cereal
1 sliced banana
1 cup skim milk

Morning Snack
½ cup low-fat fruited yogurt

Lunch
Turkey sandwich: 3 ounces turkey
breast, 2 slices whole wheat bread,
romaine lettuce, 2 thick slices tomato,
mustard

1 cup frozen broccoli pieces, steamed
with 1 tablespoon soft margarine
1 apple
1 cup skim milk

Dinner
4 ounces salmon fillet, broiled
1 cup frozen peas, microwaved
1 medium baked sweet potato
1 tablespoon soft margarine

Evening Snack
½ cup fresh or frozen raspberries

1565 calories, 91 g protein, 43 g fiber, 36 g total fat (7 g saturated fat), 1200 mg calcium

DAY TWO

Breakfast
1 whole wheat English muffin
2 tablespoons peanut butter
1 tablespoon jam
1 cup skim milk

Morning Snack
1 large pear

Lunch
Salad★: 2 cups romaine lettuce; ¼ cup
chopped green onion; 1 red bell pepper, chopped; 1 cup garbanzo beans
(chickpeas); 1 tablespoon low-calorie

French dressing
½ whole wheat bagel
1 tablespoon soft margarine

★You can purchase the salad makings from
the grocery store salad bar already chopped
up, with the exception of the garbanzo
beans, which you can purchase in a can.

Dinner
Grilled cheese sandwich: 2 ounces
cheddar cheese, 2 slices whole wheat
bread, 1 teaspoon soft margarine
6 baby carrots
1 orange

1543 calories, 92 g protein, 28 g fiber, 29 g total fat (6 g saturated fat), 1143 mg calcium

DAY THREE

Breakfast
1 slice whole wheat toast with ½ cup
2% low-fat cottage cheese
1 cup orange juice

Morning Snack
2 apricots (or 4 canned apricot halves)

Lunch
Ham sandwich: 3 ounces lean ham,
2 slices whole wheat bread

2 romaine lettuce leaves, 2 teaspoons
low-fat mayonnaise
1 cup skim milk
1 green bell pepper, sliced
1 orange

Dinner
1 serving Italian Chicken and Rice
(page 302)

1579 calories, 106 g protein, 25 g fiber, 21 g total fat (6 g saturated fat), 1082 g calcium

DAY FOUR

Breakfast

Oatmeal: Mix ½ cup oats with 1 cup skim milk. Microwave on high 2 minutes; stir and microwave for 2 minutes more. Or combine in a heavy pot and simmer 7 minutes.

1 banana

Morning Snack

1 apple

Lunch

Peanut butter and jelly sandwich: 2 tablespoons peanut butter,

1 tablespoon jam, 2 slices whole wheat bread

1 cup skim milk

Salad: 2 cups romaine lettuce, chopped; 1 tomato, chopped; 2 tablespoons low-fat French dressing

Dinner

Onion and Cheesy Tomato Soup (page 366)

Ice water

1564 calories, 65 g protein, 35 g fiber, 59 g total fat (23 g saturated fat), 1200 mg calcium

DAY FIVE★

Breakfast

1 hard-boiled egg

½ whole wheat English muffin

2 teaspoons soft margarine

1 tablespoon jam

1 cup orange juice

Morning Snack

½ cup low-fat yogurt

Lunch

3 ounces roasted lean beef (such as eye of round)

1 medium baked potato

2 teaspoons margarine

1 cup frozen peas and carrots, steamed in microwave

1 cup skim milk

1 peach (or 2 canned peach halves)

Dinner

Tuna sandwich: ½ can tuna (packed in water) with 1 tablespoon light mayonnaise, 2 slices whole wheat bread, 2 romaine lettuce leaves

1 banana

Ice water

★This has a rather large lunch, intended for a Saturday or Sunday.

1528 calories, 88 g protein, 24 g fiber, 36 g total fat (9 g saturated fat), 816 mg calcium

DAY SIX

Breakfast

1 cup Fiber One cereal (or some other high-fiber cereal)

1 cup fresh or frozen raspberries

1 cup skim milk

Morning Snack

1 large banana

Lunch

Grilled cheese sandwich: 3 ounces low-fat American cheese, 2 slices whole wheat bread, 2 teaspoons margarine

1 cup grapes

1 cup frozen vegetable blend (such as broccoli, cauliflower, red peppers), steamed in microwave

1 cup skim milk

Dinner
3 ounces roast chicken
1 medium sweet potato, baked
with 2 tablespoons brown sugar,
2 teaspoons margarine

1 cup frozen green beans, steamed in
microwave
Ice water

1472 calories, 83 g protein, 35 g fiber, 32 g total fat (9 g saturated fat), 1486 mg calcium

DAY SEVEN

Breakfast
Oatmeal: Mix ½ cup oats with 1 cup
skim milk. Microwave on high 2 minutes; stir and microwave for 2 minutes
more. Or combine in a heavy pot and
simmer 7 minutes.
2 tablespoons raisins

Morning Snack
2 crackers
2 tablespoons peanut butter
½ cup skim milk

Lunch
Scrambled Eggs for Dinner (page 254)
1 whole wheat English muffin
1 tablespoon margarine
1 orange

Dinner
Turkey sandwich: 3 ounces lean turkey,
1 slice American cheese, 2 slices
whole wheat bread, 1 tablespoon
low-calorie mayonnaise
1 large banana
Ice water

1520 calories, 90 g protein, 23 g fiber, 53 g total fat (16 g saturated fat), 972 mg calcium

References

Bennet, R. *Fibromyalgia Syndrome: An Informational Guide for FMS Patients, Their Families, Friends and Employers.* National Fibromyalgia Research Association, P.O. Box 500, Salem OR 97308. Informative pamphlet.

National Fibromyalgia Research Association. *Fibromyalgia Syndrome Diagnostic Criteria.* P.O. Box 500, Salem OR 97308. Information packet.

Romano, T.J. "Exacerbation of Soft Tissue Rheumatism by Excess Vitamin A: Case Reviews with Clinical Vignette." *West Virginia Medical Journal* 91 (1995): 147.

Russell, J. *Fibromyalgia Syndrome: A Primer.* National Fibromyalgia Research Association, P.O. Box 500, Salem OR 97308. Informative booklet.

Russell, J., et al. "Treatment of Fibromyalgia Syndrome with Super Malic: A Randomized Double Blind, Placebo Controlled, Crossover Pilot Study." *Journal of Rheumatology* 22 (1995): 953–58.

Osteoarthritis

Many people think that osteoarthritis, commonly called arthritis, is a natural consequence of aging. It's not, and there are several dietary habits you can adopt to help reduce the chances that you'll get this form of arthritis. And, if you are already afflicted, you can feel better by taking charge of several aspects of your life.

Let's review the following nutrition maneuvers you can make to help prevent osteoarthritis, or at least lessen its severity:

➤ Increase vitamin D intake.

➤ Achieve and maintain a healthy, lean body weight.

➤ Eat lots of fruits and vegetables.

➤ Eat to prevent osteoporosis.

➤ Avoid excessive vitamin A supplementation.

➤ Eat for a healthy heart.

➤ Don't take certain medications on an empty stomach.

Boost Vitamin D Intake

Vitamin D is best known for its pivotal role in building strong bones. This is because without it, the body could not absorb and use calcium to make bones more dense. Now, there's evidence that getting 400 IU of vitamin D can significantly reduce the progression of osteoarthritis in the knee.

Researchers from Boston University Medical Center studied more than 500 people with knee osteoarthritis for eight years, tracking both how much vitamin D they took in daily and the levels of vitamin D in their blood. They also followed the progression of the osteoarthritis in the knee. They found that people who took in just 200 IU were three times as likely to suffer progressive osteoarthritis as people who took in an average of 386 IU daily.

Why does vitamin D work to arrest osteoarthritis progression? The Boston researchers propose two theories. First, they think it's possible that vitamin D helps keep the cartilage in the knee healthy and strong, which is important because osteoarthritis of the knee is characterized by loss of cartilage at the ends of two bones in the knee joint. Another theory is that vitamin D helps keep the knee bones hearty and healthy. If the cartilage wears away, the bones in the knee become vulnerable to rubbing against each other and wearing away themselves. Vitamin D, however, might make the bones stronger and resistant to wearing away. Here's an analogy: if you rub two pieces of sandstone together—sandstone being a soft rock—you know that the two pieces quickly wear away and lose their shapes. However, if you rub together two pieces of granite, much stronger rocks, they are far less likely to wear down.

Get 400 IU of vitamin D daily by consuming some combination of the following:

➤ 1 cup milk (whole, 2%, 1% or skim, but skim is the healthier choice): 100 IU (note that yogurt, cheese and other dairy products have no vitamin D because they are made with unfortified milk).

➤ 1 cup canned salmon: 336 IU.

➤ 4 ounces broiled salmon fillet: 317 IU.

While it's always better to get nutrients from food, don't hesitate to turn to a supplement if you don't eat any of these foods, or if you only include them in your eating plan inconsistently. Or, use a combination of food and a supplement to meet the 400 IU daily.

While this particular study was done just on people with osteoarthritis of the knee, it's also possible that vitamin D could help stop the progression of osteoarthritis in other parts of the body, too. It just hasn't been studied.

Boosting vitamin D to 400 IU, by the way, has other benefits. There is emerging evidence that it reduces the risk of colon cancer, and other research is exploring vitamin D's ability to treat cancer.

A word to the wise: don't overdo it with vitamin D supplements. Taking just 1,000 IU daily for any length of time can quickly become toxic. Getting too much vitamin D causes excess calcium to circulate in the blood and subsequently to deposit in soft tissues, including the kidneys and heart. This can lead to irreversible kidney and heart damage.

Achieve and Maintain a Healthy Body Weight

If you're out to prevent osteoarthritis, maintaining a lean profile is your best bet. In addition, say arthritis experts, losing excess weight once you have arthritis is an aid in reducing the severity of symptoms. Some of the researchers from Boston University Medical Center that uncovered the vitamin D/arthritis connection found that when overweight women lost just eleven pounds they slashed their chances of ever developing osteoarthritis of the knee by more than one half. Losing excess weight is thought to help prevent and alleviate osteoarthritis of the hips and hands, too.

Doctors first noted the connection between arthritis and obesity as early as 1939. Over time, this connection between excess weight and arthritis has been made for just about every joint system in the body.

It makes sense that weight loss can help prevent or lessen the severity of osteoarthritis. Most obviously, carrying around excess weight puts a tremendous amount of stress on joints, especially those in the lower extremities: hips and knees. Hands, even though they don't bear weight as hips and knees do, also suffer from excess weight. This is because most of the force across a joint is the result of muscle contraction. Because plump fingers require more muscle contraction for an activity (imagine a slim hand making a fist versus a heavier hand making a fist), there is greater force on the joints in the fingers.

Another reason being too heavy increases the chances of developing osteoarthritis is that excessive weight changes the body's metabolism, which could contribute to damaging joints.

Granted, losing weight is no easy proposition. But if the payoff is less pain and greater mobility, the changes you'll have to make in the way you eat and in the exercise you get may be worth it. Refer to chapter 7 for some practical tips on shedding excess pounds.

Eat Lots of Fruits and Vegetables

Antioxidant nutrients have been in the news for a number of years. Mostly, you've heard about their possible role in helping to prevent cancer and heart disease. You may also have read that antioxidant nutrients harvested from fruits and vegetables rather than from supplements show the most promise in fighting disease. Now, there's some very preliminary evidence that antioxidant nutrients may help slow the degenerative process causing osteoarthritis.

Let's first take a look at why we need antioxidants. Every cell in the body needs oxygen to generate energy. In the process of using that oxygen, by-products are formed, free radicals among them (free radicals also enter the body when we're exposed to pollutants, such as cigarette smoke). A free radical is an atom that is missing an electron, which makes it unstable. In an attempt to stabilize itself, the free radical steals an electron from another atom. Each robbed atom, in turn, attempts to achieve stability, stealing an electron from a neighboring atom, thus creating a chain reaction.

Inside the body, free radicals steal electrons from cells, creating a chain reaction of cellular damage, or oxidation, as it's properly called. Oxidation is the same process by which metal rusts and butter turns rancid. In the body, oxidation contributes to the process of aging, heart disease, cancer, cataracts, infections and possibly osteoarthritis.

Arthritis experts from the Boston University Medical Center became interested in exploring the link between antioxidant nutrient intake and osteoarthritis after learning from laboratory studies that free radicals form in joints and can damage the tissue there, thereby contributing to the degenerative changes characteristic of osteoarthritis. They devised a study to investigate the relationship between vitamins C and E and beta-carotene (beta-carotene is the building block of vitamin A; it's the water-soluble form of vitamin A found in yellow, orange and red fruits and vegetables that the body converts into vitamin A) and both the incidence and progression of osteoarthritis. They found that people who had the highest intakes of vitamin C cut their risk of progressive cartilage loss (which means that osteoarthritis is progressing) compared to people with the lowest intake of vitamin C. They also found a slight association between the intake of beta-carotene and vitamin E intake and disease progression, but it was much less consistent. This study, though, did not find an association between antioxidant intake and the chance of getting osteoarthritis in the first place.

Even though these results are preliminary, it seems worthwhile for everyone to increase their intake of antioxidant-rich fruits and vegetables. While further studies are necessary to prove the association, there are plenty of good reasons for everyone to boost their intake of fruits and vegetables—the antioxidant nutrients may help fight cancer and heart disease, and the other vitamins, phytochemicals, and fiber packed into produce are a must for everyone to feel their best. While all fruits and vegetables have some antioxidant nutrients, some are much higher than others (see page 160).

Foods High in Antioxidant Nutrients

Beta-carotene

Pumpkin, including canned pumpkin, sweet potatoes, carrots, turnip greens, papaya, cantaloupe, spinach and apricots.

Vitamin C

Papaya, sweet red pepper, strawberries, oranges, Brussels sprouts, mango, broccoli and spinach.

Vitamin E*

Wheat germ, sunflower seeds, kale, sweet potato, papaya, turnip greens and mango.

*Also see chart on page 122.

Here are two different menu combinations that will give you 500 milligrams of vitamin C, 30 to 35 milligrams of beta-carotene and 10 IU vitamin E (just add in lean protein and whole grains for a complete diet):

DAY ONE

Breakfast
 6 ounces orange juice
 3 apricots

Lunch
 Salad: ½ grated carrot, ½ cup chopped red pepper, 1 chopped mango, 2 cups raw spinach leaves

Afternoon Snack
 6 ounces tomato juice

Dinner
 ½ cup cooked turnip greens
 ½ cup cooked cauliflower

Evening Snack
 1 orange

DAY TWO

Breakfast
 1 orange

Lunch
 Salad: 1 grated carrot, 5 cherry tomatoes, 1½ cups spinach leaves

Afternoon Snack
 1 papaya

Dinner
 ½ cup cooked kale
 5 Brussels sprouts
 1 slice watermelon

Evening Snack
 6 ounces cranberry juice
 ¼ cup peanuts

A word to the wise: get your antioxidant nutrients from real food and not supplements. A rapidly growing body of evidence points to the real thing rather than supplements as offering the most protection in other diseases—and the same will probably prove true for arthritis. While a supplement may have one or a couple of antioxidant nutrients, real food has a wide complement, including some we haven't yet discovered but that may well be responsible for part of the benefit. Finally, adding in lots of fruits and vegetable automatically means slimming down your eating style, which can help you slim down, too.

Eat to Prevent Osteoporosis

No doubt, preventing osteoporosis is important for everyone, especially women who are particularly hard hit by this bone-thinning process. But it's even more important for people with arthritis. Joints that are already weakened by the arthritic process are especially hard hit by bone-weakening osteoporosis. Refer to chapter 3, page 22 for more information on preventing osteoporosis.

Avoid Vitamin A Overdose

While a good intake of vitamin A is necessary for everyone to be healthy, getting too much can be quite dangerous. Because it is fat soluble, which means the excess is stored in fatty tissue rather than excreted, taking too much quickly builds up an excess store in the body. Among other possibly serious negative effects, excess vitamin A has been associated with rapid destructive osteoarthritis. As with all nutrients, aim to get the recommended amount, and avoid overdosing. Remember the food advantage: getting vitamin A from fruits and vegetables means getting in the previtamin, water-soluble form. Whatever the body doesn't need, we excrete. That means excess levels don't build up.

Eat for a Healthy Heart

Arthritis experts now have enough evidence to recommend exercise for all people with arthritis. Not only have specific exercise protocols been proven safe, but they've also been shown to decrease the arthritis-associated disability (as always, check with your doctor before embarking on a new exercise routine—certain forms of exercise are better for people with arthritis in specific joints). Research shows, however, that few people with arthritis do exercise. This is understandable, because it is sometimes difficult to work through the pain and limited movement to realize the benefits of exercise down the road. In addition, some people, lacking proper exercise advice, are afraid to exercise for fear they will hurt themselves.

But not exercising because of osteoarthritis places people at risk of another problem: developing artery-clogging heart disease. Research has shown that as people become more disabled by osteoarthritis, they exercise less and become more and more deconditioned overall. In one study, the chances of having heart disease was 13 percent for people without osteoarthritis but more than double, at 27 percent, for people with osteoarthritis.

The best advice is to seek guidance necessary to learn how to exercise safely—a physical therapist, after consulting with your physician, can give you the best advice. In addition, though, decrease your risk of developing heart disease by eating a heart healthy diet. Refer to pages 13–19 for the details.

Do Not Medicate on an Empty Stomach

Nonsteroidal anti-inflammatory medications are often used to treat osteoarthritis. Be careful, though, always to take these medications with food. They can be very abrasive to the lining of the stomach, causing nausea, stomach upset and even ulcer. Refer to the chapter on medications for more information.

Putting It All Together

It is indeed confusing to convert all this dietary advice into an eating plan. Here, I've taken away the guesswork by providing seven days' worth of menus. Each day has two calorie levels—1,500 calories for people who need to drop weight, and 1,800 calories for people who need to maintain weight (a few people need more calories; see pages 53–54 for ideas on adding calories if you're one of them). Each day's menu includes all the foods necessary to achieve all the dietary recommendations made in this chapter.

Menus

OSTEOARTHRITIS

Note that each day's menu (with one exception) includes three cups of skim milk—this is to ensure that you get enough vitamin D (as well as calcium). As you learned in the chapter on preventing osteoporosis, while other dairy products (cheese, yogurt, ice cream) have lots of calcium, they have no vitamin D. That's because they're made with milk before it's fortified with vitamin D. If you have a lactose intolerance, try the lactose-reduced milk, or try adding the pills that break down lactose. If you don't want to include milk in your eating plan, then make sure you take enough of a supplement of vitamin D and calcium. In place of the milk, substitute a whole grain or fruit serving.

Part 1: Weight Maintenance

DAY ONE

Breakfast

6 ounces orange juice

3 fresh apricots (or 6 canned halves)

Oatmeal: Mix ½ cup oats with 1 cup skim milk. Microwave on high 2 minutes; stir and microwave for 2 minutes more. Or combine in a heavy pot and simmer 7 minutes.

Morning Snack

1 orange

Lunch

Salad: 2 cups chopped spinach, ½ carrot, grated; ½ sweet red pepper, chopped; 1 mango, chopped; 1 cup garbanzo beans; 2 tablespoons low-fat dressing

1 whole wheat bagel

2 teaspoons margarine

1 cup skim milk

Afternoon Snack

6 ounces low-sodium tomato juice

Dinner

4 ounces broiled salmon

1 cup steamed cauliflower

1 medium sweet potato, baked with 2 tablespoons brown sugar

1779 calories, 92 g protein, 18 g fiber, 32 g total fat (5 g saturated fat), 1085 mg calcium, 1593 mg sodium

DAY TWO

Breakfast

1 cup Fiber One cereal

½ cup blueberries

1 cup skim milk

Morning Snack

1 banana

½ cup orange juice

Lunch

Sandwich: 3 ounces lean turkey, 2 slices whole wheat bread, 2 romaine lettuce leaves, 2 thick slices tomato, 1 tablespoon low-fat mayonnaise

1 apple

1 cup skim milk

Afternoon Snack

1 cup low-sodium vegetable juice

Dinner

Peppered Beef and Rice (page 324)

1 whole wheat dinner roll

1 tablespoon margarine

½ cup peas

1 cup skim milk

Evening Snack

3 fig bars

1805 calories, 100 g protein, 38 g fiber, 38 g total fat (8.7 g saturated fat), 1200 mg calcium, 1784 mg sodium

DAY THREE

Breakfast

1 whole wheat English muffin

2 teaspoons margarine

1 tablespoon jam

1 cup skim milk

Morning Snack

1 apple

Lunch

Salad: 2 cups chopped romaine lettuce, ½ medium tomato (chopped), 1 cup garbanzo (chickpeas—okay to use canned), 2 tablespoons low-fat salad dressing

1 orange

1 cup skim milk

Dinner

Apricot Chicken with Walnuts (page 290)

1 cup skim milk

Evening Snack

1 cup ice cream

1807 calories, 83 g protein, 27 g fiber, 48 g total fat (14 g saturated fat), 1464 mg calcium, 1814 mg sodium

DAY FOUR

Breakfast

Oatmeal: Mix ½ cup oats with 1 cup skim milk★. Microwave on high 2 minutes; stir and microwave for 2 minutes more. Or combine in a heavy pot and simmer 7 minutes.

1 cup orange juice

★Or make with water if you prefer and enjoy a glass of skim milk.

Morning Snack

1 cup low-fat fruited yogurt

Lunch

Peanut butter and jelly sandwich: 2 tablespoons peanut butter,

1 tablespoon jam, 2 slices whole wheat bread

3 fresh apricots (or 6 canned apricot halves)

Cucumber slices

1 cup skim milk

Afternoon Snack

1 banana

Dinner

Ruffled Crab Salad (page 276)

1 cup skim milk

Evening Snack

½ cup nonfat frozen yogurt

1840 calories, 87 g protein, 21 g fiber, 35 g total fat (8 g saturated fat), 1647 mg calcium, 2264 mg sodium

DAY FIVE

Breakfast

1 poached egg

2 slices whole wheat toast

1 tablespoon margarine

1 tablespoon jam

1 cup skim milk

Morning Snack

1 cup melon cubes

Lunch

Sandwich: 3 ounces lean turkey, 1 whole wheat bagel, 2 pieces romaine lettuce, mustard

1 cup skim milk

1 carrot

Afternoon Snack

2 oatmeal raisin cookies

1 cup skim milk

Dinner

One-Pot Chili (page 375) with 1 ounce shredded cheese

6 saltine crackers

Evening Snack

1 cup melon cubes

1773 calories, 107 g protein, 28 g fiber, 47 g total fat (17 g saturated fat), 1385 mg calcium, 2287 mg sodium

Day Six

Breakfast

Oatmeal: Mix ½ cup oats with 1 cup skim milk. Microwave on high 2 minutes; stir and microwave for 2 minutes more. Or combine in a heavy pot and simmer 7 minutes.

2 tablespoons raisins

Morning Snack

3 apricots (or 6 halves, canned in juice)

Lunch

Tuna sandwich: ½ can tuna (packed in water), 2 slices whole wheat bread, 2 pieces romaine lettuce, 2 thick slices tomato, 1 tablespoon low-fat mayonnaise

1 cup skim milk

1 orange

2 fig bars

Afternoon Snack

1 cup low-sodium vegetable juice cocktail

Dinner

Creamy Chinese Cabbage and Chicken (page 312)

1 cup steamed broccoli pieces (frozen is fine)

1 tablespoon margarine

1 cup skim milk

Evening Snack

1 cup nonfat frozen yogurt

1860 calories, 114 g protein, 30 g fiber, 36 g total fat (9 g saturated fat), 1731 mg calcium, 1741 mg sodium

Day Seven

Breakfast

1 poached egg

1 whole wheat English muffin

1 tablespoon margarine

1 tablespoon jam

1 cup skim milk

Morning Snack

1 apple

Lunch

Kielbasa Corn Chowder (page 377)

1 cup skim milk

Afternoon Snack

4 canned peach halves

Dinner

Hamburger: 3 ounces cooked extra lean ground beef patty (3½ ounces raw), 1 hamburger bun, 1 slice tomato (ketchup and mustard as desired)

1 cup cooked carrot slices

Evening Snack

1 cup ice cream

1834 calories, 95 g protein, 23 g fiber, 55 g total fat (21 g saturated fat), 1598 mg calcium, 2415 mg sodium★

★Figured with 1 tablespoon ketchup.

DAY ONE

Breakfast

6 ounces orange juice

3 fresh apricots (or 6 canned halves)

Oatmeal: Mix ½ cup oats with 1 cup
skim milk. Microwave on high
2 minutes; stir and microwave for
2 minutes more. Or combine in a
heavy pot and simmer 7 minutes.

Morning Snack

1 orange

Lunch

Salad: 2 cups chopped spinach, ½ carrot,
grated; ½ sweet red pepper, chopped;
1 mango, chopped; 1 cup garbanzo
beans (chickpeas); 2 tablespoons
low-fat dressing

½ whole wheat bagel

1 teaspoon margarine

1 cup skim milk

Afternoon Snack

6 ounces low-sodium tomato juice

Dinner

3 ounces broiled salmon

1 cup steamed cauliflower

1 medium sweet potato, baked with
1 tablespoon brown sugar

1570 calories, 82 g protein, 40 g fiber, 25 g total fat (4 g saturated fat), 1059 mg calcium, 913 mg sodium

DAY TWO

Breakfast

1 cup Fiber One cereal

½ cup blueberries

1 cup skim milk

Morning Snack

1 banana

Lunch

Sandwich: 3 ounces lean turkey, 2 slices
whole wheat bread, 2 romaine lettuce
leaves, 2 thick slices tomato, mustard

1 apple

1 cup skim milk

Afternoon Snack

1 cup low-sodium vegetable juice

Dinner

Peppered Beef and Rice (page 324)

1 whole wheat dinner roll

1 tablespoon margarine

½ cup peas

1 cup skim milk

Evening Snack

1 fig bar

1525 calories, 97 g protein, 35 g fiber, 25 g total fat (6 g saturated fat), 1174 mg calcium, 1521 mg sodium

DAY THREE

Breakfast

1 whole wheat English muffin

2 teaspoons margarine

1 tablespoon jam

1 cup skim milk

Morning Snack

1 apple

Lunch

Salad: 2 cups chopped romaine lettuce,
½ medium tomato, chopped, 1 cup
garbanzo (chickpeas—okay to use

canned), 2 tablespoons low-fat salad
dressing
1 orange
1 cup skim milk

Dinner
Apricot Chicken with Walnuts
(page 290)
1 cup skim milk

1542 calories, 78 g protein, 27 g fiber, 34 g total fat (5 g saturated fat), 1295 mg calcium, 1708 mg sodium

DAY FOUR

Breakfast
Oatmeal: Mix ½ cup oats with 1 cup
skim milk★. Microwave on high
2 minutes; stir and microwave for
2 minutes more. Or combine in a
heavy pot and simmer 7 minutes.
½ cup orange juice

★Or make with water if you prefer and
enjoy a glass of skim milk.

Morning Snack
½ cup low-fat fruited yogurt

Lunch
Peanut butter and jelly sandwich:
2 tablespoons peanut butter,

1 tablespoon jam, 2 slices whole
wheat bread
2 fresh apricots (or 4 canned apricot
halves)
Cucumber slices
½ cup skim milk

Afternoon Snack
1 banana

Dinner
Ruffled Crab Salad (page 276)
½ cup skim milk

Evening Snack
½ cup nonfat frozen yogurt

1556 calories, 74 g protein, 20 g fiber, 33 g total fat (7 g saturated fat), 1141 mg calcium, 2065 mg sodium

DAY FIVE

Breakfast
1 poached egg
2 slices whole wheat toast
1 tablespoon margarine
1 tablespoon jam
1 cup skim milk

Morning Snack
1 banana

Lunch
Sandwich: 3 ounces lean turkey, 1 whole
wheat bagel, 2 pieces romaine lettuce,
mustard

1 cup skim milk
1 carrot

Afternoon Snack
2 oatmeal raisin cookies
½ cup skim milk

Dinner
One-Pot Chili (page 375)
6 saltine crackers
½ cup skim milk

Evening Snack
1 cup melon cubes

1524 calories, 97 g protein, 27 g fiber, 35 g total fat (9.6 g saturated fat), 1142 mg calcium, 1862 mg sodium

Breakfast
Oatmeal: Mix ½ cup oats with 1 cup
    skim milk★. Microwave on high
    2 minutes; stir and microwave for
    2 minutes more. Or combine in a
    heavy pot and simmer 7 minutes.
    (Or see day four.)
2 tablespoons raisins

Morning Snack
3 apricots (or 6 halves, canned in juice)

Lunch
Tuna sandwich: ½ can tuna (packed
    in water), 2 slices whole wheat bread;
    2 pieces romaine lettuce, 2 thick
    slices tomato, 1 tablespoon low-fat
    mayonnaise
1 cup skim milk
1 orange

Afternoon Snack
1 cup low-sodium vegetable juice
    cocktail

Dinner
Creamy Chinese Cabbage and Chicken
    (page 312)
1 cup steamed broccoli pieces
    (frozen is fine)
1 tablespoon margarine
1 cup skim milk

1533 calories, 101 g protein, 25 g fiber, 31 g total fat (7 g saturated fat), 1405 mg calcium, 1498 mg sodium

DAY SEVEN

Breakfast
1 poached egg
1 whole wheat English muffin
1 tablespoon margarine
1 tablespoon jam
1 cup skim milk

Morning Snack
1 apple

Lunch
Kielbasa Corn Chowder (page 377)
1 cup skim milk

Afternoon Snack
4 canned peach halves

Dinner
Hamburger: 3 ounces cooked extra lean
    ground beef patty (3½ ounces raw),
    1 hamburger bun, 1 slice tomato
    (ketchup and mustard as desired)
1 cup cooked carrot slices

1568 calories, 91 g protein, 22 g fiber, 41 g total fat (12 g saturated fat), 1429 mg calcium, 2309 mg sodium★

★Figured with 1 tablespoon ketchup.

References

Arthritis Foundation. *Arthritis Answers: Basic Information About Arthritis.* Informative brochure. 800/283-7800.

Carman, W.J., et al. "Obesity As a Risk Factor for Osteoarthritis of the Hand and Wrist: A Prospective Study." *American Journal of Epidemiology* 139 (1994): 119–29.

Felson, D.T. "Weight and Osteoarthritis." *American Journal of Clinical Nutrition* 63 (Suppl 3) (1996): 430S–32S.

Felson, D.T. "Weight and Osteoarthritis." *Journal of Rheumatology* (Suppl 43) (1995): 7–9.

Lapadula, G., et al. "Early Ultrastructural Changes of Articular Cartilage and Synovial Membrane in Experimental Vitamin A-Induced Osteoarthritis." *Journal of Rheumatology* 22 (1995): 1,913–21.

Matkovic, V. "Nutrition, Genetics and Skeletal Development." *Journal of the American College of Nutrition* 15(6) (1996): 556–69.

McAlindon, T.E. "Relation of Dietary Intake and Serum Levels of Vitamin D to Progression of Osteoarthritis of the Knee Among Participants in the Framingham Study." *Annals of Internal Medicine* 125 (1996): 353–59.

McAlindon, T.E., et al. "Do Antioxidant Micronutrients Protect Against the Development and Progression of Knee Osteoarthritis." *Arthritis and Rheumatism* 39 (1996): 648–56.

Morrow, S. "Arthritis: Finally! Here Are the Answers to Your Questions About Arthritis." *Arthritis Today* (May/June 1995): 18–22

Philbin, E.F., et al. "Cardiovascular Fitness and Health in Patients with End-Stage Osteoarthritis." *Arthritis and Rheumatism* 38(6) (1995): 799–805.

Theiler, R., et al. "Reduced Vitamin A Tolerance in a Hyperlipidaemia Patient with Rapid Destructive and Hyperostotic Osteoarthritis of the Hip." *Clinical Rheumatology* 13 (1994): 293–98.

Rheumatoid Arthritis

Rheumatoid arthritis (RA) is the most severe type of arthritis. Fortunately, though, advances in treatment help more people with this form of arthritis lead normal lives today.

Like other autoimmune disorders, the body's immune system somehow engages in battle with some of the body's own tissues. In this case, the attack is on the lining of the joints, called the synovium. The resulting inflammation triggers the release of chemicals into the synovium. These chemicals cause thickening of the synovium, and also eat away at cartilage, bone, tendons and ligaments. This comprehensive damage gradually causes the joint to lose its shape, and even be destroyed.

The most commonly affected joints are those in the wrists, hands, feet and ankles. But even the elbows, shoulders, hips, knees, neck and jaw can be affected. The same process that causes the joint damage can also attack and set up inflammation in the membranes surrounding internal organs, especially the heart and lungs.

Women are three times more likely to be affected than men by RA, which generally strikes between the ages of twenty and fifty. Seeking an arthritis specialist to design the best treatment program for you can greatly limit the damage and therefore the pain and disability. In addition, there are several things you can do with nutrition to help yourself, including:

➤ Keep up good nutrition, even when pain and disability make it difficult and diminish your appetite.

➤ Achieve and maintain a lean body weight (but not too lean).

➤ Make fish a regular part of your eating plan.

➤ Boost intake of fruits, vegetables and selenium-containing foods.

➤ Eat to prevent osteoporosis.

➤ Eat for a healthy heart.

➤ Eat for a healthy immune system.

➤ If you take steroids, compensate for them nutritionally.

➤ If you take methotrexate, compensate for it nutritionally.

➤ Don't take certain medications on an empty stomach.

➤ If you have Sjögren's Syndrome in addition to rheumatoid arthritis, see chapter 22 for more information on this condition and how to achieve a nutrition advantage.

While not definitively proven, there is some evidence that:

➤ Following a vegetarian diet may help some patients reduce the disease process.

➤ In just a small number of rheumatoid arthritis patients, about 2 to 3 percent, eliminating certain foods may help reduce the number of disease flare-ups.

Keep Up Good Nutrition

Rheumatoid arthritis often makes it difficult to stay well nourished for several reasons. Many patients simply lose their appetite because of pain, fatigue, immobility and even depression. In addition, shopping for groceries and preparing meals can seem next to impossible for people who have difficulty standing and/or who endure severe pain when they use their hands to cook. In addition, the disease process itself uses up calories and even some nutrients at a faster rate than in healthy people, which means even little dietary deficiencies turn into big problems.

Studies have shown that the diets of people with RA are often deficient in several nutrients, including folate, vitamin B_6, magnesium, vitamin D, calcium, zinc, copper, selenium, vitamin E and dietary protein (this is especially problematic when the disease is more active and uses up more calories and nutrients). In addition, many patients lose too much weight, growing too thin: this itself can cause people to become weak and less able to fight infections. The wide range of nutrient deficiencies can compound the problem of not being able to resist infections. It can also mean that people have too little muscle mass, another factor for making someone feel weaker. In turn, growing weaker predisposes people to difficulty in getting around and also to falling. Even if someone doesn't feel weak due to a lack of essential nutrients, their bodies just don't operate as efficiently.

Indeed, keeping up good nutrition is difficult for people who suffer daily pain and movement problems. Here are some suggestions to make it easier:

➤ Make every calorie count. Instead of reaching for a can of soda pop when you're thirsty, choose more nutritious fruit juices and nectars. If you have trouble keeping weight on, opt for more of the nectars: peach, pear and apricot. They're heavier on calories as well as loaded with good nutrition. Try to use more whole wheat breads and bagels than the white version, ditto for brown rice instead of white: you'll load up on lots more nutrients and fiber, without having to eat more.

➤ When your appetite does pick up, fill up with nutrient- and calorie-heavy items. For example, when you finally feel like eating, don't choose a broth-based soup. Instead, try a creamy, milk-based soup with another good source of protein in it. Try the Onion and Cheesy Tomato Soup on page 366.

➤ If cutting up fresh fruits and vegetables is a problem for you, don't hesitate to choose precut versions from the produce section or frozen ones. Both are excellent from a nutritional point of view, and they make light work of most recipes. Most of the one-pot meals in the cookbook section of this book use frozen vegetables.

➤ Make one-pot meals a prominent part of your cooking repertoire. In this cookbook, be sure to follow the cooking instructions as given—they're designed to cut down on the number of pots and utensils you have to use to prepare a dish.

➤ When appetite is poor, don't fill up on liquids between meals—they'll only further dampen your appetite. Try not to drink for one to two hours before eating.

➤ Time your biggest meal for the time of day when you're generally most comfortable. Perhaps mornings are difficult because your hands are particularly stiff, and by evening you're worn out and your appetite is lagging. If you can, plan your biggest meal for lunch, or at least cook the dinner meal early in the day. One-pot meals are a great way to go! You can put most of them together early in the day, refrigerate, and then cook later in the day.

As difficult as it is, keeping up good nutrition is well worth it: it can give you the energy to fight the disease process and also to feel as energetic as you possibly can.

Achieve and Maintain a Lean Body Weight

The most common weight problem for people with rheumatoid arthritis is being too thin. Some people, though, pick up a few too many extra pounds. This can be a real problem for people who take steroids, for example. But shedding this extra baggage may help alleviate some of the swelling, pain and immobility. In one small study (too small, unfortunately, to make any firm conclusions), seven patients with RA who were overweight lost weight. All but one showed improvement in their arthritis symptoms. Refer to chapter 7 for some practical tips on losing weight.

Boost Intake of Fish

Scientifically speaking, the jury is still out regarding the effectiveness of fish oil in improving RA symptoms. I believe, though, that there is enough supporting information to recommend that people with RA make fish, especially fattier fish, a regular part of their eating plan.

Fish have a special type of "body fat" that helps them adapt to the cold water in which they live—the colder the water, they more of this special fat they have. This fat is called omega-3 fat. There are many types of omega-3 fat, but two in particular are high in fish fat and seem important in conferring health benefits to people, including fighting the inflammation of rheumatoid arthritis. These are eicosapentaenoic acid (EPA) and docosahexaenoic acid (DHA). Researchers have good evidence that omega-3s seem to keep the body's immune system from working overtime. Specifically, they put the brakes on the body's production of prostaglandins, leukotrienes and thromboxanes. While the body needs some of these chemicals to function normally, too-high concentrations can lead to inflammation associated with several conditions, including rheumatoid arthritis.

In one study, weekly eating about twenty-six ounces (a little over 1½ pounds) of fish significantly cut down on the number of swollen joints, the duration of morning stiffness, pain and even the amount of medication taken (the patients also received a vitamin/mineral supplement).

While you may be tempted to take fish oil, opt for the real fillet instead. First of all, fish oil capsules are pure fat, introducing lots of extra calories. The fish oil can fill you up on just fat calories, leaving no room for foods containing protein and other nutrients. If you tend to pick up weight easily, the fish oil can put you over the edge. In addition, some people who take fish oil drive up levels of blood fat to unhealthy levels, which can increase their risk of artery-clogging heart disease. Finally, some people who take lots of fish oil capsules end up thinning their blood too much, which can be dangerous.

Eating fish is a great way to boost protein, as well as to get the omega-3s that may help fight RA. It's a great source of lean protein, too, which is a help if you're trying to drop excess weight—even the fattier fishes are still leaner than beef.

Fish highest in omega-3 include salmon, tuna, mackerel, herring and sardines—including the canned versions (canned salmon with bones is loaded with calcium, too). Try to include two fish meals weekly. Even if further studies don't prove omega-3s helpful in reducing RA symptoms, you'll be doing your heart a big favor!

Boost Intake of Fruits, Vegetables and Selenium-Containing Foods

Antioxidant nutrients have been in the news for a number of years. Mostly, you've heard about their possible role in helping to prevent cancer and heart disease. You may also have read that antioxidant nutrients harvested from fruits and vegetables rather than from supplements show the most promise in fighting disease. Now there's some preliminary evidence that antioxidant nutrients may help slow the inflammatory process causing rheumatoid arthritis.

Let's first take a look at why we need antioxidants. Every cell in the body needs oxygen to generate energy. In the process of using that oxygen, by-products, including free radicals, are formed. The body is also exposed to free radicals from other sources, including environmental pollutants such as cigarette smoke. A free radical is an atom that is missing an electron, which makes it unstable. In an attempt to stabilize itself, the free radical steals an electron from another atom. Each robbed atom, in turn, attempts to achieve stability, stealing an electron from a neighboring atom, thus creating a chain reaction.

Inside the body, free radicals steal electrons from cells, creating a chain reaction of cellular damage, or oxidation, as it's properly called. Oxidation is the same process by which metal rusts and butter turns rancid. In the body, oxidation contributes to the process of aging, heart disease, cancer, cataracts, infections and possibly rheumatoid arthritis.

For more than two decades, arthritis experts have known that the products of free radical damage are present in synovial fluid, with the amount increasing in joints inflamed by rheumatoid arthritis. Other research has shown that patients with rheumatoid arthritis have lower blood levels of the antioxidant vitamins A and E and beta-carotene. (While we don't often think of vitamin A itself as an antioxidant, it does have some antioxidant properties, albeit distinct from its precursor, beta-carotene. While beta-carotene is thought to disable free radicals, vitamin A is thought to repair damage after it has already occurred.)

Researchers from Finland, studying 1,419 adult men and women, found that people with the lowest intakes of beta-carotene and selenium—two antioxidant nutrients—were 8.3 times more likely to develop rheumatoid arthritis than people with the highest intake.

New research from Johns Hopkins University suggests that low-antioxidant blood levels may actually increase a person's risk of coming down with rheumatoid arthritis.

Taking advantage of blood samples drawn (and frozen) from an entire community in Washington County, Maryland, in 1974, the Johns Hopkins researchers restudied people who developed rheumatoid arthritis or lupus two to fifteen years later. Researchers then compared blood levels of antioxidant vitamins of people who came down with the disease to those of people who gave blood but who remained healthy. People who later developed either disease had lower blood levels of vitamin E, beta-carotene and vitamin A than their matched controls. Among people who had rheumatoid arthritis, the predisease beta-carotene levels were 29 percent lower, a difference that was statistically significant.

"While the only statistically significant association was for beta-carotene, we suspect that the vitamins A and E associations would have been significant if our numbers had been greater," says George W. Comstock, M.D., Ph.D., professor of epidemiology at Johns Hopkins School of Hygiene and Public Health.

Foods Containing Antioxident Nutrients

Beta-carotene
Pumpkin, including canned pumpkin, sweet potatoes, carrots, turnip greens, papaya, cantaloupe, spinach and apricots.

Vitamin C
Papaya, sweet red pepper, strawberries, oranges, Brussels sprouts, mango, broccoli and spinach.

Vitamin E*
Wheat germ, sunflower seeds, kale, sweet potato, papaya, turnip greens and mango

Selenium
Brazil nuts (one of the best sources), seafoods, meats, eggs, whole grains and legumes (such as lentils, black beans, split peas).

*Also see chart on page 122.

The best way to increase blood levels of antioxidant nutrients is to consume a diet high in fruits and vegetables. Indeed, says Dr. Comstock, "People should interpret this study to mean that they should eat more fruits and vegetables, not consume beta-carotene supplements."

While a minimum of five servings are recommended daily, aiming for closer to nine to ten might be a good idea. Red, orange and yellow produce—cantaloupe, carrots, tomatoes—are particularly high in beta-carotene, and dark green leafy vegetables are rich in other carotenoids. While people often think of fatty foods as the best sources of vitamin E, several fruits and vegetables are good sources, including blueberries, Swiss chard, turnip greens, spinach, prunes and papaya.

While further studies are necessary to prove the association, there are plenty of good reasons for everyone to boost their intake of fruits and vegetables—the antioxidant nutrients may help fight cancer and heart disease, and the other vitamins, phytochemicals and fiber packed into produce are a must for everyone to feel their best. While all fruits and vegetables have some antioxidant nutrients, some are much higher than others (see page 160).

Here are two different combinations that will give you 500 milligrams of vitamin D, 30 to 35 milligrams of beta-carotene and 10 IU vitamin E (just add in lean protein and whole grains for a complete diet):

DAY ONE

Breakfast
    6 ounces orange juice
    3 apricots

Lunch
    Salad: ½ cup raw spinach leaves, ½ grated
    carrot, ½ cup chopped red pepper,
    1 chopped mango

Afternoon Snack
    6 ounces tomato juice

Dinner
    ½ cup cooked turnip greens
    ½ cup cooked cauliflower

Evening Snack
    1 orange

DAY TWO

Breakfast
    1 orange

Lunch
    Salad: 1½ cups spinach leaves, 1 grated
    carrot, 5 cherry tomatoes

Afternoon Snack
    1 papaya

Dinner
    ½ cup cooked kale
    5 Brussels sprouts
    1 slice watermelon

Evening Snack
    6 ounces cranberry juice
    ¼ cup peanuts

A word to the wise: get your antioxidant nutrients from real food and not supplements. A rapidly growing body of evidence points to the real thing rather than supplements as offering the most protection in other diseases—and the same will probably prove true for rheumatoid arthritis. While a supplement may have one of a couple of antioxidant nutrients, real food has a wide complement—including some we haven't yet discovered but that may well be responsible for part of the benefit. Finally, adding in lots of fruits and vegetables automatically means slimming down your eating style, which can help you slim down, too.

Eat to Prevent Osteoporosis

No doubt, preventing osteoporosis is important for everyone, particularly women who are especially hard hit by this bone-thinning disease. But it's even more important for people with rheumatoid arthritis. Joints that are already weakened by the arthritic process are especially hard hit by bone-weakening osteoporosis. Refer to chapter 3 for more information on preventing osteoporosis.

Eat for a Healthy Heart

It is understandable that many people with rheumatoid arthritis don't exercise, or at least don't exercise vigorously. Sometimes, it's just too painful and difficult. In addition, some people, lacking proper exercise advice, are afraid to exercise for fear they will hurt themselves.

But not exercising because of RA places people at risk of another problem: developing artery-clogging heart disease. Try to seek the advice of a physical therapist for ideas on how you can exercise to help keep heart disease risk down, as well as to improve mobility.

In addition, make a commitment to follow a heart-healthy diet. Because of limited mobility, it may be even more important for you than for other people. Eating for a healthy heart becomes of even greater importance if you take steroids, which can increase the chances of developing artery-clogging heart disease. Refer to pages 13–19 for the details on adopting a heart-healthy eating plan.

Eat for a Healthy Immune System

The immune system is the body's way of fighting off foreign invaders, such as bacteria, viruses and allergens. In people with autoimmune diseases, though, the immune system somehow goes awry. While taking large amounts of certain nutrients isn't a way to boost the immune system, making sure you are well nourished in general is an excellent way to make sure the immune system is as healthy as it can be. Some of the nutrients that are especially important to a healthy immune system (as well as foods high in that nutrient) include:

- ➤ PROTEIN: Milk, cheese, meat, legumes (such as lentils).
- ➤ ZINC: Good sources include seafoods, meats, whole grains, legumes.
- ➤ IRON: Red meat (the best source), fish, poultry, legumes, nuts and seeds, whole grains.
- ➤ MANGANESE: Rice cakes, brown rice, whole wheat bread, oatmeal, wheat germ, tea.
- ➤ COPPER: Legumes, meats, seafood, shellfish, whole grains, nuts and seeds.
- ➤ MAGNESIUM: Foods that are a good source of protein are generally a good source of magnesium; in addition, whole grains, legumes, nuts and seeds, green vegetables, avocados, bananas are good sources.

➤ SELENIUM: Protein-rich foods and whole grains are also a good source of selenium. One of the richest sources is Brazil nuts.

➤ VITAMIN B_6: Chicken, fish, pork, eggs, liver, whole grains, legumes, avocados, bananas.

➤ RIBOFLAVIN: Meat, poultry, fish, eggs, and dairy products.

➤ FOLIC ACID: Dark green leafy vegetables, such as romaine lettuce and spinach; orange juice.

➤ VITAMIN B_{12}: This vitamin is found only in foods of animal origin, including meats, seafood, dairy products and eggs.

➤ THIAMIN: Whole grains, legumes, seeds, pork and brewer's yeast.

➤ VITAMIN C: Citrus fruits, tomatoes, broccoli, cantaloupe, berries, cabbage, asparagus, green and red sweet peppers.

➤ VITAMIN A: Sweet potatoes, carrots, evaporated skim milk, apricot nectar, liver, part skim ricotta cheese, cantaloupe, tomatoes, squash, spinach.

➤ VITAMIN E: Asparagus, beet greens, broccoli, cabbage, mustard greens, soybeans, spinach, tomatoes, hams, almonds, peanut butter, sunflower seeds, blueberries, papaya, quinoa, wheat germ, tuna steak, salmon, sole, shrimp.

➤ FATTY ACIDS: The human body needs a certain amount of special fats called essential fatty acids; most people get enough fatty acids if they get just 15 grams of fat per day. On the other hand, diets that have too much fat are thought to suppress the immune system. Therefore, it is suggested that people with autoimmune diseases eat a low-fat diet, or one in which no more than 20 to 30 percent (with the low end more commonly recommended) of calories as fat.

As you can see, the list of nutrients important to the immune system is quite long! That's why it is so important to eat a diet that supplies all essential nutrients, including plenty of whole grains, fruits, vegetables, protein foods and dairy foods.

A word to the wise: just because some is good, it doesn't mean that a little more is better. While you may be tempted to load up on vitamins in an attempt to "boost" your immune system, consider the results of studies with zinc. Researchers know that zinc is an essential ingredient in a healthy immune system. In one study, research subjects were given high doses of zinc (many times the RDA). Instead of boosting the immune system, these high doses actually suppressed it (as measured by the population of lymphocytes in the bloodstream, one type of white blood cell). Similarly, in animal studies, the right amount of manganese helped study animals have a normal immune response, but an overdose suppressed their immune system. The best advice? Stick to the RDA for nutrients, concentrating on getting these nutrients from a healthy diet rather than from supplements.

Nutritionally Compensating for Steroids

As wonderful as they are in alleviating the symptoms of RA and granting people greater mobility, steroid medications (such as cortisone) can have significant side effects. Some of these side effects include interfering with the way the body uses certain nutrients. Please refer to chapter 11 for more information on how to compensate for the effect steroids have on nutritional status.

Nutritionally Compensating for Methotrexate

Sometimes, physicians prescribe methotrexate to relieve rheumatoid arthritis symptoms; in some people it works particularly well. It can break down an important B vitamin, folate. That's why people who take methotrexate are advised to boost intake of folate. Ask your physician how much folate you should be getting; this is often dependent on your dose of methotrexate. In all cases, though, you'll need to make sure you get at least 400 micrograms. Turn to the following foods for folate:

Foods Rich in Folate

Food	Folate (mcg)
1 cup cooked black beans	256
¼ cup wheat germ	99
½ cup cooked spinach	102
8 ounces fresh orange juice	69
2 cups chopped romaine lettuce	152

But be careful not to overdose on folate. Taking too much can mask the symptoms of deficiency of another B vitamin, B_{12}, which can lead to irreversible nerve damage. Remember, just because some is good, it doesn't mean that a lot more is better!

Do Not Medicate on an Empty Stomach

Nonsteroidal anti-inflammatory medications are often used to treat rheumatoid arthritis. Be careful, though, to always take these medications with food. They can be very abrasive to the lining of the stomach, causing nausea, stomach upset and even ulcer. Refer to the chapter on medications for more information.

Follow a Vegetarian Diet

There are more than 400 kinds of bacteria that live in the intestine and are necessary for a healthy intestinal tract. Because these bacteria are truly necessary to life, we call them healthy or good bacteria. Without them, we're likely to develop diarrhea and other maladies. And now, there is evidence that the type and amounts of bacteria in the intestinal tract influence the immune system throughout the entire body. There is mounting research indicating that a vegetarian diet may change the type of bacteria living in the intestinal tract, which in turn may help turn down the immunological response responsible for RA. Note, however, that this is one of the more uncertain dietary connections.

Norwegian researchers studied fifty-three people with RA who, before the study, were omnivorous—or included meat in their diet. Some were assigned to the vegetarian group, and some to the control group, or a group that would continue eating meat for the duration of the study. During a "cleansing period," the vegetarian group first fasted for seven to ten days, and then followed a strict vegan diet for three months. A vegan diet includes only fruits, vegetables, grains and legumes, and no dairy foods or eggs. After three months on the vegan diet, they followed a lactovegetarian diet, adding dairy foods to their eating plan, for the remaining nine months of the study.

At the end of the year study period, the people in the vegetarian group fared considerably better. They showed improvement in several laboratory measures of disease activity— rheumatoid factor and complement components C3 and C4. In addition, they reported less pain and inflammatory activity.

I'm the first to admit that following a vegetarian diet is a real commitment, which means it is just not practical for some people. But if it means a difference between being in pain and having reduced mobility or not being in pain and able to move better, perhaps the payoff is worth it. There are several vegetarian recipes in this cookbook; refer to chapter 23. *Caution:* the vegan diets mentioned above are difficult to make nutritionally complete. If you elect to try this—which I don't recommend—do it only under the care of a registered dietitian.

Certainly, though, everyone can augment the intake of healthy gut bacteria by boosting their intake of complex carbohydrates. To get complex carbohydrates, eat plant foods as close to the way they come from nature as possible. For example:

➤ Use whole wheat products over white flour products, including whole wheat bread and bagels (better yet, seven- or ten-grain bread over their white counterparts).

➤ Opt for brown rice instead of white rice.

➤ Peel and enjoy a whole orange at breakfast instead of just the orange juice; similarly, munch an apple instead of drinking apple juice.

➤ Nibble on a whole carrot instead of "juicing" carrots and drinking the juice.

➤ Include legumes (lentils, soybeans, tofu, split peas, garbanzo beans) in your diet at least a couple of times per week, preferably daily. Try the easy recipes on pages 370–74.

Eliminate Certain Foods

Rarely, a certain food seems to cause RA symptoms to flare up. While there are only limited data, some research indicates that in about 2 to 3 percent of RA patients, symptoms become worse after eating a specific food. The most commonly reported foods are milk, shrimp, wheat products and certain meats.

Remember, though, just a very small proportion of RA patients are affected. Unnecessarily restricting foods can actually do more harm than good. As you read above, it is common for RA patients to come up short on several nutrients—and restricting the diet can only make this worse. Therefore, always check with your doctor before restricting your diet. He or she will help you figure out how to determine if a specific dietary item does indeed seem to make your disease worse. If you do restrict your diet, it's wise to meet with a registered dietitian to make sure that you can make up for the nutrients in the foods you eliminate by eating other foods or by turning to a supplement. If, for example, you eliminate milk products, you have to find alternative ways of getting enough calcium and vitamin D.

Putting It All Together

Don't be overwhelmed by all this dietary advice. The most important thing to know is how to convert it to an eating plan that will give you the edge on feeling better.

There are two different sets of week-long menus. The first, for the person who does not wish to adopt a vegetarian lifestyle, accommodates all the dietary modifications recommended in this chapter. The second is the vegetarian version. Both provide 1,800 calories per day.

Menus

RHEUMATOID ARTHRITIS

Part 1: Nonvegetarian

DAY ONE

Breakfast
   1 cup Fiber One cereal
   1 cup skim milk
   1 cup fresh or frozen raspberries

Morning Snack
   1 banana

Lunch
   Lentil Vegetable Soup (page 371)
   1 cup skim milk
   3 fresh apricots (or 6 halves, canned in
      juice)

Afternoon Snack
   1 apple

Dinner
   3 ounces roasted chicken
   1 large baked potato
   1 cup frozen broccoli, steamed
   1 tablespoon margarine
   1 cup skim milk

Evening Snack
   1 cup low-fat frozen yogurt or fruited
      low-fat yogurt

1784 calories, 96 g protein, 45 g fiber, 34 g total fat (8 g saturated fat), 1693 mg calcium, 1605 mg sodium

DAY TWO

Breakfast

    Oatmeal: Mix ½ cup oats with 1 cup skim milk. Microwave on high 2 minutes; stir and microwave for 2 minutes more. Or combine in a heavy pot and simmer 7 minutes.

    3 tablespoons raisins

Morning Snack

    1 peach (or 2 canned peach halves)

Lunch

    Peanut butter and jelly sandwich:

        2 tablespoons peanut butter, 1 tablespoon jam, 2 slices whole wheat bread

    10 baby carrots

    1 cup skim milk

Afternoon Snack

    1 cup low-fat fruited yogurt

Dinner

    Italian Chicken and Rice (page 302)

    ½ cup skim milk

Evening Snack

    3 fig bars

    ½ cup skim milk

1805 calories, 98 g protein, 27 g fiber, 35 g total fat (10 g saturated fat), 1586 mg calcium, 1651 mg sodium

DAY THREE

Breakfast

    1 poached egg

    1 whole wheat English muffin

    1 tablespoon margarine

    1 tablespoon jam

    1 cup skim milk

Morning Snack

    1 banana

Lunch

    Grilled cheese sandwich: 3 ounces low-fat cheese, 2 slices whole wheat bread, 2 teaspoons margarine

    1 cup frozen peas, steamed in microwave

    1 peach

    1 cup skim milk

Afternoon Snack

    5 cherry tomatoes

Dinner

    Penne Pasta with Tuna in a Garlic Cream Sauce (page 285)

    ½ cup skim milk

Evening Snack

    1 oatmeal raisin cookie

    ½ cup skim milk

1783 calories, 112 g protein, 25 g fiber, 47 g total fat (13 g saturated fat), 1983 mg calcium, 3431 mg sodium

DAY FOUR

Breakfast

    1 whole wheat bagel

    1 tablespoon margarine

    1 tablespoon jam

    1 cup skim milk

Morning Snack

    1 apple

Lunch

    Barley and Bacon Soup (page 370)

    1 skim milk

    1 peach

Afternoon Snack

    1 apple

Dinner
   4 ounces grilled salmon
   1 medium sweet potato,
      baked
   1 tablespoon margarine

1 cup frozen cauliflower (steamed in
   microwave)
1 cup skim milk

Evening Snack
   ½ cup ice cream

1754 calories, 98 g protein, 34 g fiber, 48 g total fat (16 g saturated fat), 1359 mg calcium, 1666 mg sodium

DAY FIVE

Breakfast
   1 cup Fiber One cereal
   1 cup skim milk
   1 cup fresh or frozen raspberries

Morning Snack
   1 apple

Lunch
   Salad: 2 cups chopped romaine lettuce,
      ½ medium tomato, 1 cup cooked gar-
      banzo beans (chickpeas), 2 tablespoons
      low-fat salad dressing

6 whole wheat crackers
1 cup skim milk
3 apricots (or 6 canned apricot halves)

Afternoon Snack
   1 cup low-fat fruited yogurt

Dinner
   Pot Roast (page 339)
   1 cup skim milk

Evening Snack
   2 fig bars

1804 calories, 94 g protein, 42 g fiber, 29 g total fat (8 g saturated fat), 1596 mg calcium, 1628 mg sodium

DAY SIX

Breakfast
   1 poached egg
   2 slices whole wheat toast
   1 tablespoon margarine
   1 cup skim milk

Morning Snack
   1 peach

Lunch
   3-Bean Pasta Salad (page 272)
   1 cup skim milk

Afternoon Snack
   2 chocolate chip cookies

Dinner
   4 ounces broiled sole
   1 medium sweet potato, baked
   1 tablespoon margarine
   1 cup frozen peas, steamed in microwave
   1 cup skim milk

Evening Snack
   1 cup low-fat fruited yogurt

1904 calories, 104 g protein, 33 g fiber, 53 g total fat (12 g saturated fat), 1525 mg calcium, 1637 mg sodium

DAY SEVEN

Breakfast
   Oatmeal: Mix ½ cup oats with 1 cup
      skim milk. Microwave on high 2 min-
      utes; stir and microwave for 2 minutes
      more. Or combine in a heavy pot and
      simmer 7 minutes.
   2 tablespoons raisins

Morning Snack
   1 apple

Lunch
   Peanut butter and jelly sandwich:
      2 tablespoons peanut butter, 1 table-
      spoon jam, 2 slices whole wheat bread

1 cup skim milk
3 apricots (or 6 canned halves)
6 baby carrots

Afternoon Snack
1 cup low-sodium vegetable juice cocktail

Dinner
Jamaican Chicken (page 294)
1 cup skim milk

Evening Snack
1 cup ice cream

1786 calories, 93 g protein, 26 g fiber, 52 g total fat (18 g saturated fat), 1315 mg calcium, 1637 mg sodium

Part 2: Vegetarian

DAY ONE

Breakfast
1 cup Fiber One cereal
1 cup skim milk
1 cup fresh or frozen raspberries

Morning Snack
1 banana

Lunch
Lentil Vegetable Soup (page 371)
1 cup skim milk
3 fresh apricots (or 6 halves, canned in juice)

Afternoon Snack
1 apple

Dinner
1 large baked potato, with 3 ounces 50% reduced fat cheese melted on top
1 cup frozen broccoli, steamed
1 tablespoon margarine
1 cup skim milk

Evening Snack
1 cup low-fat frozen yogurt or fruited low-fat yogurt

1861 calories, 95 g protein, 45 g fiber, 34 g total fat (8 g saturated fat), 1693 mg calcium, 1605 mg sodium

DAY TWO

Breakfast
Oatmeal: Mix ½ cup oats with 1 cup skim milk. Microwave on high 2 minutes; stir and microwave for 2 minutes more. Or combine in a heavy pot and simmer 7 minutes.
3 tablespoons raisins

Morning Snack
1 peach (or 2 canned peach halves)

Lunch
Peanut butter and jelly sandwich:
2 tablespoons peanut butter, 1 tablespoon jam, 2 slices whole wheat bread

10 baby carrots
1 cup skim milk

Afternoon Snack
1 cup low-fat fruited yogurt

Dinner
Egg Salad Sandwich (page 381)
Cream of Broccoli Soup (page 368)
1 cup skim milk

Evening Snack
3 fig bars
½ cup skim milk

1819 calories, 96 g protein, 24 g fiber, 52 g total fat (17 g saturated fat), 1737 mg calcium, 3094 mg sodium

DAY THREE

Breakfast
1 poached egg
1 whole wheat English muffin
1 tablespoon margarine
1 tablespoon jam
1 cup skim milk

Morning Snack
1 banana

Lunch
Grilled cheese sandwich: 3 ounces low-fat cheese, 2 slices whole wheat bread, 2 teaspoons margarine

1 cup frozen peas, steamed in microwave
1 peach
1 cup skim milk

Afternoon Snack
5 cherry tomatoes

Dinner
Basil Tomato Pasta Salad—Vegetarian Style (page 268)
1 cup skim milk

Evening Snack
1 oatmeal raisin cookie
½ cup skim milk

1850 calories, 96 g protein, 33 g fiber, 58 g total fat (13 g saturated), 1950 mg calcium, 3081 mg sodium

DAY FOUR

Breakfast
1 whole wheat bagel
1 tablespoon margarine
1 tablespoon jam
1 cup skim milk

Morning Snack
1 apple

Lunch
Tofu Chow Mein (page 392)
1 cup skim milk
1 peach

Afternoon Snack
1 apple

Dinner
4 ounces grilled salmon
1 medium sweet potato, baked
1 tablespoon margarine
1 cup frozen cauliflower (steamed in microwave)
1 cup skim milk

Evening Snack
½ cup ice cream

1780 calories, 88 g protein, 26 g fiber, 44 g total fat (12 g saturated fat), 1159 mg calcium, 2440 mg sodium

DAY FIVE

Breakfast
1 cup Fiber One cereal
1 cup skim milk
1 cup fresh or frozen raspberries

Morning Snack
1 apple

Lunch
Salad: 2 cups chopped romaine lettuce, ½ medium tomato, 1 cup cooked garbanzo beans (chickpeas), 2 tablespoons low-fat salad dressing

6 whole wheat crackers
1 cup skim milk
3 apricots (or 6 canned apricot halves)

Afternoon Snack
1 cup low-fat fruited yogurt

Dinner
Bean Enchiladas (page 388)
1 cup skim milk

Evening Snack
2 fig bars

1840 calories, 81 g protein, 47 g fiber, 31 g total fat (11 g saturated fat), 1822 mg calcium, 2212 mg sodium

Breakfast
1 poached egg
2 slices whole wheat toast
1 tablespoon margarine
1 cup skim milk

Morning Snack
1 peach

Lunch
3-Bean Pasta Salad (page 272)
1 cup skim milk

Afternoon Snack
2 chocolate chip cookies

Dinner
4 ounces broiled sole
1 medium sweet potato, baked
1 tablespoon margarine
1 cup frozen peas, steamed in microwave
1 cup skim milk

Evening Snack
1 cup low-fat fruited yogurt

1904 calories, 104 g protein, 33 g fiber, 53 g total fat (12 g saturated fat), 1525 mg calcium, 1637 mg sodium

DAY SEVEN

Breakfast
Oatmeal: Mix ½ cup oats with 1 cup skim
milk. Microwave on high 2 minutes;
stir and microwave for 2 minutes
more. Or combine in a heavy pot and
simmer 7 minutes.
2 tablespoons raisins

Morning Snack
1 apple
1 cup low-sodium vegetable juice cocktail

Lunch
Peanut butter and jelly sandwich:
2 tablespoons peanut butter,

1 tablespoon jam, 2 slices whole
wheat bread
1 cup skim milk
3 apricots (or 6 canned halves)
6 baby carrots

Afternoon Snack
1 cup low-fat fruited yogurt

Dinner
Lentil Vegetable Soup (leftover from
day two)
1 cup skim milk

Evening Snack
1 cup ice cream

1748 calories, 75 g protein, 28 g fiber, 46 g total fat (15 g saturated fat), 1597 mg calcium, 1592 mg sodium

References

Fortin, P.R., et al. "Validation of a Meta-Analysis: The Effects of Fish Oil in Rheumatoid Arthritis." *Journal of Clinical Epidemiology* 48 (1995): 1379–90.

Geusens, P., et al. "Long-term Effect of Omega-3 Fatty Acid Supplementation in Active Rheumatoid Arthritis: A 12-Month, Double-Blind, Controlled Study." *Arthritis and Rheumatology* 37(6) (1994): 824–29.

Hansen, G.V.O., et al. "Nutritional Status of Danish Rheumatoid Arthritis Patients and Effects of a Diet Adjusted in Energy Intake, Fish-Meal, and Antioxidants." *Scandinavian Journal of Rheumatology* 25 (1996): 325–30.

Heliovaara, M., et al. "Serum Antioxidants and Risk of Rheumatoid Arthritis." *Annals of Rheumatic Disease* 53 (1994): 51–53.

Hernandez-Beriain, J.A., et al. "Undernutrition in Rheumatoid Arthritis Patients with Disability." *Scandinavian Journal of Rheumatology* 25 (1996): 383–87.

Kjeldsen-Kragh, J. "Vegetarian Diet for Patients with Rheumatoid Arthritis: Can the Clinical Effects Be Explained by the Psychological Characteristics of the Patients." *British Journal of Rheumatology* 33 (1994): 569–75.

Kjeldsen-Kragh, J., et al. "Controlled Trial of Fasting and One-Year Vegetarian Diet in Rheumatoid Arthritis." *The Lancet* 338 (1991): 899–902.

———. "Changes in Laboratory Variables in Rheumatoid Arthritis Patients During a Trial of Fasting and One-Year Vegetarian Diet." *Scandinavian Journal of Rheumatology* 24 (1995): 85–93.

———. "Decrease in Anti-Proteus Mirabilis But Not Anti-Escherichia Coli Antibody Levels in Rheumatoid Arthritis Patients Treated with Fasting and a One Year Vegetarian Diet." *Annals of Rheumatic Disease* 54 (1995): 221–24.

Leventhal, L.J., et al. "Treatment of Rheumatoid Arthritis with Blackcurrant Seed Oil." *British Journal of Rheumatology* 33 (1994): 847–53.

Peltonen, R., et al. "Changes of Faecal Flora in Rheumatoid Arthritis During Fasting and One-Year Vegetarian Diet." *British Journal of Rheumatology* 33 (1994): 638–34.

Purdy, K.S., et al. "You Are What You Eat: Healthy Food Choices, Nutrition, and the Child with Juvenile Rheumatoid Arthritis." *Pediatric Nursing* 22(5) (1996): 391–98.

Ryan, S. "Nutrition and the Rheumatoid Patient." *British Journal of Nursing* 4(3) (1995): 132–36.

Roubenoff, R., et al. "Abnormal Vitamin B_6 Status in Rheumatoid Cachexia: Association with Spontaneous Tumor Necrosis Factor Alpha Production and Markers of Inflammation." *Arthritis & Rheumatism* 38 (1995): 105–09.

Slotkoff, A.T., and P. Katz. "Approach to the Patient with Rheumatoid Arthritis." *Advances in Internal Medicine* 39 (1994): 197–240.

Strano, C.G., et al. "Nutritional Status in Active Juvenile Chronic Arthritis Not Treated with Steroids." *Acta Paediatrica* 84 (1995): 1010–13.

Reactive Arthritis and Reiter's Syndrome

Safe food handling is important for everyone—foodborne illness (often called food poisoning) cannot only make you miserable with diarrhea and nausea, but it can also be dangerous for people with chronic illness who are often a little weaker than others.

Now, there's evidence that certain types of bacteria that cause foodborne illness may bring on a type of arthritis called reactive arthritis. Researchers know that the bacteria Salmonella and Campylobacter, as well as some other less-common ones, can cause this chronic form of arthritis in about 2 percent of people who come down with the foodborne illness they cause.

The symptoms of this arthritis begin about one week to one month after eating the contaminated food. The most common sites of the painful joint inflammation are the knees and ankles, but the sacroiliac joint can also be affected (causing lower back pain). Fortunately, the arthritic symptoms generally go away after about six months. Some people, though, develop Reiter's syndrome—in addition to the arthritis, they also suffer inflammation of the mucous membrane covering the eyeball (conjunctivitis) and also inflammation of the urethra, resulting in painful urination.

To prevent all food contamination, even the type that doesn't result in the obvious symptoms of vomiting, nausea and/or diarrhea:

➤ Cook all food thoroughly; while we've always known this to be critical for poultry and pork, now we know that it's necessary for ground beef, too.

➤ Store raw foods separate from cooked foods.

➤ Store raw fruits and vegetables separate from uncooked meat (so that meat juices don't contaminate the produce).

➤ Refrigerate leftovers promptly (within two hours of cooking; preferably sooner), doing so in shallow containers so that they chill quickly—it's an old wives' tale, and a dangerous one at that, that you have to let food come to room temperature before putting it in the refrigerator.

➤ Wash all produce well before using—this includes washing melons before cutting into them, as bacteria on their surfaces can be carried into the fleshy interior on the cutting knife.

➤ Thaw meat in the refrigerator rather than at room temperature.

Lupus

17

Lupus (Latin for "wolf") erythematosus (Greek for "reddish") was the name nineteenth-century physicians gave to a mysterious disease that often caused a rash on the face that resembled the bite of a wolf. Systemic lupus erythematosus (SLE), commonly shortened to lupus, is an autoimmune disease in which the immune system turns inward, harming the body's own tissues. Another form of the disease that affects only the skin is called cutaneous or discoid lupus.

Lupus is a case of the body not recognizing itself. For some as yet unknown reason, the immune system goes awry and begins manufacturing substances called antibodies against its own tissues. These autoantibodies, as they are called, cause a complex sequence of immune responses. They combine with other immune substances to form immune complexes, which become lodged in selective tissues, frequently connective tissue, causing painful and sometimes dangerous inflammation.

Connective tissue is found throughout the body. It binds cells and tissues together; some examples are tissues around joints and tissue lining the heart and lungs. The immune complexes can also deposit in the kidneys, interfering with kidney function, or in the tissues of the brain, causing headaches and/or seizures. Tissues are also damaged as the body attempts to destroy the immune complexes, a process that releases harmful chemicals.

Lupus is as voracious as it is mysterious. It can ravage not just one, but a host of sites within the body, producing a multitude of symptoms. As a result of this inflammatory process, lupus can cause a number of seemingly unrelated symptoms: fatigue, fever (not related to infection), joint pain (similar to arthritis), skin rash, chest pain (from inflammation around the heart and lungs) and headaches. Many types of blood abnormalities, including anemia, low white count, which in turn impairs the body's ability to fight infections, and low platelet count, which impairs the blood's clotting ability, can also occur.

In some cases doctors know what triggers increased disease activity, called flares. In some lupus patients, for example, infections, ultraviolet light (including sunlight), various medications and pregnancy can cause flares. In other cases, however, the disease flares for no readily apparent reason.

More common than cystic fibrosis, multiple sclerosis, muscular dystrophy, leukemia or cerebral palsy, lupus affects at least 500,000 Americans, and possibly as many as 1.4 million. It is nine times more common among women than among men and three times as common among black women as it is among white women. Women are thought to be affected more frequently because of their distinctive combination of sex hormones; this is also thought to explain why the disease commonly flares during pregnancy, after childbirth and even around the time of a woman's monthly period.

While it can be diagnosed at any age, it strikes most commonly during the childbearing years. Most people with lupus have at least one of six genes thought to play a role in causing lupus; some have all six. Even though genetics are involved in lupus, there is only about a 4 percent chance of passing on the disease to offspring.

The Nutrition Advantage

Several symptoms can interfere with eating a nutritious diet, including sores forming in the mouth, nausea, and lack of appetite. Sometimes, just being in pain takes away appetite or even the ability to prepare nutritious food.

There are several nutrition strategies lupus patients can use to feel the best they can and to prevent other health troubles that are associated with the disease and/or the medications used to treat it.

The primary nutrition concerns of people with lupus include:

- Designing and consuming a diet lower in fat, both to prevent flares and to prevent atherosclerosis (artery-clogging heart disease).

- Eating more fruits and vegetables.

- For lupus patients who take glucocorticosteroid medications, preventing osteoporosis and excessive weight gain and getting enough protein and potassium.

- Maintaining a healthy body weight: Because people who have lupus often have prolonged periods of inactivity, weight gain can be a problem. For others (or even for the same people at different times in their illness), eating enough and keeping weight on can be a problem.

- For lupus patients who take methotrexate, boosting dietary intake of the nutrient folate.

- Dispelling myths about foods that cause lupus to flare, and figuring out if any of these foods cause you to flare.

- Understanding the potential benefits and possible dangers of various supplements often touted for lupus, including flaxseed and fish oil, including fish oil capsules.

- Modifying the diet significantly if disease activity in the kidneys compromises kidney function. This topic will not be covered in here because diets for kidney disease are highly specialized according to each patient's disease state; ask your physician to refer you to a renal dietitian, or a dietitian specializing in diets for patients with kidney disease.

- Eating for a healthy immune system.

Let's take a look at each of these.

Design and Consume a Low-Fat Diet

There are two critical reasons why lupus patients should consume a low-fat diet. First, preliminary research suggests that a diet too high in fat may cause lupus to flare. Second, lupus patients have to have a heightened concern for preventing atherosclerosis. Some research suggests that steroid medications contribute to the artery-clogging process, and other research suggests that lupus itself may cause earlier onset heart disease.

There's at least some evidence that everyone's good dietary advice—eating a low-fat diet and maintaining a trim build—may be especially important for lupus patients. While this dual strategy decreases heart disease and cancer risk in everyone, it may help reduce disease activity in lupus patients.

In laboratory animals fed too much fat, especially unsaturated fat, and allowed to grow too heavy, the immune system doesn't work properly. This is especially relevant to lupus, as the disease occurs because the immune system somehow goes awry.

And in the strain of mice bred to develop lupus, it seems especially important to reduce the amount of polyunsaturated fat. When researchers did, disease activity was lessened and lupus symptoms reduced.

In another study of 156 Japanese women, researchers found that frequent meat consumption (especially beef and pork) increased the risk of developing lupus by nearly 3½ times. While this is only one study, bear in mind that having too much meat isn't healthy for anyone, as it's such a heavy contributor to artery-clogging saturated fat that, as we said above, may hamper normal immune system functioning, as well as contributing to heart disease risk.

Here's how to reduce overall dietary fat:

➤ Reduce meat to one 2- to 3-ounce portion per day and bake, broil or grill it.

➤ Substitute vegetarian meals (such as grains and legumes) for at least two meat meals weekly.

➤ Substitute at least one fish meal each week, preferably featuring a fish that is high in omega-3 fatty acids (such as salmon, mackerel or tuna).

➤ Cut or eliminate butter, margarine, sour cream and cream cheese, enjoying vegetables with herbs and lemon juice; breads and muffins as they are; baked potatoes with fat-free sour cream.

➤ Substitute pretzels and fresh fruit for such high-fat snacks as chips and tortilla chips; nonfat frozen yogurt and sorbets for ice creams and regular frozen yogurts.

➤ Fill up on fruits, vegetables and whole grains.

The best way to cut polyunsaturated fats in the diet is to:

➤ Use olive or canola oils (both are high in monounsaturated fats) in cooking and baking instead of corn, safflower, sunflower or peanut oils.

➤ Use fewer frozen and convenience foods, made largely with high-polyunsaturated fat soy and cottonseed oils.

Fortunately, consuming a diet with lots of fruits, vegetables and grains with the appropriate sprinkling of lean meat, poultry and fish translates into consuming a diet that is low in polyunsaturated fats, low in saturated fats and low in total fat.

Eat More Fruits and Vegetables

Preliminary evidence suggests that people with low blood levels of antioxidant nutrients—vitamin E, beta-carotene and vitamin A—are more likely to get lupus.

Taking advantage of blood samples drawn (and frozen) from an entire community in Washington County, Maryland, in 1974, researchers from Johns Hopkins University traced people who later developed lupus or rheumatoid arthritis. They compared blood levels of antioxidant vitamins of people who gave blood but remained healthy. People who later developed either diseases had lower blood levels of vitamin E, beta-carotene and vitamin A (although the only statistically significant difference was for beta-carotene in rheumatoid arthritis. Researchers speculate that too few people with lupus were studied to achieve statistical significance).

Further studies are needed to verify the association. In the meantime, there's no harm in boosting fruit and vegetable intake, the safest and best way to increase the amount of antioxidant nutrients in the bloodstream. Indeed says chief researcher of the study, George W. Comstock, M.D., Ph.D., professor of epidemiology at Johns Hopkins School of Hygiene and Public Health, "people should interpret this study to mean they should eat more fruits and vegetables, not consume supplements."

Glucocorticosteroid Medications: Nutritional Concerns

Prednisone and other glucocorticosteroid medications are almost magical for people with lupus, relieving the pain, alleviating the crippling fatigue and quieting potentially dangerous disease activity. But this powerful medication can have devastating side effects. Please turn to chapter 11 to find out more about the nutritional concerns of people who take glucocorticosteroid medications.

Maintain a Healthy Body Weight

It's frustrating, indeed: sometimes, you can barely eat enough to keep weight on and to fight your disease. Whether increased disease activity erases your appetite, medications make you nauseous and/or you have sores in your mouth from lupus, eating enough can be a problem. On the other hand, you may feel like sewing your mouth shut to keep yourself from cleaning out the refrigerator. Generally, this happens when you're on steroid medications like prednisone for any length of time. And then there are times when your disease keeps you from being active and you have to cut down on calories while still trying to harvest plenty of protein and nutrients from food to fight disease and replenish your energy stores. This combination of challenges means that maintaining an "ideal" body weight is often difficult: many lupus patients are either too thin or too heavy.

Refer to chapter 7 for what to do if you have trouble eating enough to keep weight on. You can battle excess pounds and reduce calorie intake, and yet harvest loads of nutrients and protein.

Dispel Myths

Many lupus patients are convinced that certain foods cause their disease to be more active. Currently, there is no proof that any particular food really does cause the disease to flare. This doesn't mean that certain foods don't cause flares, just that there hasn't been a study to confirm the association.

One food that lupus patients are told can cause a flare is alfalfa sprouts (and alfalfa supplements); some people believe that alfalfa brings on the disease in people not previously diagnosed. Interestingly, though, folklore has it that alfalfa is good for arthritis. What's the truth?

Physician-nutrition expert Victor Herbert, M.D., of the Nutrition Center at Mount Sinai and Bronx Veterans' Affairs Medical Centers, cuts through the confusion: "For every case in which it is recognized that alfalfa in one form or another induced an autoimmune disease, there are probably a thousand cases in which a patient with autoimmune disease had been taking alfalfa, in one form or another, and was never recognized for side effects." In addition, there are also countless cases in which alfalfa may have helped the disease (although there is no proof that it is effective).

The best advice for now? If you're a lupus patient, it's important to keep a diary of what happened around the time your disease flared up. Whether it's alfalfa or some other food, if you find that that food is associated with a time of greater disease activity, avoid it in the future.

A word of caution: it's never wise, and almost never necessary, to put yourself on a highly restrictive diet in which whole food groups are eliminated. While it's okay to cut out one or two foods, do consult your physician before embarking on a restrictive diet. Remember, while eating certain foods seems to precipitate a flare, it may just be that you ate the food at a time when you would have flared anyway.

Benefits and Dangers of Supplements

You may have heard about the study involving nine patients with lupus-caused kidney disease who were given flaxseed and who showed some improvement. Here are the details.

Flaxseed is the seed of the linen plant; you might know it as linseed. Although not commonly eaten in the United States, people in many other parts of the world start their day with a flaxseed-based breakfast cereal.

Encouraged by preliminary testing of flaxseed in mice that had lupus-caused kidney troubles, researchers at the University of Western Ontario went one step further. They gave varying doses of flaxseed to nine patients with lupus nephritis, a common form of lupus-induced kidney disease. Several measurements of kidney function improved with a dose of thirty grams of flaxseed per day (about one-quarter cup of raw flaxseed), which they stirred into juice or breakfast cereal. (One group of patients was given forty-five grams, but they showed no further improvement, and many suffered unpleasant side effects, such as bloating and gas.)

While this study is too small to draw any firm conclusions, it is encouraging. But, like any research, it must be replicated by other researchers to prove that it really is a help. In the meantime, lupus patients with kidney disease should not stop the medication and diet schedule recommended by their physicians. Because flaxseed is such a great food for many reasons other than its ability to help lupus patients, it might be a good idea to work some into the diet. For one, it's high in fiber, and it is also loaded with phytochemicals. Phytochemicals are naturally occurring substances in plants that are thought to be an aid in fighting cancer and heart disease.

As with any product you can use as a potential therapy, always ask your physician first. If you do decide to work some flaxseed into your eating plan, do so gradually. Because it's so high in fiber, adding large amounts quickly (such as the one-quarter cup consumed by the lupus kidney patients) can cause unpleasant gastrointestinal side effects. Start with no more than one tablespoon per day, adding another tablespoon every four to five days if you tolerate it. You can stir flaxseed into juice, sprinkle it over salad, bake it into bread and muffins (see the recipes on pages 260–61), sprinkle it over your cold breakfast cereal or cook it with hot cereal (see the recipe on page 248). You can purchase flaxseed in some health food stores or purchase it from mail-order baker's catalogs. Always buy milled or cracked flaxseed. The body cannot break down the whole seed, so it (and its goodness) just passes through the body.

One more word to the wise: avoid the flaxseed oil, which is becoming a popular product in many health food stores. The most important reason to avoid it is that it is pure fat, and therefore very high in calories. Many lupus patients, because of steroid medications and limited activity, have a tough time controlling weight, and taking flaxseed oil can compound this problem. In addition, it is thought that the majority of the phytochemicals are found in portions of the flaxseed other than the oil. This is an important reason to try to work flaxseed into the diet, to benefit from the portion of flaxseed thought responsible for some of the improvement in lupus kidney patients.

Many lupus research teams have studied the effect of fish oil supplements (either as capsules or as the liquid itself) on lupus. At best, results have been mixed. That means that while some studies found fish oil supplements helpful in alleviating lupus-related symptoms, many others found no benefit.

Researchers probed fish oil's ability to help lupus patients because it is high in omega-3 fatty acids, a type of fat that is fairly unique to fish (although there is also some in flaxseed and a select few other plant foods). Omega-3 fatty acids have anti-inflammatory properties, which could theoretically be a help in reducing lupus symptoms. The best advice for now? Steer clear of the fish oil supplements and reel in the whole fillet. Like flaxseed oil, fish oil is very high in calories. It, too, can quickly lead to weight gain. In addition, because fish oil may thin the blood in some people, it may increase the risk of abnormal bleeding.

Including more fish in the diet is always a great idea, as fish is an excellent source of lean, low-calorie protein, which is a welcome addition to anyone's eating plan. And, if the omega-3 fatty acids are eventually proven to be helpful, you will have been eating them for years. In any case, heart disease researchers are fairly convinced that omega-3 fatty acids may help cut down on the process by which arteries become clogged (atherosclerosis). Putting a halt to this process may be especially important in lupus patients, as research reveals that lupus patients are at high risk of developing atherosclerosis earlier in life than people without lupus.

Types of fish that are particularly high in omega-3 fatty acids are salmon, mackerel and tuna with canned tuna one of the most inexpensive sources of omega-3s.

Eat for a Healthy Immune System

The immune system is the body's way of fighting off foreign invaders, such as bacteria, viruses and allergens. In people with autoimmune diseases, though, the immune system somehow goes awry. While taking large amounts of certain nutrients isn't a way to boost the immune system, making sure you are well nourished in general is an excellent way to make sure the immune system is as healthy as it can be. Some of the nutrients that are especially important to a healthy immune system (as well as foods high in that nutrient) include:

➜ PROTEIN: Milk, cheese, meat, legumes (such as lentils).

➜ ZINC: Good sources include seafoods, meats, whole grains, legumes.

➜ IRON: Red meat (the best source), fish, poultry, legumes, nuts and seeds, whole grains.

➜ MANGANESE: Rice cakes, brown rice, whole wheat bread, oatmeal wheat germ, tea.

➜ COPPER: Legumes, meats, seafood, shellfish, whole grains, nuts and seeds.

➜ MAGNESIUM: Foods that are a good source of protein are generally a good source of magnesium; in addition, whole grains, legumes, nuts and seeds, green vegetables, avocados, bananas are good sources.

➜ SELENIUM: Protein-rich foods are also a good source of selenium, as are whole grains. One of the richest sources is Brazil nuts.

➜ VITAMIN B_6: Chicken, fish, pork, eggs, liver, whole grains, legumes, avocados, bananas.

➜ RIBOFLAVIN: Meat, poultry, fish, eggs and dairy products.

➜ FOLIC ACID: Dark green leafy vegetables, such as romaine lettuce and spinach; orange juice.

➜ VITAMIN B_{12}: This vitamin is found only in foods of animal origin, including meats, seafood, dairy products and eggs.

➜ THIAMIN: Whole grains, legumes, seeds, pork and brewer's yeast.

➤ VITAMIN C: Citrus fruits, tomatoes, broccoli, cantaloupe, berries, cabbage, asparagus, green and red sweet peppers.

➤ VITAMIN A: Sweet potatoes, carrots, evaporated skim milk, apricot nectar, liver, part skim ricotta cheese, cantaloupe, tomatoes, squash, spinach.

➤ VITAMIN E: Asparagus, beet greens, broccoli, cabbage, mustard greens, soybeans, spinach, tomatoes, hams, almonds, peanut butter, sunflower seeds, blueberries, papaya, quinoa, wheat germ, tuna steak, salmon, sole, shrimp.

➤ FATTY ACIDS: The human body needs a certain amount of special fats called essential fatty acids; most people get enough fatty acids if they get just fifteen grams of fat per day. On the other hand, diets that have too much fat are thought to suppress the immune system. Therefore, it is suggested that people with autoimmune diseases eat a low-fat diet, or one in which no more than 20 to 30 percent (with the low end more commonly recommended) of calories as fat.

As you can see, the list of nutrients important to the immune system is quite long! That's why it is so important to eat a diet that supplies all essential nutrients, including whole grains, fruits, vegetables, protein foods and dairy foods.

A word to the wise: just because some is good, it doesn't mean that a little more is better. While you may be tempted to load up on vitamins in an attempt to "boost" your immune system, consider the results of studies with zinc. Researchers know that zinc is an essential ingredient in a healthy immune system. In one study, research subjects were given high doses of zinc (many times the Recommended Dietary Allowance [RDA]). Instead of boosting the immune system, these high doses actually suppressed it (as measured by the population of lymphocytes in the blood stream, one type of white blood cell). Similarly, in animal studies, the right amount of manganese helped study animals have a normal immune response, but an overdose suppressed their immune system. The best advice? Stick to the RDA for nutrients, concentrating on getting these nutrients from a healthy diet rather than from supplements.

Menus

LUPUS

You'll find two sets of menus here: one with daily menus totaling around 1,500 calories, and one with daily menus of around 1,800 calories. If you need to drop a few pounds, try the 1,500-calorie level; if you're at a healthy body weight, try the higher level.

As recommended, each menu is low in total fat, low in saturated fat and low in polyunsaturated fat. Each day's menu supplies at least 100 percent of the RDA for all nutrients, with a few minor exceptions, and, in many cases, there is more than 100 percent of the RDA for several nutrients. You'll notice several meals with tuna or salmon, both great sources of lean protein and also omega-3 fatty acids; at the same time, there is not a lot of red meat in these menus.

Do try to drink the milk recommended in these menus. It's a great source of protein and, more importantly, the calcium and vitamin D you need to keep strong bones, especially if you take steroid medications. It also helps keep you feeling full longer after each meal—a help if you're trying to drop a few pounds.

I've loaded these menus with fruits and vegetables, to help give you the edge on fighting off cancer and heart disease, as well as lupus. Always think of the total picture!

If you'd like, try adding two tablespoons of flaxseed to your diet daily. Stir it into half a cup of orange juice (it tends to settle, so stir or swirl as you drink it). Even if further studies don't find it helpful in lupus, it is a great high-fiber, high-nutrient and high-phytochemical item to include in your diet. If you do this, take out half of a bread serving (such as half a piece of bread, half a potato, and so on) and one fruit serving.

Part 1: Weight Loss

DAY ONE

Breakfast
  2 slices whole wheat toast
  1 tablespoon peanut butter
  1 tablespoon jam
  1 cup skim milk

Morning Snack
  1 orange

Lunch
  Tuna sandwich: ½ can tuna (packed in water), 2 slices whole wheat bread, 2 leaves romaine lettuce, 2 slices tomato, 1 tablespoon low-fat mayonnaise
  1 apple
  1 cup skim milk

Afternoon Snack
  1 banana

Dinner
  One-Pot Chili (page 375)
  1 cup steamed broccoli
  1 cup skim milk

1569 calories, 97 g protein, 37 g fiber, 33 g total fat (18% of calories), 9 g saturated fat (5% of calories), 1286 mg calcium, 1981 mg sodium

DAY TWO

Breakfast
  ½ cup nonfat cottage cheese
  1 whole wheat English muffin
  1 tablespoon jam
  1 cup skim milk

Morning Snack
  ½ cup low-fat fruited yogurt

Lunch
  Salad: 2 cups chopped romaine lettuce, 1 tomato (sliced), ½ cup garbanzo beans (chickpeas—okay to use canned, just drain and rinse to reduce sodium), 2 tablespoons low-fat dressing
  1 ounce whole wheat pretzel sticks
  Ice water

Dinner
  Honey Glazed Carrots and Parsnips with Chicken Thighs (page 298)
  1 cup skim milk

Evening Snack
  1 cup fruit cocktail, packed in juice

1561 calories, 85 g protein, 23 g fiber, 23 g total fat (13% of calories), 6 g saturated fat (3% of calories), 1188 mg calcium, 2040 mg sodium

DAY THREE

Breakfast

Creamy Breakfast Barley with Banana and Dried Cranberries (page 247)

Lunch

Peanut butter and jelly sandwich:
2 tablespoons peanut butter, 1 tablespoon jam, 2 slices whole wheat bread
1 cup skim milk
1 orange
6 baby carrots

Afternoon Snack

1 fig bar
½ cup skim milk

Dinner

Lentil Vegetable Soup (page 371)
½ cup skim milk

Evening Snack

1 cup fresh or frozen raspberries with ½ cup milk and a sprinkle of sugar if you desire

1586 calories, 73 g protein, 40 g fiber, 32 g total fat (17% fat), 6 g saturated fat (4% fat), 1420 mg calcium, 1111 mg sodium

DAY FOUR

Breakfast

1 poached egg
2 slices whole wheat toast
2 teaspoons margarine
1 cup skim milk

Morning Snack

1 apple

Lunch

Favorite Tuna Pasta Salad (page 275)
1 cup skim milk

Afternoon Snack

2 chocolate chip cookies
½ cup skim milk

Dinner

5 ounces grilled salmon
1 medium sweet potato, baked
2 teaspoons margarine
1 cup steamed broccoli

Evening Snack

½ cup nonfat frozen yogurt

1581 calories, 109 g protein, 21 g fiber, 48 g total fat (27% of calories), 10 g saturated fat (6% of calories), 1392 mg calcium, 1695 mg sodium

DAY FIVE

Breakfast

Oatmeal: Mix ½ cup oats plus 1 skim milk. Microwave on high for 2 minutes; stir and microwave for 2 minutes more. Or combine in a heavy pot and simmer for 7 minutes.
1 sliced banana
1 cup orange juice

Lunch

Turkey sandwich: 3 ounces lean turkey, 2 slices whole wheat bread, 2 leaves romaine lettuce, 2 slices tomato, 1 tablespoon light mayonnaise

1 orange
1 cup skim milk

Afternoon Snack

20 thin pretzel sticks

Dinner

Chicken and Zucchini Spaghetti (page 283)
1 peach
1 cup skim milk

Evening Snack

½ cup ice cream

1520 calories, 91 g protein, 17 g fiber, 29 g total fat (17% of calories), 10 g saturated fat (6% of calories), 1197 mg calcium, 1582 mg sodium

DAY SIX

Breakfast
½ cup nonfat cottage cheese
1 whole wheat English muffin
1 tablespoon jam
1 cup skim milk

Morning Snack
1 peach

Lunch
Barley and Bacon Soup (page 370)
6 baby carrots
1 cup skim milk

Afternoon Snack
1 chocolate chip cookie
½ cup skim milk

Dinner
Hamburger: 3 ounces very lean ground
beef, 1 hamburger bun, 1 slice tomato
(ketchup and mustard as desired)
½ cup frozen corn, steamed in
microwave
1 cup skim milk

Evening Snack
1 orange

*1496 calories, 101 g protein, 30 g fiber, 31 g total fat (18% of calories), 10 g saturated fat (6% of calories),
1279 mg calcium, 3130 mg sodium*

DAY SEVEN

Breakfast
1 poached egg
2 slices whole wheat toast
1 tablespoon jam
½ cup skim milk

Morning Snack
½ cup orange juice

Lunch
Cream of Broccoli Soup (page 368)
4 crackers
½ cup skim milk

Afternoon Snack
2 fig bars
½ cup skim milk

Dinner
5 ounces grilled tuna
1 baked potato
2 tablespoons nonfat sour cream
1 cup frozen peas and carrots, steamed
in microwave
Ice water

Evening Snack
½ cup nonfat frozen yogurt with a sliced
banana

*1559 calories, 106 g protein, 22 g fiber, 29 g total fat (17% of calories), 11 g saturated fat (6% of calories),
1117 mg calcium, 1592 mg sodium*

Part 2: Weight Maintenance

DAY ONE

Breakfast
2 slices whole wheat toast
2 tablespoons peanut butter
1 tablespoon jam
1 cup skim milk

Morning Snack
1 orange

Lunch
Tuna sandwich: ½ can tuna (packed in
water), 2 slices whole wheat bread, 2
leaves romaine lettuce, 2 slices tomato,
1 tablespoon low-fat mayonnaise

1 apple
1 cup skim milk

Afternoon Snack
1 banana

Dinner
One-Pot Chili (page 375)
1 cup steamed broccoli
1 cup skim milk

Evening Snack
2 chocolate chip cookies
½ cup skim milk

1802 calories, 106 g protein, 38 g fiber, 46 g total fat (22% of calories), 12 g saturated fat (6% of calories), 1446 mg calcium, 2189 mg sodium

DAY TWO

Breakfast
½ cup nonfat cottage cheese
1 whole wheat English muffin
1 tablespoon jam
1 cup skim milk

Morning Snack
1 cup low-fat fruited yogurt

Lunch
Salad: 2 cups chopped romaine lettuce,
1 tomato (sliced), 1 cup garbanzo
beans (chickpeas—okay to use

canned, just drain and rinse to
reduce sodium), 2 tablespoons low-
fat dressing
1 ounce whole wheat pretzel sticks
Ice water

Dinner
Honey Glazed Carrots and Parsnips
with Chicken Thighs (page 298)
1 cup skim milk

Evening Snack
½ cup ice cream

1882 calories, 101 g protein, 30 g fiber, 34 g total fat (16% of calories), 11 g saturated fat (5% of calories), 1487 mg calcium, 2372 mg sodium

DAY THREE

Breakfast
Creamy Breakfast Barley with Banana
and Dried Cranberries (page 247)
1 cup apple juice

Lunch
Peanut butter and jelly sandwich:
2 tablespoons peanut butter, 1 tablespoon jam, 2 slices whole wheat bread

1 cup skim milk

1 orange

6 baby carrots

Afternoon Snack

2 fig bars

½ cup skim milk

Dinner

Lentil Vegetable Soup (page 371)

1 cup skim milk

Evening Snack

1 cup fresh or frozen raspberries with ½ cup milk and a sprinkle of sugar if you desire

1794 calories, 77 g protein, 41 g fiber, 33 g total fat (16% of calories), 7 g saturated fat (3% of calories), 1597 mg calcium, 1231 mg sodium

DAY FOUR

Breakfast

1 poached egg

2 slices whole wheat toast

2 teaspoons margarine

1 cup skim milk

Morning Snack

1 apple

Lunch

Favorite Tuna Pasta Salad (page 275)

5 whole grain Rye Krisp

1 cup skim milk

Afternoon Snack

2 chocolate chip cookies

½ cup skim milk

Dinner

5 ounces grilled salmon

1 medium sweet potato, baked

2 teaspoons margarine

1 cup steamed broccoli

Evening Snack

1 cup nonfat frozen yogurt

1802 calories, 118 g protein, 28 g fiber, 49 g total fat (24% of calories), 11 g saturated fat (6% of calories), 1373 mg calcium, 2143 mg sodium

DAY FIVE

Breakfast

Oatmeal: Mix ½ cup oats with 1 cup skim milk. Microwave on high for 2 minutes; stir and microwave for 2 minutes more. Or combine in a heavy pot and simmer for 7 minutes.

1 sliced banana

1 cup orange juice

Lunch

Turkey sandwich: 3 ounces lean turkey, 2 slices whole wheat bread, 1 slice American cheese, 2 leaves romaine lettuce, 2 slices tomato, 1 tablespoon light mayonnaise

1 orange

1 cup skim milk

Afternoon Snack

20 thin pretzel sticks

Dinner

Chicken and Zucchini Spaghetti (page 283)

1 peach

1 cup skim milk

Evening Snack

1 cup ice cream

1830 calories, 101 g protein, 18 g fiber, 44 g total fat (21% of calories), 18 g saturated fat (9% of calories), 1415 mg calcium, 1936 mg sodium

DAY SIX

Breakfast
½ cup nonfat cottage cheese
1 whole wheat English muffin
1 tablespoon jam
1 cup skim milk

Morning Snack
1 peach

Lunch
Barley and Bacon Soup (page 370)
6 baby carrots
1 cup skim milk

Afternoon Snack
1 chocolate chip cookie
½ cup skim milk

Dinner
Hamburger: 3 ounces very lean ground
beef, 1 hamburger bun, 1 slice tomato
(ketchup and mustard as desired)
½ cup frozen corn, steamed in
microwave
1 cup skim milk

Evening Snack
1 orange

1799 calories, 116 g protein, 29 g fiber, 36 g total fat (18% of calories), 13 g saturated fat (6% of calories), 1216 mg calcium, 3370 mg sodium

DAY SEVEN

Breakfast
1 poached egg
2 slices whole wheat toast
1 tablespoon jam
½ cup skim milk

Morning Snack
1 cup orange juice

Lunch
Cream of Broccoli Soup (page 368)
1 whole wheat bagel
2 teaspoons margarine
1 cup skim milk

Afternoon Snack
2 fig bars
½ cup skim milk

Dinner
5 ounces grilled tuna
1 baked potato
2 tablespoons nonfat sour cream
1 cup frozen peas and carrots, steamed
in microwave
Ice water

Evening Snack
½ cup nonfat frozen yogurt with a sliced
banana

1818 calories, 116 g protein, 27 g fiber, 36 g total fat (18% of calories), 12 g saturated fat (6% of calories), 1297 mg calcium, 1872 mg sodium

References

Clark W.F., et al. "Fish oil in lupus nephritis: clinical findings and methodological implications." *Kidney International* 44 (1993): 75–86.

Clark W.F., et al. "Flaxseed: a potential treatment for lupus nephritis." *Kidney International* 48 (1995): 475–80.

Clark W.F., Parbtani A. :"Omega-3 fatty acid supplementation in clinical and experimental lupus nephritis." *American Journal of Kidney Disease* 23 (1994): 644–7.

Corman L.C. "The role of diet in animal models of systemic lupus erythematosus: possible implications for human lupus." *Seminars in Arthritis and Rheumatism* 15 (1985): 61–9.

Endres S., et al. "N-3 polyunsaturated fatty acids: update 1995." *European Journal of Clinical Investigation* 25 (1995): 629–638.

Hearth-Holmes M., et al. "Dietary treatment of hyperlipidemia in patients with systemic lupus erythematosus." *Journal of Rheumatology* 22 (1995): 450–454.

Herbert V., Kasdan T.S. "Alfalfa, vitamin E and autoimmune disorders." *American Journal of Clinical Nutrition* 60 (1994): 639–42.

Ilowite N.T., et al. "Effects of dietary modification and fish oil supplementation on dyslipoproteinemia in pediatric systemic lupus erythematosus." *Journal of Rheumatology* 22 (1995): 1347–51.

Komatireddy G.R., et al. "Association of systemic lupus erythematosus and gluten enteropathy." *Southern Medical Journal* 88 (1995): 673–676.

Maki P.A., Newberne P.M., "Dietary lipids and immune function." *Journal of Nutrition* 122 (3 suppl) (1992): 610–4.

Minami Y., et al. "Female systemic lupus erythematosus in Miyagi Prefecture, Japan: a case–control study of dietary and reproductive factors." *Tohoku Journal of Experimental Medicine* 169 (1993): 245–52.

Molad Y., et al. "Serum cobalamin and transcobalamin levels in systemic lupus erythematosus." *American Journal of Medicine* 88 (1990): 141–4.

Obermeyer W.R., et al. "Chemical studies of phytoestrogens and related compounds in dietary supplements: flax and chaparral.": PSEBM 208 (1995): 6–12.

Serraino M., Thompson L.U. "Flaxseed supplementation and early markers of colon carcinogenesis." *Cancer Letters* 63 (1992): 159–165.

Shigemasa C., et al. "Effect of vegetarian diet on systemic lupus erythematosus." *The Lancet* 339 (1992): 1177.

Swanson C.A., et al. "Effect of low dietary lipid on the development of sjogren's syndrome and hematological abnormalities in NZB mix NZW-F-1 mice." *Annals of the Rheumatic Diseases* (1989): 765–770.

Thompson L.U. "Antioxidants and hormone-mediated health benefits of whole grains." *Critical Reviews in Food Science and Nutrition* 34 (1994): 473–497.

Westberg G., et al. "Effect of MaxEPA in patients with SLE. A double–blind, crossover study." *Scandinavian Journal of Rheumatology* 19 (1990): 137–43.

Yell J.A., et al. "Vitamin E and discoid lupus erythematosus." *Lupus* 1 (1992): 303–5.

Multiple Sclerosis 18

Some 350,000 to 500,000 Americans have multiple sclerosis, another autoimmune disease, or a condition in which the immune system somehow gets misdirected and attacks part of the body's own tissues. In the case of multiple sclerosis, the immune system starts battling myelin. Myelin is the tissue that covers and protects nerve fibers throughout the body. A healthy myelin coat is necessary for nerve cells to communicate with each other. As a result, when myelin becomes destroyed in multiple sclerosis (which it does in patches), the nerve cells cannot communicate properly. Because of disrupted nerve-to-nerve communication, people with multiple sclerosis can suffer a wide range of neurological symptoms, including fatigue, loss of coordination, muscle weakness, numbness, slurred speech, dizziness, memory lapses and visual difficulties.

Multiple sclerosis often strikes between ages thirty and fifty, and occurs more often in women than men and more commonly in the Caucasian population. Researchers have also discovered that the closer people are to the equator the less like they are to develop multiple sclerosis. Like many autoimmune diseases, multiple sclerosis is a somewhat mysterious disease. Doctors don't know what causes it, why it progresses and which patients diagnosed with it will become disabled.

The Nutrition Advantage

Although no one diet has been proven definitively to improve the course of disease in people with multiple sclerosis, there is encouraging evidence that a low-fat diet may help. While the efficacy of this diet has not been proven, note that it just happens to be an exceptionally healthy diet! Remember the low total fat and low saturated diet you read about earlier in this book—the type of diet that nearly every person can benefit from? This type of diet might be even more important for people with multiple sclerosis. Read on to learn more.

The most common recommended dietary modification for multiple sclerosis patients is a diet low in fat, especially saturated fat, and one that includes a higher percentage than normal of polyunsaturated fatty acids, especially the type found in fish. It is also important to get enough vitamin D and calcium and eat for a healthy immune system. Other nutrition issues that deserve mentioning are vitamin B_{12} and vitamin E.

Dietary regimens that are less commonly recommended and may not be supported by scientific evidence are diets free of gluten, allergens, and sucrose; diets with restrictions on pectin and fructose; and diets that include raw foods and high levels of manganese.

Low-Fat Diet

After noticing that people in China, Japan and Korea get multiple sclerosis (MS) much less often than people in the United States, researchers thought that these Asian populations might be protected by their heavy rice consumption. Delving further, researchers changed their thinking, believing that the relatively lower fat consumption in the Orient is more likely responsible for the lower rate of multiple sclerosis there.

Multiple sclerosis researchers in Norway have also made some interesting observations about the fat level of the diet and the incidence of multiple sclerosis. They have noted that the rates of multiple sclerosis in coastal fishing communities are lower than in inland, agricultural communities, leading them to believe that people who eat more fish (and therefore less dietary fat) seem to have a lower risk of MS. They've also noticed that people who eat more animal fat are more likely to develop multiple sclerosis. Researchers from other parts of the world have made similar observations. The rate of MS is relatively low among southern Europeans and Eskimos, who are known for eating diets low in saturated fat and relatively high in polyunsaturated fats. On the other hand, people from northern Europe have relatively higher rates of MS, and they are known to consume a diet higher in saturated fat.

Note that a low-fat diet (which is also called the Swank Diet) has never undergone the rigorous testing that proves that it does indeed help people with multiple sclerosis. The only diet endorsed by the International Federation of Multiple Sclerosis Societies Therapeutics Claims Committee, a panel of physicians who review claims for the treatment of MS, is a well-balanced, nutrient-rich one devoid of excess calories.

That said, it makes sense to review dietary maneuvers that may help MS, as long as they cannot do any harm. A low-fat diet that is also low in saturated fat is a healthy diet for everyone, so it definitely is prudent to take a look at the theory behind why it could work in MS. This is the way I look at it: if you could do something that is healthy for you anyway, and that may at least reduce the symptoms or the frequency of MS symptoms, it's worth a try.

Theoretically, it makes sense that fat could affect the course of multiple sclerosis. Researchers have shown that by-products (metabolites) of a certain kind of fat called omega-3 fats are immunomodulatory. That means that they can modulate, or affect the immune system. Some of the them seem to fight inflammation and some seem to encourage inflammation. A diet too high in fat would no doubt have too much of the fats that stimulate inflammation. On the other hand, a low-fat diet, and one that stresses omega-3 fats, is more likely to have more of the inflammation-fighting fats and less of the inflammation-inducing fats.

Two specific omega-3 fatty acids are thought to be especially important in terms of how they affect the immune system: eicosapentaenoic acid (EPA) and docosahexaenoic acid (DHA). They are quite abundant in certain fatty fish. These omega-3 fatty acids are thought to fight inflammation, including the type that occurs in MS. While this has not been proven, there is epidemiological evidence that it may be true—that is, the evidence that people who eat more fish are less likely to get MS.

Even if a low-fat diet (with an emphasis on using omega-3 fat) does not prove to be helpful for people with multiple sclerosis, there is good reason to stick with this type of diet. For one, heart disease experts know that reducing total fat and saturated fat is the best type of diet to fight artery-clogging heart disease, which is important for everyone. We also know that a low-fat diet is a help in fighting cancer. A lower-fat diet makes keeping a trim figure much easier, which is important for everyone—especially people with limited mobility. And in eating a lower-fat diet, people generally greatly boost their intake of fresh fruits and vegetables, which is another aid in fighting cancer and heart disease—and also in harvesting the vitamins, minerals, phytochemicals and fiber that help you feel your best. Incidentally, while there has only been a suggestion that dietary antioxidants may help in fighting the inflammation of MS, consuming large amounts of fresh fruits and vegetables is the absolute best way to take in a wide variety of these dietary antioxidants.

Vitamin D and Calcium

A person with multiple sclerosis who can remain active and who doesn't take steroid medications has the normal risk of osteoporosis—which, for a woman, is fairly high (especially at menopause and after). But if your disease occasionally imposes periods of relative inactivity, necessitates the use of steroid medications or requires that you use a wheelchair, your risk of osteoporosis is greatly enhanced. Experts estimate that immobility—bed rest, lying on the couch, having to use a wheelchair—can result in losing as much as 1 percent of bone mass per week. With prolonged inactivity, you can imagine how quickly this compounds. In one study, multiple sclerosis experts estimated that MS patients have a two- to threefold increased risk of fractures which result from osteoporosis.

Fortunately, though, there is a way to fight this bone loss: increase the amount of calcium and vitamin D in the diet. While all women should take in between 1,000 and 1,500 milligrams of calcium, women and men who are inactive and/or on steroid medications should aim for 1,500 to 2,000 milligrams. Vitamin D intake should be around 400 IU, and 800 IU for people on steroid medications. Drinking about four glasses of milk per day tallies a quick 1,200 milligrams calcium and 400 IU vitamin D. If you don't like milk, rely on calcium supplements; just make sure they include vitamin D.

Eat for a Healthy Immune System

The immune system is the body's way of fighting off foreign invaders, such as bacteria, viruses and allergens. In people with autoimmune diseases, though, the immune system somehow goes awry. While taking large amounts of certain nutrients isn't a way to boost the immune system, making sure you are well nourished in general is an excellent way to make sure the immune system is as healthy as it can be. Some of the nutrients that are especially important to a healthy immune system (as well as foods high in that nutrient) include:

- → PROTEIN: Milk, cheese, meat, legumes (such as lentils).

- → ZINC: Good sources include seafoods, meats, whole grains, legumes.

- → IRON: Red meat (the best source), fish, poultry, legumes, nuts and seeds, whole grains.

- → MANGANESE: Rice cakes, brown rice, whole wheat bread, oatmeal, wheat germ, tea.

- → COPPER: Legumes, meats, seafood, shellfish, whole grains, nuts and seeds.

- → MAGNESIUM: Foods that are a good source of protein are generally a good source of magnesium; in addition, whole grains, legumes, nuts and seeds, green vegetables, avocados, bananas are good sources.

- → SELENIUM: Protein-rich foods are also a good source of selenium, as are whole grains. One of the richest sources is Brazil nuts.

- → VITAMIN B_6: Chicken, fish, pork, eggs, liver, whole grains, legumes, avocados, bananas.

- → RIBOFLAVIN: Meat, poultry, fish, eggs, and dairy products.

- → FOLIC ACID: Dark green leafy vegetables, such as romaine lettuce and spinach; orange juice.

- → VITAMIN B_{12}: This vitamin is found only in foods of animal origin, including meats, seafood, dairy products and eggs.

- → THIAMIN: Whole grains, legumes, seeds, pork and brewer's yeast.

- → VITAMIN C: Citrus fruits, tomatoes, broccoli, cantaloupe, berries, cabbage, asparagus, green and red sweet peppers.

- → VITAMIN A: Sweet potatoes, carrots, evaporated skim milk, apricot nectar, liver, part skim ricotta cheese, cantaloupe, tomatoes, squash, spinach.

- → VITAMIN E: Asparagus, beet greens, broccoli, cabbage, mustard greens, soybeans, spinach, tomatoes, hams, almonds, peanut butter, sunflower seeds, blueberries, papaya, quinoa, wheat germ, tuna steak, salmon, sole, shrimp.

- → FATTY ACIDS: The human body needs a certain amount of special fats called essential fatty acids; most people get enough fatty acids if they get just fifteen grams of fat per day. On the other hand, diets that have too much fat are thought to suppress the immune system. Therefore, it is suggested that people with autoimmune diseases eat a low-fat diet, or one in which no more than 20 to 30 percent (with the low end more commonly recommended) of calories as fat.

As you can see, the list of nutrients important to the immune system is quite long! That's why it is so important to eat a diet that supplies all essential nutrients, including plenty of whole grains, fruits, vegetables, protein foods and dairy foods.

A word to the wise: just because some is good, it doesn't mean that a little more is better. While you may be tempted to load up on vitamins in an attempt to "boost" your immune system, consider the results of studies with zinc. Researchers know that zinc is an essential ingredient in a healthy immune system. In one study, research subjects were given high doses of zinc (many times the recommended dietary allowance). Instead of boosting the immune system, these high doses actually suppressed it (as measured by the population of lymphocytes, one type of white blood cell, in the bloodstream). Similarly, in animal studies, the right amount of manganese helped study animals have a normal immune response, but an overdose suppressed their immune system. The best advice? Stick to the RDA for nutrients, concentrating on getting these nutrients from a healthy diet rather than from supplements.

Vitamin B_{12}

You may have read about an association between multiple sclerosis and vitamin B_{12}. Here's the scoop. Doctors have noticed that multiple sclerosis patients seem to have a higher than expected chance of having low blood levels of vitamin B_{12}, a vitamin necessary, among other things, for normal nervous system functioning. Boosting intake of B_{12}, though, has not proven helpful in reducing the symptoms of MS.

When MS is diagnosed initially, most physicians do check blood levels of vitamin B_{12}. This makes sense, as symptoms of a true vitamin B_{12} deficiency can cause a condition that mimics multiple sclerosis.

While current research doesn't support the idea that B_{12} supplements can help multiple sclerosis patients, taking in the RDA for this nutrient does make sense. Only foods of animal origin have vitamin B_{12}. To get the RDA of two micrograms of vitamin B_{12}, try to work in the following foods (note that one of the best sources is salmon, which is also rich in omega-3 fatty acids):

> *5 ounces broiled salmon = 4 mcg*
> *½ can (3 ounces) tuna = 2*
> *3 ounces cooked pork loin = 0.49*
> *3 ounces cooked chicken breast = 0.27*
> *3 ounces cooked beef = 1.85*
> *8 ounces nonfat skim milk = 0.93*

Vitamin E

Vitamin E is an important antioxidant vitamin, protecting cells throughout the body from oxygen-free radicals and pollutants. (Vitamin E is also necessary for normal cell structure and for the formation of red blood cells.) MS patients should be concerned about getting enough vitamin E because of the emphasis in their diets on omega-3 fats as the main type of dietary fat consumed. This is because omega-3 fats use up more vitamin E in the metabolic process. There is another potential reason to get a healthy intake of vitamin E: preliminary research indicates that antioxidants may be a help in attenuating the multiple sclerosis disease process.

Try to get around 10 IU of vitamin E, which will give you the Recommended Dietary Allowance (RDA) for this nutrient. Some experts think that everyone should get no less than 30 IU daily. Refer to the table for dietary sources of vitamin E; it's generally necessary to take a supplement to get 30 IU.

Foods Rich in Vitamin E

It is possible to get at least 10 IU of vitamin E without eating a lot of high-fat foods. Use this table to boost your intake of vitamin E and yet follow a diet that limits fat, especially saturated fat. Another benefit: you'll also be reaping lots of other key nutrients that may help fight heart disease and cancer and keep you healthy in general. Remember the key: lots of fruits, vegetables, and whole grains.

Food	Serving Size	IU Vitamin E Per Serving	Other Nutrients
Asparagus, steamed	1 cup	2.7	fiber, vitamin C, folate, iron, potassium
Beet greens, boiled	1 cup	3.0	fiber, beta–carotene, vitamin C, calcium, iron, potassium
Broccoli, boiled	1 cup	2.6	fiber, vitamin C, folate, calcium, iron, potassium
Cabbage, raw, shredded	1 cup	1.7	fiber, vitamin C
Cabbage, boiled	1 cup	3.7	fiber, vitamin C
Dandelion greens, boiled	1 cup	3.1	fiber, beta–carotene, calcium, iron, potassium, vitamin C
Mustard greens, boiled	1 cup	4.2	fiber, beta–carotene, vitamin C, folate, calcium, iron, potassium
Soybeans, boiled	1 cup	5.0	fiber, calcium, iron, folate, potassium
Spinach, boiled	1 cup	3.5	beta–carotene, folate, calcium, iron, potassium, vitamin C
Spinach, raw	1 cup	1.5	beta–carotene, folate, calcium, iron, potassium, vitamin C
Sweet potato	1 each	0.7	fiber, beta–carotene, vitamin C, potassium
Swiss chard, cooked	1 cup	1.8	fiber, beta–carotene, vitamin C, calcium iron, potassium
Tomato paste, canned	¼ cup	1.6	vitamin C, iron, potassium
Tomato, raw	1 medium	1.5	vitamin C, beta–carotene, potassium
Turnip green, boiled	1 cup	3.7	fiber, beta–carotene, vitamin C, folate, calcium, iron, potassium
Yam, white boiled	1 cup	9.2	fiber, vitamin C, potassium
Almonds, whole, toasted	1 ounce	10.2	fiber, calcium, iron
Filberts, dry or oil roasted	1 ounce	10.6	fiber, calcium, iron
Peanut butter	2 tablespoons	3.6	iron
Sunflower seeds	1 tablespoon	6.7	iron
Blueberries	1 cup	2.2	fiber, vitamin C, potassium
Guava	1 each	1.5	fiber, vitamin C, potassium
Kiwi	1 each	1.3	vitamin C, fiber, potassium
Papaya	1 each	5.1	vitamin C, fiber, potassium

Food	Serving Size	IU Vitamin E Per Serving	Other Nutrients
Prunes	10 each	1.7	fiber, vitamin C, potassium
Barley	1 cup	1.8	B vitamins, minerals, fiber
Quinoa, uncooked	½ cup	6.2	B vitamins, minerals, fiber
Wheat germ, toasted	2 tablespoons	4.2	B vitamins, minerals, fiber
Catfish, steamed	3 ounces	1.9	
Crab, broiled, baked	3 ounces	2.1	
Halibut, baked or broiled	3 ounces	0.9	
Salmon, steamed	3 ounces	2.4	Omega-3 fatty acids
Shrimp, steamed	3 ounces	2.2	
Sole, poached	3 ounces	3.0	
Tuna steak, baked or broiled	3 ounces	2.5	
Chicken breast, skinless, baked	3 ounces	0.2	
Chicken thigh, skinless, baked	3 ounces	0.6	
Turkey meat, dark, baked	3 ounces	8	
Corn oil	1 tablespoon	4.3	
Sunflower oil	1 tablespoon	12.2	

How to Devise a Low-Fat Diet

It takes a huge commitment to follow a low-fat diet, but the payoff could be a big one. The easiest way to devise a low-fat diet that is also high in omega-3 fatty acids is to include lots of fruits and vegetables, very little added fat (such as margarine, mayonnaise, oil), relatively more fish—especially salmon, tuna and other fish high in omega-3 fatty acids—than other meat sources of protein and few convenience snack foods, because they are generally high in saturated fat. This type of eating plan will automatically decrease saturated fat, which has also been implicated (but not proven) as increasing the disease process. In addition, your MS eating plan should be very high in calcium, as the lifestyle sometimes imposed by MS and some of the medications used to treat the disease can place patients at heightened risk of developing osteoporosis. Finally, try to consume a high-fiber diet. While it's healthy for everyone, it may be a tremendous help during periods of relative inactivity, when constipation can make you miserable.

In general, try to include:

➤ Ten servings of fruits and vegetables, where a serving is one piece of fruit (such as one banana), ½ cup of fruit (such as ½ cup raspberries), ½ cup of raw vegetable (such as ½ cup of chopped green pepper), 1 cup cooked vegetable (such as 1 cup cooked spinach).

➤ Six to eight bread/starch servings, where a serving is one slice of bread, ½ bagel, ½ cup of rice or other grain (such as barley), 1 small potato, or 1 plain cookie.

➤ Four to six lean protein servings, where a serving is one ounce after cooking, emphasizing fish, chicken, turkey, and occasionally very lean beef and very lean pork. If you want to take a more vegetarian approach, use more legumes, such as kidney beans and lentils.

➤ Four nonfat milk servings, where a serving is 1 cup of skim milk or 1 cup of nonfat or low-fat yogurt.

Menus

MULTIPLE SCLEROSIS

These menus achieve several dietary goals that may be a help for people with multiple sclerosis (MS): they are low in total fat, containing 15 to 20 percent of calories as total fat; they are low in saturated fat, with a maximum of 5 percent of calories as saturated fat. These eating plans are also high in fiber and high in dietary antioxidants, which have been implicated (but never proven) as helping to ameliorate MS.

In addition, these menus contain more fish than meat, and several vegetarian dishes—both may be very important in achieving the nutrition advantage.

Each day has about 1,800 calories—a good calorie level for most women. If you need more calories (either because you are more active or a man), try to add them as whole grain, fruit or vegetable servings, as these are very low fat or fat-free.

Each day's menu contains at least 100 percent of the RDA for all nutrients, with a few minor exceptions (but generally another day makes up for a lag of 3 or 4 percent in reaching 100 percent). All menus are exceptionally healthy, and help you achieve the nutrition advantage in fighting osteoporosis, cancer and heart disease, as well as your disease.

When margarine is included in the menu, please be sure and measure carefully. Also, choose a soft tub margarine, such as Fleishman's. The softer the margarine, the lower the saturated fat and transfatty acids, the latter of which may act somewhat like saturated fat in the body.

DAY ONE

Breakfast
Apple oatmeal: cook together ½ cup oats, 1 cup skim milk, and 1 diced apple

Morning Snack
1 cup low-fat, fruited yogurt

Lunch
Lentil Vegetable Soup (page 371)
1 cup skim milk

Afternoon Snack
½ sweet potato: bake at 350°F for 45 minutes, or until a fork inserted indicates tenderness; chill and slice

Dinner
3 ounces lean roast (such as eye of round)
1 baked potato with 1 teaspoon tub corn oil margarine★
1 carrot
1 cup steamed broccoli
1 pear
1 cup skim milk
★such as Fleishman's

Evening Snack
1 fig bar

1843 calories, 100 g protein, 35 g fiber, 31 g total fat (15% of calories); 11 g saturated fat (5% of calories), 1928 mg calcium

Breakfast
  Scrambled eggs: 1 egg plus 1 egg white
    scrambled in nonstick pan with veg-
    etable oil spray
  ½ whole wheat bagel
  1 teaspoon corn oil tub margarine
  1 cup skim milk

Morning Snack
  1 apple

Lunch
  Tuna sandwich: ½ can tuna (packed
    in water), 2 slices whole wheat bread,
    2 teaspoons light Miracle Whip plus
    pickle relish, if desired, romaine
    lettuce leaves, 1 thick slice
    of tomato

  1 banana
  1 cup skim milk

Afternoon Snack
  1 cup low-fat yogurt with 2 tablespoons
    wheat germ

Dinner
  4 ounces roasted chicken (skin removed
    before eating)
  1 cup cooked rice (try cooking it with
    an herbal tea bag, such as orange
    spice, to lend a rich flavor)
  1 cup cooked spinach
  1 orange
  1 cup skim milk

Evening Snack
  ½ cup low-fat frozen yogurt

1833 calories, 139 g protein, 24 g fiber, 31 g total fat (15% of calories); 10 g saturated fat (5% of calories); 1972 mg calcium

DAY THREE

Breakfast
  1 bagel
  2 tablespoons peanut butter
  1 cup skim milk

Morning Snack
  ½ cup orange juice

Lunch
  Salad: 2 cups romaine lettuce, 1 cup
    garbanzo beans (chickpeas—okay to
    use canned), 1 small tomato, 2 table-
    spoons fat-free salad dressing
  1 cup skim milk

Afternoon Snack
  1 apple

Dinner
  5 ounces grilled or baked salmon
  1 cup cooked pasta
  8 asparagus spears, steamed, served with
    a squeeze of lemon juice
  1 cup skim milk

Evening Snack
  1 cup skim milk
  1 oatmeal-raisin cookie

1826 calories, 114 g protein, 22 g fiber, 40 g total fat (19% of calories); 9 g saturated fat (4% of calories), 1400 mg calcium

DAY FOUR

Breakfast
  1 poached egg
  2 slices whole wheat toast
  1 teaspoon corn oil tub margarine
  6 ounces pear nectar

Morning Snack
  1 orange

Lunch
  Ham sandwich: 3 ounces very lean ham,
    2 slices rye bread, romaine lettuce
    leaves, 2 teaspoons light Miracle Whip
  ½ sweet potato as cold slices
  1 cup skim milk

Afternoon Snack
  1 cup fresh or frozen raspberries
  1 cup skim milk

Dinner
  8 large shrimp, steamed or stir-fried
  1 cup cooked winter squash
  1 cup brown rice
  1 cup skim milk

Evening Snack
  1 large baked apple: core apple, insert
    1 tablespoon brown sugar in core;
    place 2 tablespoons water per apple in
    bottom of baking dish, bake uncov-
    ered at 350°F for 30 to 40 minutes

1785 calories, 87 g protein, 35 g fiber, 31 g total fat (15% of calories), 8 g saturated fat (4% of calories), 1422 mg calcium

DAY FIVE

Breakfast
  2 slices whole wheat toast
  1 tablespoons peanut butter
  2 teaspoons jam
  1 cup skim milk

Morning Snack
  1 banana

Lunch
  Salad: 2 cups romaine lettuce, 1 can tuna
    (packed in water), ½ tomato, 2 table-
    spoons fat-free salad dressing
  1 whole wheat bagel
  1 cup fresh or frozen strawberries
  1 cup skim milk

Afternoon Snack
  1 cup low-fat vanilla yogurt with
    1 apple sliced and sprinkled with
    1 teaspoon brown sugar

Dinner
  Salmon Loaf (page 352)
  1 baked sweet potato
  1 cup steamed cauliflower
  ½ cup peas
  ½ cup skim milk

Evening Snack
  2 fig bars
  ½ cup skim milk

1842 calories, 134 g protein, 30 g fiber, 36 g total fat (17% of calories); 11 g saturated fat (5% of calories), 1728 mg calcium

Breakfast

Oatmeal: Mix ½ cup oats with 1 cup skim milk. Microwave for 2 minutes on high; stir and microwave for 2 more minutes. Or combine in a heavy pot and simmer for 7 minutes.

2 tablespoons raisins

Morning Snack

1 cup orange juice

Lunch

Barley and Bacon Soup (page 370)

1 cup skim milk

1 banana

Afternoon Snack

Raspberry Cream Gelatin (page 397)

Dinner

4 ounces grilled tuna steak

1 cup cooked pasta with 2 teaspoons margarine

1 cup green peas

1 cup skim milk

1843 calories, 120 g protein, 33 g fiber, 31 g total fat (15% of calories); 8 g saturated fat (4% of calories); 1288 mg calcium

Day Seven

Breakfast

½ cup nonfat cottage cheese

2 slices whole wheat toast

1 tablespoon jam

1 cup skim milk

Morning Snack

1 banana

Lunch

Black Bean and Barley Stew with Mushrooms (page 379)

1 cup red grapes

1 cup skim milk

Dinner

Chicken Parmesan and Linguine (page 282)

1 cup steamed broccoli

1 cup skim milk

Evening Snack

Easy as Pie Apple Pie (page 267)

1826 calories; 110 g protein; g fiber; 33 g total fat (16% of calories); 10 g saturated fat (5% of calories); 1234 mg calcium

References

Fawcett, J., et al. "Use of Alternative Health Therapies by People with Multiple Sclerosis: An Exploratory Study." *Holistic Nurse Practitioner* 8(2) (1994): 36–42.

Harbige, L.S., et al. "Nutritional Management in Multiple Sclerosis with Reference to Experimental Models." *Upsala Journal of Medical Science* 48 (Suppl) (1990): 189–207.

Hutter, C.D.D., and P. Laing. "Multiple Sclerosis: Sunlight, Diet, Immunology and Aetiology." *Medical Hypotheses* 46 (1996): 67–74.

Kruger, P.G., and H.I. Nyland. "The Role of Mast Cells and Diet in the Onset and Maintenance of Multiple Sclerosis: A Hypothesis." *Medical Hypotheses* 44 (1995): 66–69.

Multiple Sclerosis Foundation. *MS Facts* (information packet). 350 North Andrews Ave., Fort Lauderdale, FL 33309-2130. 954/776-6805 or 800/441-7055.

Newcombe, J., et al. "Low Density Lipoprotein Uptake by Macrophages in Multiple Sclerosis Plaques: Implications for Pathogenesis." *Neuropathology and Applied Neurobiology* 20 (1994): 152–62.

Nieves, J., et al. "High Prevalence of Vitamin D Deficiency and Reduced Bone Mass in Multiple Sclerosis." *Neurology* 44 (1994): 1,687–92.

Ransohoff, R.M., et al. "The Immunology of Multiple Sclerosis: New Intricacies and New Insights." *Current Opinions in Neurology* 7(3) (1994): 242–49.

———. "Vitamin B_{12} Deficiency and Multiple Sclerosis." *The Lancet* 335 (1990): 1,285–86.

Myasthenia Gravis

19

Another autoimmune disease, myasthenia gravis, affects the neuromuscular system. That means that it "attacks" the nerves that tell muscles what to do. The most prominent symptom of myasthenia gravis, which often first strikes in the second and third decades of life, is muscular weakness. People with this disease often have worse muscular weakness when they are up and about, but this improves with rest. It is also common to have diurnal muscle weakness—or muscle weakness that fluctuates according to the time of day. While patients with myasthenia gravis may feel normal in the morning, they may have severe muscle weakness in the evening. Resting, though, may help relieve this weakness.

While it can affect many different muscle groups, it often affects the muscles that control breathing and those that control swallowing. Overall, this can interfere with the ability to get good nutrition. Indeed, patients with myasthenia may have difficulty with chewing and choking during meals. Over time, this can lead to weight loss. Severe weight loss can contribute to the feeling of weakness.

While there is very little research on nutritional maneuvers that may help in myasthenia gravis, the following may be helpful for patients with this disease:

➤ Plan menus with foods that are easier to swallow when flare-ups make this difficult.

➤ Eat to prevent weight loss, especially during disease flare-ups.

➤ Eat to maximize energy.

➤ Accommodate the nutritional problems that can occur when you take steroid medications.

Plan Menus with Easy-to-Swallow Foods

When muscular weakness strikes the muscles that affect breathing and swallowing, eating can become a real chore. This is especially true when the foods are drier and harder. Many people turn to softer, more liquid foods during these difficult-to-swallow times. The trouble with this, though, is that many of these foods are low in calories and nutrients. That's why careful nutrition planning is so important. As with any disease, it is during these flare-ups that good nutrition is even more critical—it can give you the nutrition advantage to better battle your disease and improve your health.

Try to choose soft foods that are dense in nutrients. Many of the recipes in the back of this book fit that bill, and I've included them in the menus at the end of this chapter. In general, though, here are some tricks to increase the nutrients and calories in softer foods:

→ Avoid empty-calorie liquids, such as soda, opting instead for juices.

→ Choose more calorie-dense juices, such as nectars. They're also higher in nutrients.

→ Find recipes that use pureed or mashed vegetables, which are often the most difficult foods to work into your diet when swallowing becomes difficult. For example, the custards in the recipe portion of this book include pureed sweet potatoes (one of the most nutritionally powerful vegetables) and applesauce. There are also recipes for mashed carrots, and you can mash sweet potatoes. Look for recipes that include other powerhouse nutrition, such as spinach, in a quiche or casserole. It's a great way to boost nutrient intake in an easy-to-swallow form.

→ Include recipes in which meat is cut into smaller pieces and in a sauce, which makes it easier to swallow.

→ Plan small, frequent meals instead of three larger ones.

Because myasthenia gravis is a lifelong disease, try not to boost calories by simply loading up on butter or margarine or other fatty foods. While this is okay on the rare occasion, over the long run, dietary habits like this can drive up the fats in the bloodstream and get you into trouble with heart disease. Striking a balance of what might help in the short term versus what is healthy over the long run is often difficult in chronic illness like myasthenia, but certainly not impossible. Eating to avoid heart disease is especially important for people who must take steroid medications, which can also drive up the chances of getting artery-clogging heart disease.

Eat to Prevent Weight Loss

Disease flare-ups make it especially difficult to keep weight on. Refer to chapter 7, "Maintaining a Healthy Weight," for lots of ideas that will help you prevent the weight loss that increases muscular weakness. Pay particular attention to the last section in that chapter called "Overall Diet Quality."

Eat to Maximize Energy

Take advantage of the fact that many times you wake up feeling your best—it's a time of day when muscular weakness is often the least noticeable (or at least not as bad as it is at the end of the day). Use this time to prepare a healthy and hearty breakfast. Remember, your "tank" is on empty after an all-night fast. Load it up with lots of good nutrition to maximize your energy for the rest of the day, especially in preparation for later in the day when weakness and fatigue generally strike. Remember, everyone (including people without disease) feels more fatigued and weak when they haven't eaten properly throughout the day, and this is no doubt even more true for people with myasthenia.

If you can, also use your maximum-energy time of the day to prepare meals and snacks for the rest of the day. Fix dinner, for example, and pop it in the refrigerator—that way you just have to heat it up at dinnertime. Try to prepare leftovers on purpose, especially those you can freeze, so you always have a nutritious meal on days when you don't feel like cooking.

Steroid Medications: Nutritional Problems

Steroid medications remain one of the mainstays of therapy for people with myasthenia—they are literally a life-saver. They are often used in fairly large doses during disease flare-ups, doses that can affect nutritional status. To minimize side effects of the drug, do what you can nutritionally, including:

➤ Get plenty of protein.

➤ Balance sodium and potassium.

➤ Plan for healthy, strong bones.

➤ Get enough zinc.

➤ Eat to prevent hyperlipidemia, or too-high levels of fats in the bloodstream—commonly known as hardening of the arteries or atherosclerosis.

➤ Watch out for diabetes, which can crop up when you take high doses of steroid medications.

➤ Watch out for the "steroid appetite," or your appetite kicked into high gear by this medication, and try not to gain weight while on the medication. While many people with myasthenia often have trouble keeping weight on, those on long-term steroids may battle excess weight while on higher steroid doses. Or it may be that your weight is like a yo-yo, going down when disease strikes, and then going back up as steroids abate symptoms and the steroid appetite kicks in.

For more detail on these points, refer to chapter 11.

Menus

MYASTHENIA GRAVIS

DAY ONE

Breakfast
Creamy Oatmeal (page 249)
½ cup apricot nectar

Morning Snack
Pumpkin Custard (page 400)

Lunch
Kielbasa Corn Chowder (page 377)
1 cup cranberry juice

Dinner
Grilled sole
The Best Mashed Potatoes (page 394)
½ cup apricot nectar

Evening Snack
1 cup ice cream
1 cup sliced strawberries

1877 calories, 96 g protein, 20 g fiber, 30 g total fat (14% of calories), 13 g saturated fat (6% of calories), 1192 mg calcium, 1795 mg sodium

DAY TWO

Breakfast
Bread Pudding (page 264)
1 cup skim milk

Morning Snack
Strawberry–Mandarin Orange Gelatin
(page 396)

Lunch
Chicken Rice and Mushroom Casserole
(page 305)
½ cup peach nectar

Afternoon Snack
½ cup peach nectar
1 banana

Dinner
Tuna Quiche (page 352)
½ cup skim milk
1 cup low-fat vanilla yogurt
1 cup sliced strawberries

Evening Snack
Pumpkin Custard (page 400)
½ cup skim milk

1992 calories, 112 g protein, 20 g fiber, 41 g total fat (18% of calories), 13 g saturated fat (6% of calories), 1886 mg calcium, 2787 mg sodium

DAY THREE

Breakfast
Creamy Scrambled Eggs (page 250)
1 cup peach nectar

Morning Snack
Banana Custard (page 400)

Lunch
White Cheddar Macaroni and Cheese
(page 278)
1 cup apricot nectar

Afternoon Snack
1 cup vegetable juice

Dinner
Best-Loved Ground Beef Casserole
(page 328)
1 cup skim milk

Evening Snack
1 cup ice cream

1681 calories, 81 g protein, 16 g fiber, 47 g total fat (25% of calories), 25 g saturated fat (13% of calories), 1260 mg calcium, 2479 mg sodium

DAY FOUR

Breakfast
Creamy Breakfast Barley with Bananas and Dried Cranberries (page 247)
½ cup pear nectar

Morning Snack
Strawberry-Mandarin Orange Gelatin (leftover from day two)

Lunch
Tuna Quiche (leftover from day two)
1 cup skim milk

Afternoon Snack
½ cup pear nectar

Dinner
Creamed Spinach and Chicken over English muffin (page 296)
1 cup cranberry juice

Evening Snack
Bread Pudding (leftover from day two)

1733 calories, 90 g protein, 24 g fiber, 27 g total fat (14% of calories), 8 g saturated fat (4% of calories), 1332 mg calcium, 1832 mg sodium

DAY FIVE

Breakfast
Tex–Mex Scrambled Eggs (page 253)
1 cup skim milk

Morning Snack
Banana Custard (leftover from day three)

Lunch
White Cheddar Macaroni and Cheese (leftover from day three)
1 cup cranberry juice

Afternoon Snack
2 fig bars
1 cup skim milk

Dinner
Chicken Rice and Mushroom Casserole (leftover from day two)
1 cup skim milk

Evening Snack
Strawberry-Mandarin Orange Gelatin (leftover from day two)
1 cup pear nectar

1901 calories, 106 g protein, 11 g fiber, 42 g total fat (20% of calories), 19 g saturated fat (9% of calories), 1844 mg calcium, 2292 mg sodium

DAY SIX

Breakfast
Banana Custard (leftover from day three)
1 cup apricot nectar

Morning Snack
Creamy Strawberry–Banana Gelatin (page 396)

Lunch
Lemon Fresh Salmon Patties with Creamed Peas (page 350)
The Best Mashed Potatoes (leftover from day one)

1 banana
½ cup skim milk

Afternoon Snack
1 cup ice cream
1 cup sliced strawberries

Dinner
Kielbasa Corn Chowder (leftover from day one)
15 oyster crackers
½ cup skim milk

Evening Snack
Pumpkin Custard (leftover from day one)

2042 calories, 107 g protein, 29 g fiber, 44 g total fat (19% of calories), 20 g saturated fat (8% of calories), 1970 mg calcium, 2744 mg sodium

DAY SEVEN

Breakfast
  Creamy Scrambled Eggs (page 250)
  1 cup peach nectar

Morning Snack
  Bread Pudding (leftover from day four)
  ½ cup skim milk

Lunch
  Creamed Spinach and Chicken
  over English Muffin (leftover from
  day four)
  1 cup skim milk

Afternoon Snack
  1 cup vegetable juice

Dinner
  Best-Loved Ground Beef Casserole
  (leftover from day three)
  1 cup skim milk

Evening Snack
  Creamy Strawberry-Banana Gelatin
  (leftover from day six)

1577 calories, 113 g protein, 17 g fiber, 27 g total fat (15% of calories), 9 g saturated fat (5% of calories), 1532 mg calcium, 2651 mg sodium

References

Donohoe, K.M. "Nursing Care of the Patient with Myasthenia Gravis." *Neurology Clinics* 12(2) (1994): 369–85.

Drachman, D.B., et al. "Oral Tolerance in Myasthenia Gravis." *Annals of the New York Academy of Science* 778 (1996): 258–72.

Garcia, Rio F., et al. "Breathing Pattern and Central Ventilatory Drive in Mild and Moderate Generalised Myasthenia Gravis." *Thorax* 49(7) (1994): 703–6.

Hopkins, L.C. "Clinical Features of Myasthenia Gravis." *Neurology Clinics* 12(2) (1994): 243–61.

Khan, O.A., and W.W. Campbell. "Myasthenia Gravis Presenting As Dysphagia: Clinical Considerations." *American Journal of Gastroenterology* 89(7) (1994): 1,083–85.

Sanders, D.B., and C. Scoppetta. "The Treatment of Patients with Myasthenia Gravis." *Neurology Clinics* 12(2) (1994): 343–68.

Schon, F., et al. "Myasthenia Gravis and Elderly People." *Age and Ageing* 25 (1996): 56–58.

Parkinson's Syndrome

20

One out of every hundred people over the age of sixty is diagnosed with Parkinson's Syndrome (PS), making it one of the most common ailments in the United States. Each year, some fifty thousand Americans learn they have this slowly progressive neurological disease.

Parkinson's Syndrome (PS) affects a small area of cells in the middle part of the brain, causing them to degenerate and eventually die. The loss of these brain cells causes a reduction in a vital brain chemical called dopamine, which is needed to carry messages from the brain to the muscles to tell them to move. Ultimately, this lack of dopamine causes tremors, muscle stiffness (also called rigidity), slowness of movement (bradykinesia), and loss of balance (postural dysfunction). Typically, PS patients have a stooped posture and they walk with a slow shuffling gait; sometimes, they "freeze" or have a sudden inability to walk. They can also have memory troubles and difficulty in controlling fine hand movements.

Good nutrition can play several roles in bettering the lives of people with Parkinson's. For all patients, modifying foods, eating utensils and menus appropriately can make eating easier and therefore help Parkinson's patients achieve the optimal nutrition that will give them the edge to fight their disease and to feel as strong as they can possibly feel.

All patients can benefit from a diet that helps them fight constipation. Whether due to inactivity or the Parkinson's disease process itself (causing decreased intestinal motility), constipation can be a tremendous problem, creating discomfort and decreasing appetite.

All patients can maximize the effectiveness of levodopa, a drug used to treat Parkinson's, by timing the medication properly. In addition, there is now evidence that modifying the protein content of the diet can help maximize the therapeutic benefit of levodopa in a select portion of PS patients.

The Nutrition Advantage

For many reasons, eating can be a real chore for people with PS. Sometimes, depression brought on by the disease can decrease appetite; in addition, appetite can lag just from the inactivity or as a result of the medication used to treat the disease. To make food more appealing to small appetites:

➤ Don't overfill the plate. The sight of too much food can be overwhelming, crushing whatever appetite someone may have.

➤ Arrange the table setting in a pretty and interesting manner. For example, set out a pretty place mat and napkin, even add a flower in a vase if that is convenient. In addition, arrange the food on the plate attractively.

➤ Offer smaller servings, but more frequently. Instead of serving cereal and juice at breakfast, serve the cereal alone and then offer juice an hour or two later.

➤ Consider serving food in an insulated dish (also available from the catalogs, page 403) to keep food warm. It often takes longer for people with PS to eat, and food can become cold and unappetizing.

To help people with Parkinson's feel more independent and maintain pride that they don't have to make a mess when eating (which they are more likely to do because their hands shake or their arms don't cooperate with moving their hands), try the following ideas. Note that some people with this condition don't like to eat just because they are afraid of making a mess or simply because they have a difficult time doing so independently.

➤ Purchase a rocker knife, which requires less coordination, but still allows a person with Parkinson's to cut her own food, an important step in feeling independent. Similarly, purchase forks and spoons with built-up handles, or make them yourself by using foam rubber.

➤ When using even a special knife becomes difficult, cut food into very small pieces for the person you care for.

➤ Arrange food toward the middle of the plate. This prevents the person with PS from spilling food onto the table, which can be very unappetizing and demoralizing.

➤ Alternatively, purchase high-sided plates, which help prevent spills. Food guards are also available to achieve the same purpose. These items are available from the catalogs (see page 403).

➤ Serve all liquids with a straw, which is a tremendous help in preventing the liquids from spilling. Similarly, fill glasses only partway. Also, add a couple of rubber bands to the center of the glass to facilitate holding on to it.

➤ Serve soup from a mug, allowing the person to drink it rather than eat it with a spoon.

➤ Encourage the person to use a spoon rather than a fork to eat foods that might roll around, such as peas.

If eating becomes more difficult, also modify food appropriately to make chewing and swallowing easier. For example:

➤ Serve creamy hot breakfast cereals rather than cold, crunchier versions. If the person you care for isn't on a protein-modified diet (see the later part of this chapter), make the oatmeal or cream of wheat with milk instead of water to boost protein, calories and nutrients (see the recipe on page 249).

→ Serve thicker beverages. Try nectars rather than juices, serving apricot, peach and pear nectars instead of apple or orange juice. This has another advantage: the nectars have more calories than the juices, which is important when eating is difficult and appetite is poor. In addition, always serve beverages with a straw.

→ Try finger foods when eating utensils become too difficult to use: soft peanut butter and jelly sandwiches cut into finger-sized pieces; gelatin squares made with extra plain gelatin to make them harder and "beefed up" with cottage cheese; tuna fish sandwiches cut into finger-sized pieces; soft cooked carrot coins; soft cooked broccoli pieces and other vegetables; cheese cubes.

→ Keep mealtime peaceful and quiet, helping the person you care for to concentrate on eating. Eating and speaking at the same time can be very difficult and can induce spasms that might cause choking.

Fight Constipation

Constipation can be quite uncomfortable; in addition, it can greatly reduce appetite. There are two ways to fight constipation, most importantly:

→ Ensuring adequate fluid intake.

→ Increasing the fiber content of the diet.

A high-fiber diet is critical to help the intestinal tract function normally. The indigestible portion of plant foods, fiber soaks up water in the intestinal tract. This makes intestinal wastes much heavier, speeding up their journey through the intestinal tract. Drinking enough liquids is key, as even with enough dietary fiber but too little fluid, fiber cannot do its job of battling constipation.

In addition to fighting constipation, fiber has other health benefits—depending on the type of fiber it is. There are two main types of fiber: soluble and insoluble. All plant foods generally have some soluble and some insoluble fiber, with some foods being better sources of one or the other. Soluble fiber, which is particularly abundant in oats and dried beans, dissolves in the watery contents of the gastrointestinal tract to form a gel. This gel corrals fats and chemicals in the intestinal tract that otherwise get absorbed and transformed into blood cholesterol. That's why foods high in soluble fiber lower blood cholesterol levels.

Insoluble fiber seems to fight colon cancer. One of the main ways is by cutting down on the number of polyps that form in the gastrointestinal tract. Polyps are small, pre-cancerous growths may grow larger and turn cancerous if left alone. There are at least two other avenues by which insoluble fiber decreases colon cancer risk. First, it shuttles wastes much faster through the intestinal tract. Cancer researchers think that translates into ushering out cancer-causing substances more rapidly, too, leaving them less time to exert their toxic influences on intestinal tissues.

Insoluble fiber thwarts another cancer-causing process. Bacteria normally present in the intestine produce enzymes that convert bile acids, body chemicals needed for digestion, into a more sinister form, secondary bile acids. Insoluble fiber soaks up and eliminates secondary bile acids and disables enzymes, rendering them less able to do their dirty work.

Maximize Medications

The most common medication used to treat PS is called levodopa, often called L-dopa for short and sold under the trade names Larodopa and Dopar; Sinemet contains levodopa and another drug called carbidopa. Levodopa helps make up for the loss of dopamine responsible for PS symptoms. Here's how. The drug enters the brain, where it is converted to dopamine, and is chemically indistinguishable from the dopamine naturally produced by the body. This extra hit of dopamine improves the communication between the brain and the muscles, alleviating some of the movement and coordination problems.

After about five years of taking levodopa, though, some one-half of Parkinson's patients start experiencing the "on-off" syndrome. During the "off" phase, they have erratic, uncontrollable tremors, rigidity and/or loss of movement. But during the "on" phase, they feel in control of their muscles. These alternating on-off phases are due to the fluctuating dopamine levels. When most people start taking dopamine, their disease is in such a state that that their brains still make some dopamine; therefore, the rate at which the medication reaches the brain isn't that critical. However, about five years into taking the medication, the disease in about half the people has progressed to the point where natural dopamine production has dramatically diminished. Because of this, the dopamine boost from the medication becomes increasingly important.

There are two ways to use diet to maximize levodopa's positive effect. The first is quite simple: take levodopa on an empty stomach. If taken with food, the amount of levodopa reaching the brain can be decreased, or at least delayed. If taken with food, some of the drug is broken down and inactivated by the greatly increased amount of stomach acid that is produced to digest the food. In addition, the remaining levodopa leaves the stomach much more slowly when food is present, which means it takes longer for the medication to reach the brain.

Many Parkinson's experts also believe that following a fairly strict diet and meal schedule can help prolong levodopa's positive effects and thereby decrease symptoms. In particular, the most critical dietary factor to control is protein.

Protein

Dietary protein is broken down by the body's digestive machinery into its constituent building blocks called amino acids. Eventually, the amino acids find their way into the bloodstream and are carried to every cell throughout the body, where they are used for many purposes (to repair tissues, make body chemicals, fight infections). In order to travel through the bloodstream, the amino acids have to have a form of transportation. Brain cells, like other cells, need a regular supply of protein to function properly. To get to the brain, amino acids attach to the same carriers that transport levodopa to the brain to be converted to dopamine. There is only a finite number of these carriers. As a result, after a meal that includes protein, the carriers become jam packed, leaving no mode of transportation for the dopamine to reach the brain. When a person's own dopamine production has fallen off so dramatically the result is the "off" phase described above.

The theory, then, is that restricting dietary protein all day while a person is up and active can help keep dopamine levels in the brain fairly constant and therefore prevent the on-off fluctuations. The bulk of dietary protein is given late in the day, just before bed. This way, the on-off period should occur one to three hours after eating, while the person sleeps.

A note of caution: some people ask if they can just go on a very low protein diet, and try to avoid the on-off phase all together. This, however, would be quite dangerous. *Dietary protein is an absolutely essential ingredient to good health, helping to repair tissues, fight infections, make hormones and manufacture thousands of other body chemicals necessary to live.* A person who doesn't eat enough protein would ultimately feel quite weak, and then begin to suffer many other consequences.

While the protein modified diet doesn't work in all Parkinson's patients who experience the on-off syndrome, it probably works in more people than not. Sometimes, patients think they are on the appropriate dietary modifications, but they really aren't. Protein is found in many foods, including breads, pastas, cakes and cookies and so all of these items must be restricted and timed accordingly. The following information should make it easier to follow the protein modified eating plan. *Note once again that this special diet is only intended for people who take levodopa and who are experiencing on-off fluctuations. This diet cannot prevent Parkinson's from occurring or from advancing.*

How Much Protein?

While many Americans eat close to 80 to 100 grams of protein daily, adults need only about 50 to 60 grams for good health. The protein-modified diet for people with the on-off syndrome in Parkinson's has a total of 50 grams of protein. But it is the way in which the protein is distributed that is so critical to preventing the on-off fluctuations.

When to Eat Protein

From morning until late in the day, restrict protein intake to just 10 grams. During this time, people can eat the following foods freely, as they are either protein free or very low in protein:

➤ All fresh, canned and dried fruits.

➤ All green and yellow vegetables, raw or cooked (except corn and peas, which are higher in protein and so are among the restricted foods).

➤ Lettuce, tomatoes, cucumbers, onions, pickles and avocado.

➤ Condiments, including oil, vinegar, margarine, butter, herbs, spices, salt, pepper, sugar, honey, jam, jelly and nondairy creamer.

➤ Coffee, tea, soda, all fruit and vegetable juices, water.

During the day, some people can eat foods containing small amounts of protein, including breads, bagels, breakfast cereal, rice, pasta, potatoes, popcorn, corn and peas. Some people can choose one serving of just one of these foods at each the breakfast and lunch meals. Refer to the chart for choices at each breakfast and lunch, as well as the appropriate serving sizes. *It is essential to measure accurately, as otherwise you'll end up getting too much protein and end up jeopardizing the success of the diet.* Also note that although the protein content of these foods is low, it is still enough to interfere with the amount of dopamine reaching the brain and cause the on-off problem in some people. You'll have to experiment to see if you tolerate these moderate protein foods during the day.

Breakfast: Choose One Serving of One Food*

Food	Serving Size
Bran cereal★★	
concentrated (such as Fiber One)	⅓ cup
flaked, such as All Bran	½ cup
Other breakfast cereal	Read the label and determine what portion will provide no more than 2 to 3 grams of protein total; in most cases, this is ½ to ¾ cup.
Cooked cereal, made with water instead of milk	Read the label and determine the portion that will provide no more than 2 to 3 grams of protein total; generally, ½ to ¾ cup.
Bread or toast	1 ounce slice (the size of most slices from commercial loaves).
English muffin	½
Bagel	⅓ or ½, depending on size of bagel; note that most bagels from bagel shops are generally 3 ounces.

Serve breakfast cereals with up to ½ cup of nondairy creamer, but not milk.

**Bran cereal is recommended because many people with Parkinson's experience constipation from their disease and/or relative inactivity.*

Lunch: Choose One Serving of One Food

Food	Portion Size Per Serving
Rice, white or brown	½ cup cooked
Pasta, plain	½ cup cooked
Potatoes, mashed with water	½ cup
Potatoes, baked or boiled	One 3-ounce potato
Potatoes, french fried	10 (1.5 ounce)
Popcorn, not flavored	3 cups
Corn or peas	½ cup

Late Dinner: Choose High-Protein Foods

The following foods contain the indicated amount of protein for the serving size listed. These foods should be reserved for a late dinner, and should total no more than 40 grams at this dinner meal. In addition, portion sizes should be measured carefully.

Food	Serving size	Protein (grams)
Chicken, turkey, beef, pork, lamb, fish	1 ounce	7
Cheese	1 ounce	7
Cottage cheese	¼ cup	8
Luncheon meats	1 ounce	5 to 7
Hot dogs, sausage	1 (2 ounces)	7
Tofu	1 ounce	2
Peanut butter	1 tablespoon	4
Lentils and other dried beans and peas, such as black beans, split peas, navy beans	½ cup	9
Milk (skim, 1%, 2%, whole)	8 ounces	8
Yogurt	1 cup	13
Ice cream	½ cup	2.5
Ice milk	½ cup	2.5
Custard	½ cup	7
Pudding	½ cup	4.5
Combination foods		
Pizza	⅛ of a 15-inch pie	15
Chili	1 cup	15
Macaroni and cheese	1 cup	13
Lasagna	4-ounce piece	10

Please note that chocolates, pies, cakes, cookies, pastries and other desserts are considered higher protein foods, and you should read labels to determine their protein content.

Calories

Following such a restricted eating plan, it can be hard to take in enough calories. In addition, it can be difficult to get in enough calories without going overboard on dietary fat. To help you get started on this eating plan, I've devised five days of menus, each totaling around two thousand calories. If you need more calories, add more protein-free foods, such as juices, nectars, fruit ices, margarine and olive oil.

Making Calories Count

As you read over the menus, note that they contain as many nutrient-heavy foods as possible, limiting the number of empty-calorie foods such as sherbets, jellies and fruit ices. For examples, notice that there is generally a couple of different types of nectars on each day's menus—these beverages are not only high in calories, but they're also loaded with nutrients. Similarly, I've included canned fruits, which are softer and generally easier to eat than fresh fruits, but still more nutritious than gelatins and sherbets. Making calories count means achieving better nutrition and therefore using nutrition to your greatest advantage.

In addition, I've used healthier fats throughout the menus. For example, instead of butter, I've used corn oil tub margarine; the calories are the same, teaspoon for teaspoon, but the fat in corn oil tub margarine is short on both saturated fat and the probably dangerous transfatty acids. Similarly, I've used olive oil where oil would be used, as it is high in monounsaturated fats, another better type of fat to include in the diet (see chapter 3 for more information on dietary fats).

Go for Variety

Notice that each day's menus contain several different types of juice, rather than just one type. Similarly, I've included a couple of different types of canned fruits and several different types of vegetables. Adding in such wonderful variety not only makes the diet more interesting but also helps ensure getting a wider variety of nutrients.

Supplement

Because foods from the bread group are limited in this diet, it is sometimes difficult to get all nutrients. These eating plans come quite close to getting in all essential nutrients at the recommended levels, but do fall a little short here and there. Taking a one-a-day vitamin/mineral supplement that supplies no more than 100 percent of the recommended dietary allowance (RDA) for all nutrients is good insurance for those days when you may fall a little short on some nutrients. Do remember, though, it's still a great idea to include foods in the eating plans that are nutrient-dense, and not to rely totally on the supplement.

Menus

PARKINSON'S SYNDROME

This eating plan is recommended only for people who take levodopa and who experience the on-off difficulties. Weighing and measuring foods that contain any significant quantity of protein is necessary to make sure you don't go overboard on protein. *I have placed a † after those foods that you should measure carefully.* Note that all dinners should be eaten late in the day, preferably about one-half to one hour before going to bed. Because of this late dinner time, I have included two snacks after lunch.

DAY ONE

Breakfast
½ English muffin
1 tablespoon corn oil tub
 margarine
1 tablespoon of jam or preserves
1 cup peach nectar

Morning Snack
1 cup canned apricots in heavy syrup

Lunch
Corn Chowder (see below)
1 cup canned peaches in heavy syrup

Afternoon Snack
1 cup grape juice

Afternoon Snack
1 cup sherbet

Dinner
8 ounce slice of lasagna (with cheese
 and meat)†
½ cup frozen green peas†
½ cup vanilla ice cream†

2015 calories, 43 g protein, 28 g fiber, 45 g total fat (19% of calories), 20 g saturated fat (8% of calories)

½ cup nondairy creamer
 (such as Rich's)
½ cup frozen corn

1 cup frozen green beans
1 cup frozen carrot slices
salt and pepper to taste

Corn Chowder

Combine all ingredients in microwave-safe bowl and microwave for 3 to 5 minutes, stopping to stir after two minutes, or until all vegetables are tender and heated through.

DAY TWO

Breakfast
⅓ cup Fiber One cereal†
½ cup nondairy creamer†
5 whole dates, chopped

Morning Snack
1 cup pear nectar

Lunch
Pasta Primavera (see below)
1 cup canned apricots in heavy syrup

Afternoon Snack
1 cup sherbet

Afternoon Snack
1 cup prune juice

Dinner
1 cup mashed potatoes† (mashed with
 margarine and milk)
4 ounces fried chicken†
4 tablespoons chicken gravy
1 cup pineapple juice

2000 calories, 57 g protein, 35 g fiber, 40 g total fat (17% of calories), 9.5 g saturated fat (4% of calories)

---

1 tablespoon olive oil
1 cup frozen broccoli pieces
1 cup frozen carrot coins

½ cup cooked small sea shell pasta
garlic, salt and pepper as desired

Pasta Primavera

Heat olive oil over medium heat; add frozen broccoli and frozen carrot coins, stir-frying until vegetables are hot. Add cooked pasta and spices as desired.

DAY THREE

Breakfast
  Apple oatmeal: ⅓ cup cooked oatmeal†
    (made with water, not milk) plus
    1 cup applesauce
  1 cup grape juice

Morning Snack
  1 cup apple juice

Lunch
  Rice Stir-Fry (see below)
  1 cup canned pears in heavy syrup

Afternoon Snack
  1 cup orange sherbet

Afternoon Snack
  ½ cup fruit ice or frozen juice bar

Dinner
  4 ounces grilled salmon†
  1 small boiled potato†, with 1 table-
    spoon corn oil tub margarine and
    fresh parsley
  1 cup broccoli pieces with 1 tablespoon
    corn oil tub margarine

1954 calories, 51 g protein, 24 g fiber, 67 g total fat (30% of calories), 12 g saturated fat (5% of calories)

Rice Stir-Fry

2 tablespoons olive oil
¼ cup chopped onion
1 cup frozen chopped spinach, thawed
1 cup frozen carrot coins

½ cup cooked brown rice†
salt, pepper and other spices as desired;
  soy sauce is an excellent addition

Heat oil over medium heat; add onions, spinach and carrots; stir-fry until vegetables are heated through; stir in rice and spices and stir-fry until all is heated through.

DAY FOUR

Breakfast
  ⅓ cup Fiber One cereal†
  1 banana, sliced
  ¼ cup nondairy creamer†
  1 cup pear nectar

Morning Snack
  1 cup apricot nectar

Lunch
  Salad: 2 cups chopped romaine lettuce;
    1 tomato, chopped; ½ cucumber,
    chopped; 3 tablespoons regular salad
    dressing (not low fat)

1 small baked potato† with 1 tablespoon
  corn oil tub margarine

Afternoon Snack
  1 cup sherbet

Afternoon Snack
  1 cup applesauce

Dinner
  4 ounce lean hamburger patty† on
    hamburger bun†
  1 cup grape juice

1990 calories, 51 g protein, 24 g fat, 67 g total fat (29% of calories), 16 g saturated fat (7% of calories)

References

Abbott, R.A., et al. "Diet, Body Size and Micronutrient Status in Parkinson's Disease." *European Journal of Clinical Nutrition* 46 (1992): 879–84.

Carlton, L. "Practical Pointers for Parkinsonians." *National Parkinson Foundation* (June 1996).

Davies, K.N., et al. "A Study of the Nutritional Status of Elderly Patients with Parkinson's Disease." *Age and Ageing* 23 (1994): 142–45.

Karstaedt, P.J., et al. "Standard and Controlled-Release Levodopa/Carbidopa in Patients with Fluctuating Parkinson's Disease on a Protein Redistribution Diet." *Archives of Neurology* 48 (1991): 402–05.

King, D., et al. "Concentrations of Vitamins A, C and E in Elderly Patients with Parkinson's Disease." *Postgraduate Medical Journal* 68 (1992): 634–37.

Morens, D.M., et al. "Case-Control Study of Idiopathic Parkinson's Disease and Dietary Vitamin E Intake." *Neurology* 46 (1996):1270–74.

National Parkinson Foundation. *The Parkinson's Handbook: A Guide for Parkinson Patients and Their Families.* Informative booklet. The National Parkinson Foundation, 1501 NW 9th Ave., Bob Hope Road, Miami Florida 33136, 305/547-6666.

National Parkinson Foundation. *The Parkinson's Patient: What You and Your Family Should Know.* Informative brochure. The National Parkinson Foundation, 1501 NW 9th Ave., Bob Hope Road, Miami Florida 33136, 305/547-6666.

Pengilly, K. "Introduction to Speech and Swallowing Problems Associated with Parkinson's Disease." National Parkinson Foundation, 3rd printing (October 1996).

Persson, M., et al. "Influence of Parkinson's Disease on Oral Health." *Acta Odontologica Scandinavia* 50 (1992): 37–42.

Pincus, J.H. "Nutritional Considerations of Parkinson's Disease: The Route of Better Management of Parkinson's Disease." National Parkinson Foundation, 7th printing (July 1996).

Yen, Peggy Kloster. "Does a Low-Protein Diet Help with Parkinson's?" *Geriatric Nursing* 11 (1990): 48.

Psoriasis

21

From the Greek work meaning "to itch," psoriasis can be a devastating skin condition—not because it kills, but because of the embarrassment and emotional stress induced by the disfiguring lesions it causes.

Fortunately, taking charge of diet in a few important ways may help some of the four to six million Americans (about 2 percent of the population) affected by psoriasis to control the condition.

What It Is: Too Many Skin Cells

A normal skin cell lives about one month. Every day, millions of skin cells die, are shed and then replaced by healthy ones. With psoriasis, however, the blueprint for normal skin cell reproduction is somehow damaged or lost. As a result, the body makes far too many skin cells—some thousand times more than is necessary. Dead cells pile up on top of each other, creating thick, reddened patches of skin covered with flaky, silver scales. These skin lesions are called plaques. Pain and itching results when this "horny" layer dries and cracks. While the skin over the knees, elbows, back and buttocks is most commonly affected, every inch of skin is susceptible. Even the scalp and fingernails can be affected.

There are many treatments for psoriasis that are highly effective. Some, however, have unpleasant side effects—that's why psoriasis patients and doctors alike have always searched for alternative therapies, including dietary solutions.

E. William Rosenberg, M.D., chairman of the department of dermatology at the University of Tennessee in Memphis, says that many dietary treatments have been tried, "But few have been definitively proven effective." He does acknowledge, though, that there is plenty of indirect evidence that something about certain diets does indeed improve psoriasis symptoms.

Some of the evidence goes back a few decades. Dutch psoriasis patients interned in Japanese prison camps during World War II, for example, experienced significant improvement in their psoriasis. No one knows, though, what dietary factor or factors is responsible for the improvement. It could be a particular food, such as the rice that was the dietary staple in the Japanese prison camps. Or it could have been just eating a calorie-restricted diet. The calorie-restricted theory gains support from the observation that some people with psoriasis who go on certain calorie-restricted diets for weight loss or to lower their cholesterol also coincidentally have some lessening of their psoriatic skin lesions.

For now, psoriasis experts recommend several dietary maneuvers that may help, including:

➤ Eat plenty of fruits and veggies.

➤ Eat for a healthy intestinal tract.

➤ Maintain a healthy, lean body weight, avoiding picking up excess pounds.

➤ Consume plenty of folic acid and protein.

➤ Avoid alcohol.

➤ Eat for a healthy immune system.

We'll review each of these factors, and also the effect of fish oil supplements and vitamin D supplements on psoriasis.

Eat Plenty of Fruits and Vegetables

In 1996, Italian researchers released the results of a large study that examined the effects of eating fruits and vegetables on psoriatic skin lesions. The results were promising, and should encourage people with psoriasis to load up their diet with plenty of nature's bounty.

These researchers studied 316 psoriatic patients and compared them to 366 people without psoriasis. They found that patients who ate more carrots, tomatoes, fresh fruit and green vegetables decreased the chances of getting psoriasis. In particular, certain fruits and vegetables reduced the risk of psoriasis by varying degrees:

➤ Eating at least three carrots per week decreased the risk 40 percent.

➤ Eating seven or more tomatoes weekly decreased the risk 60 percent.

➤ Consuming fourteen or more servings of fresh fruit weekly was associated with a 50 percent decreased risk.

➤ Eating at least ten servings of green vegetables weekly dropped the risk 30 percent.

While the Italian researchers have not nailed down the exact mechanism by which more fruits and vegetables decrease psoriasis symptoms, they theorize that it could be the antioxidant nutrients, or possibly the folic acid. By the way, don't take the point about antioxidant nutrients out of context: while consuming lots of fruits and vegetables helped, there's absolutely no evidence that taking antioxidant supplements would. Remember that antioxidant nutrients, being responsible for the improvement is just a theory—it could be something else in the fruits and vegetables. Better to stick with the real foods—it's the healthiest way to eat, anyway!

While other groups have not done formal studies, some have noticed an association between eating more produce and an improvement in psoriasis symptoms. "We have noticed that our psoriasis patients do better when they eat more fruits and vegetables," says

Dr. Rosenberg. "We definitely recommend including plenty of fruits and vegetables in the daily diet."

Eat for a Healthy Intestinal Tract

There are more than 400 kinds of bacteria that live in the intestine and that are necessary for a healthy intestinal tract. Because these bacteria are truly necessary to life, we call them healthy or good bacteria. Without them, we're likely to develop diarrhea and other maladies. And now, says Dr. Rosenberg, "there is evidence that the type and amounts of bacteria in the intestinal tract influence the immune system throughout the entire body. Because psoriasis is an immune system disease, there is mounting evidence that maintaining good levels of healthy gut bacteria may help lessen the severity of psoriasis."

So, how do you boost the population of healthy bacteria in the intestinal tract? The best way is to eat one cup of yogurt daily—just make sure that the yogurt has active yogurt cultures. While many yogurt brands are made with active yogurt cultures (and print this on the label), some are further processed in such a way that the active yogurt cultures are deactivated. Read that product label carefully to make sure that the product *has* active yogurt cultures, and wasn't just made with active cultures.

There is also some evidence that a diet high in complex carbohydrates boosts levels of good gut bacteria. To get complex carbohydrates, eat plant foods as close as possible to the way they come from nature. For example:

➤ Choose whole wheat products over white flour products, including whole wheat bread and bagels over their white counterparts.

➤ Opt for brown rice instead of white rice.

➤ Peel and enjoy a whole orange at breakfast instead of just the orange juice; similarly, crunch down an apple instead of drinking apple juice.

➤ Nibble on a whole carrot instead of "juicing" carrots and drinking the juice.

➤ Include legumes (lentils, soybeans, split peas, garbanzo beans) in your diet at least a couple of times per week, preferably daily.

Avoid Being Overweight

Since World War II, when people were held captive in prison camps and faced semi-starvation, dermatologists have noticed that psoriasis patients who stay on the lean side often have fewer relapses of their skin lesion.

Mark Lebwohl, M.D., chairman of department of dermatology at New York's Mt. Sinai Medical Center adds, "Patients who are overweight relapse sooner after some psoriasis treatments." In addition, studies have verified that being too heavy contributes to the chances of getting psoriasis in the first place. Refer to chapter 7 for ideas on how to trim down weight.

Boost Protein and Folic Acid

According to dermatologists at New York's Columbia University Medical Center, people with widespread psoriasis are at risk of losing precious protein and folic acid, one of the B vitamins. This is because protein and folic acid are important ingredients in the vast numbers of skin cells that psoriasis patients lose at such a rapid rate: the more active the disease, the more skin cells lost, and the more protein and folic acid lost.

The Columbia University Researchers used blood tests to analyze the nutritional status of fifty patients with severe psoriasis, testing for levels of protein and folic acid in their blood (blood tests that measure protein and folic acids reflect whether or not people have enough of these important nutritional factors in their bodies). They found that 18 percent were low on protein and 38 percent came up short on folic acid. Although folic acid and protein may not help you fight psoriasis, getting enough will help you be healthier overall. Incidentally, if you take methotrexate for your psoriasis, you may want to increase folic acid intake; this medication tends to deplete the body's stores of folic acid. Always try to get folic acid from food; when you do, you'll be eating an exceptionally healthy diet, as the good sources of folic acid are foods that are nutritional powerhouses. If you do take supplements, take care not to overload. If you take too much folic acid and you have a deficiency of another B vitamin, B_{12}, you can actually develop some irreversible neurological problems.

Refer to the sidebars below for how to get enough protein and folic acid.

Good Sources of Folic Acid

Although the recommended daily allowance for folic acid is only 180 mcg for adults (although many experts recommend raising it to 400 mcg), try to get at least 400 mcg.

2 cups romaine lettuce = 152 mcg
½ cup cooked spinach = 131 mcg
¼ cup toasted wheat germ = 99 mcg★
1 cup cooked lentils = 358 mcg★
1 cup cooked black beans = 256 mcg★

★Also a good source of protein and complex carbohydrates.

Good Sources of Protein

While all meats are good sources of protein, we've just included the lean varieties. Avoiding the fattier varieties is a help in maintaining a lean body weight, another advantage in reducing psoriasis symptoms. Try to get 50 to 60 grams of protein daily.

¼ cup toasted wheat germ = 8 grams★
1 cup cooked lentils = 18 grams★
1 cup cooked black beans = 15 grams★
3 ounces roasted, skinless chicken breast = 26 grams

3 ounces salmon = 22 grams
3 ounces pork tenderloin = 24 grams
3 ounces beef eye of round = 25 grams
1 cup skim milk = 8 grams
1 cup 1% (low-fat) cottage cheese = 28 grams
1 cup low-fat yogurt = 13 grams★★

★This is also a good source of complex carbohydrates, which helps boost the population of "good" intestinal bacteria.

★★A great way to boost the population of "good" intestinal bacteria, as long as the yogurt contains active yogurt cultures.

Avoid Alcohol

Consuming too much alcohol also worsens psoriasis, says Dr. Lebwohl. What's too much? "For some people, any alcohol at all worsens psoriasis; others can drink modest amounts, such as one or two drinks per day"; a drink is defined as 12 ounces of regular beer, 5 ounces of wine, and 1.5 ounces of 90-proof distilled spirits. The best way to tell how much alcohol is too much for you and your psoriasis is to keep track of what happens to your skin after drinking. Then, modify your intake accordingly, either decreasing alcohol intake or cutting it out altogether.

Fish Oil: An Uncertain Benefit

Greenland Eskimos, who eat lots of fish high in omega-3 fatty acids, rarely have psoriasis. Because of this observation, psoriasis researchers have searched for a role of fish oil in preventing or treating psoriasis. Before we continue, let's understand what fish oil is, and why it (theoretically) could help.

While the word *fat* almost always conjures up negative connotations, the fat in fish is definitely a healthier type of fat. This is largely because it contains a special type of polyunsaturated fatty acids called omega-3s. In particular, fish fat is especially abundant in two of these omega-3s: eicosapentaenoic acid and docosahexaenoic acid. Fish have this type of fat because it helps them adapt to the cold water in which they live, much more than other types of fat. And now we know that this special type of fat may confer health benefits to people who include fish in their diet.

Here's how. Omega-3s seem to keep the body's immune system from working overtime. Specifically, they cut down on the body's production of natural (and necessary) chemicals called prostaglandins, leukotrienes and thromboxanes. While the body needs some of these chemicals to function normally, too-high concentrations can lead to inflammation associated with several conditions, including possibly psoriasis. It might also cut down on the inflammation associated with arthritis and asthma.

According to the National Psoriasis Foundation, though, study results on the effects of fish oil supplements are mixed, with most studies, unfortunately, finding that the supplements had no benefit. Encouragingly, one British study of people who ate fish to get fish oil instead of taking supplements produced encouraging results. Psoriasis patients who ate 5½ ounces of fatty fish daily experienced modest improvement of psoriasis symptoms. Among the fattier fishes are mackerel, salmon, sardines and herring.

Avoid Vitamin D Supplements

You may have heard that downing lots of vitamin D helps alleviate psoriasis. "Indeed, that is the case," says Dr. Lebwohl, "but the amount you have to ingest orally is toxic." Taking high levels of vitamin D causes hypercalcemia, or too much calcium in the blood. In turn, this leads to calcium deposits in certain tissues, especially in the heart and kidneys—which causes irreversible damage.

Eat for a Healthy Immune System

The immune system is the body's way of fighting off foreign invaders, such as bacteria, viruses and allergens. In people with autoimmune diseases, though, the immune system somehow goes awry. While taking large amounts of certain nutrients isn't a way to boost the immune system, making sure you are well nourished in general is an excellent way to make sure the immune system is as healthy as it can be. Some of the nutrients that are especially important to a healthy immune system (as well as foods high in that nutrient) include:

- → PROTEIN: Milk, cheese, meat, legumes (such as lentils).

- → ZINC: Seafoods, meats, whole grains, legumes.

- → IRON: Red meat (the best source), fish, poultry, legumes, nuts and seeds, whole grains.

- → MANGANESE: Whole grains.

- → COPPER: Legumes, meats, seafood, shellfish, whole grains, nuts and seeds.

- → MAGNESIUM: Foods that are a good source of protein are generally a good source of magnesium; in addition, whole grains, legumes, nuts and seeds, green vegetables, avocados, bananas.

- → SELENIUM: Protein-rich foods including lean meat, poultry, fish, lentils, split peas and other legumes, milk, tofu, and cheese; whole grains are also a good source. One of the richest sources is Brazil nuts.

- → VITAMIN B$_6$: Chicken, fish, pork, eggs, liver, whole grains, legumes, avocados, bananas.

- → RIBOFLAVIN: Meat, poultry, fish, eggs and dairy products.

- → FOLIC ACID: Dark green leafy vegetables, such as romaine lettuce and spinach; orange juice.

- → VITAMIN B$_{12}$: Found only in foods of animal origin, including meats, seafood, dairy products and eggs.

- → THIAMIN: Whole grains, legumes, seeds, pork and brewer's yeast.

- → VITAMIN C: Citrus fruits, tomatoes, broccoli, cantaloupe, berries, cabbage, asparagus, green and red sweet peppers.

- → VITAMIN A: Sweet potatoes, carrots, evaporated skim milk, apricot nectar, liver, part skim ricotta cheese, cantaloupe, tomatoes, squash, spinach.

- → VITAMIN E: Asparagus, beet greens, broccoli, cabbage, mustard greens, soybeans, spinach, tomatoes, hams, almonds, peanut butter, sunflower seeds, blueberries, papaya, quinoa, wheat germ, tuna steak, salmon, sole, shrimp.

- → FATTY ACIDS: The human body needs a certain amount of special fats called essential fatty acids; most people get enough fatty acids if they get just 15 grams of fat per day. On the other hand, diets that have too much fat are thought to suppress the immune system. Therefore, it is suggested that people with autoimmune diseases eat a low-fat diet, or one in which no more than 20 to 30 percent (with the low end more commonly recommended) of calories as fat.

As you can see, the list of nutrients important to the immune system is quite long! That's why it is so important to eat a diet that supplies all essential nutrients, including plenty of whole grains, fruits, vegetables, protein foods and dairy foods.

A word to the wise: just because some is good, it doesn't mean that a little more is better. While you may be tempted to load up on vitamins in an attempt to "boost" your immune system, consider the results of studies with zinc. Researchers know that zinc is an essential ingredient in a healthy immune system. In one study, research subjects were given high doses of zinc (many times the RDA). Instead of boosting the immune system, these high doses actually suppressed it (as measured by the population of lymphocytes in the blood stream, one type of white blood cell). Similarly, in animal studies, the right amount of manganese helped study animals have a normal immune response, but an overdose suppressed their immune system. The best advice? Stick to the RDA for nutrients, concentrating on getting these nutrients from a healthy diet rather than from supplements.

Menus
PSORIASIS

The following menus for people with psoriasis are exceptionally high in dietary antioxidants—not the least of which are vitamin A, beta-carotene and vitamin C. More than that, though, the meal plans are high in a very wide variety of other dietary antioxidants that come from such a rich intake of fruits and vegetables.

The high fiber content of these menus will help make your intestinal tract healthier, which may be important in psoriasis. Choose the calorie level that helps you drop any excess weight you may carrying, another move that will give you the nutrition advantage in healing your skin. If 1,800 calories (the higher of the two levels given) aren't enough for you, add more grains, fruits, vegetables or nonfat dairy products.

Part 1: Weight Loss
DAY ONE

Breakfast
  2 slices whole wheat toast
  1 tablespoon peanut butter
  1 tablespoon jam
  1 cup skim milk

Morning Snack
  1 orange

Lunch
  Tuna sandwich: ½ can tuna (packed in water), 2 slices whole wheat bread, 2 leaves romaine lettuce, 2 slices tomato, 1 tablespoon low-fat mayonnaise
  1 apple
  1 cup skim milk

Afternoon Snack
  1 cup vegetable juice or tomato juice

Dinner
  One-Pot Chili (page 375)
  1 cup steamed broccoli
  1 cup skim milk

1523 calories, 98 g protein, 36 g fiber, 32 g total fat (18% of calories), 9 g saturated fat (5% of calories), 1309 mg calcium, 2329 mg sodium

Supplies over 120% of the (adult) RDA for the following nutrients: vitamin A, thiamin, riboflavin, niacin, vitamin B_6, vitamin C (494%!), folate, magnesium, manganese, phosphorus and selenium.

Day Two

Breakfast
½ cup nonfat cottage cheese
1 whole wheat English muffin
1 tablespoon jam
1 cup skim milk

Morning Snack
½ cup plain low-fat yogurt with 1 sliced peach

Lunch
Salad: 2 cups chopped romaine lettuce,
1 tomato (sliced), ½ cup garbanzo
beans (chickpeas—okay to use canned,
just drain and rinse to reduce sodium),
2 tablespoons low-fat dressing
1 ounce whole wheat pretzel sticks
1 cup vegetable juice

Dinner
Honey Glazed Carrots and Parsnips
with Chicken Thighs (page 298)
1 cup skim milk

Evening Snack
3 apricots, or 6 apricot halves (canned in juice)

1660 calories, 89 g protein, 28 g fiber, 24 g total fat (13% of calories), 6 g saturated fat (3% of calories), 1274 mg calcium, 2405 mg sodium

Supplies over 120% of the (adult) RDA for the following nutrients: vitamin E, thiamin, riboflavin, niacin, vitamin B₁₂, vitamin C, folate, magnesium, manganese, phosphorous and selenium.

Day Three

Breakfast
Creamy Breakfast Barley with Bananas
and Dried Cranberries (page 247)

Lunch
Peanut butter and jelly sandwich:
2 tablespoons peanut butter,
1 tablespoon jam, 2 slices whole
wheat bread
1 cup skim milk
1 orange
6 baby carrots

Afternoon Snack
1 fig bar
1 cup skim milk

Dinner
Lentil Vegetable Soup (page 371)
Salad: 2 cups romaine lettuce, ½ tomato
(chopped), 2 tablespoons fat-free salad
dressing
Ice water

Evening Snack
1 cup fresh or frozen raspberries

1604 calories, 71 g protein, 42 g fiber, 32 g total fat (17% fat), 6 g saturated fat (3% of calories), 1312 mg calcium, 1422 mg sodium

Supplies over 120% of the (adult) RDA for the following nutrients: vitamin A, thiamin, riboflavin, niacin, vitamin B₆, vitamin B₁₂, folate, magnesium, manganese, phosphorus and selenium.

Day Four

Breakfast
1 poached egg
2 slices whole wheat toast
1 teaspoon margarine
1 cup skim milk

Morning Snack
1 cup cantaloupe pieces
1 cup vegetable juice or tomato juice

Lunch
Favorite Tuna Pasta Salad (page 275)
1 cup skim milk

Afternoon Snack
    1 chocolate chip cookie
    ½ cup skim milk
    1 peach

Dinner
    5 ounces grilled salmon
    1 medium sweet potato, baked

1 teaspoon margarine
1 cup steamed broccoli

Evening Snack
    ½ cup nonfat frozen yogurt

1535 calories, 112 g protein, 22 g fiber, 46 g total fat (22% of calories), 8 g saturated fat (5% of calories)

Supplies over 120% of the (adult) RDA for the following nutrients: vitamin A, thiamin, riboflavin, niacin, vitamin B$_6$, vitamin B$_{12}$ (554%!), vitamin C (504%!), folate, magnesium, phosphorus and selenium.

DAY FIVE

Breakfast
    Oatmeal: Mix ½ cup oats with 1 cup
    skim milk. Microwave on high for
    2 minutes; stir and microwave 2 min-
    utes more. Or combine in a heavy pot
    and simmer for 7 minutes.
    1 sliced banana
    1 cup orange juice

Lunch
    Turkey sandwich: 3 ounces lean turkey,
    2 slices whole wheat bread, 2 leaves
    romaine lettuce, 2 slices tomato,
    1 tablespoon light mayonnaise

1 orange
1 cup skim milk

Afternoon Snack
    10 thin pretzel sticks
    1 cup peach or apricot nectar

Dinner
    Chicken and Zucchini Spaghetti
       (page 283)
    1 peach
    1 cup skim milk

Evening Snack
    ½ cup ice cream

1539 calories, 91 g protein, 18 g fiber, 29 g total fat (17% of calories), 10 g saturated fat (6% of calories), 1197 mg calcium, 1496 mg sodium

Supplies more than 120% of the (adult) RDA for the following nutrients: vitamin A, thiamin, riboflavin, niacin, vitamin B$_6$, vitamin B$_{12}$, vitamin C, folate, magnesium, phosphorus and selenium.

DAY SIX

Breakfast
    ½ cup nonfat cottage cheese
    1 whole wheat English muffin
    1 tablespoon jam
    1 cup skim milk

Morning Snack
    1 peach

Lunch
    Barley and Bacon Soup
       (page 370)

6 baby carrots
1 cup skim milk

Afternoon Snack
    1 chocolate chip cookie
    ½ cup skim milk

Dinner
    Hamburger: 3 ounces very lean
       ground beef, 1 hamburger bun,
       1 slice tomato (ketchup and mustard
       as desired)

Salad: 2 cups chopped romaine lettuce,
  1 tomato (chopped), ¼ cup grated
  carrot, ½ red bell pepper (chopped),
  2 tablespoons fat-free dressing
1 cup skim milk

Evening Snack
1 orange
1 cup vegetable or tomato juice

1516 calories, 102 g protein, 32 g fiber, 31 g total fat (18% of calories), 10 g saturated fat (6% of calories), 1333 mg calcium, 3511 mg sodium

Supplies more than 120% of the (adult) RDA for the following nutrients: vitamin A, thiamin, riboflavin, niacin, vitamin B_6, vitamin B_{12}, vitamin C, folate, magnesium, manganese, selenium and zinc.

DAY SEVEN

Breakfast
1 poached egg
2 slices whole wheat toast
1 tablespoon jam
½ cup skim milk

Morning Snack
½ cup orange juice

Lunch
Cream of Broccoli Soup (page 368)
4 crackers
1 tomato sliced, sprinkled with balsamic
  vinegar and basil (dried or fresh)
½ cup skim milk

Afternoon Snack
2 fig bars
½ cup skim milk

Dinner
5 ounces grilled tuna
1 baked potato
2 tablespoons nonfat sour cream
1 cup frozen peas and carrots, steamed
  in microwave
½ cup apricot nectar

Evening Snack
½ cup nonfat frozen yogurt with a sliced
  banana

1687 calories, 106 g protein, 22 g fiber, 29 g total fat (15% of calories), 11 g saturated fat (6% of calories), 1117 mg calcium, 1592 mg sodium

Supplies more than 120% of the (adult) RDA for the following nutrients: vitamin A, thiamin, riboflavin, niacin, vitamin B_6, vitamin B_{12}, vitamin C, folate, magnesium and selenium.

DAY ONE

Breakfast
2 slices whole wheat toast
2 tablespoons peanut butter
1 tablespoon jam
1 cup skim milk

Morning Snack
1 orange

Lunch
Tuna sandwich: ½ can tuna (packed in water), 2 slices whole wheat bread, 2 leaves romaine lettuce, 2 slices tomato, 1 tablespoon low-fat mayonnaise

1 apple
1 cup skim milk

Afternoon Snack
1 cup vegetable juice

Dinner
One-Pot Chili (page 375)
1 cup steamed broccoli
1 cup skim milk

Evening Snack
2 chocolate chip cookies
½ cup skim milk

1756 calories, 107 g protein, 38 g fiber, 46 g total fat (23% of calories), 12 g saturated fat (6% of calories), 1468 mg calcium, 2537 mg sodium

Supplies more than 120% of the (adult) RDA for the following nutrients: vitamin A, thiamin, riboflavin, niacin, vitamin B_6, vitamin B_{12}, vitamin C, folate, magnesium, manganese, selenium and zinc.

DAY TWO

Breakfast
½ cup nonfat cottage cheese
1 whole wheat English muffin
1 tablespoon jam
1 cup skim milk

Morning Snack
½ cup low-fat fruited yogurt
1 peach

Lunch
Salad: 2 cups chopped romaine lettuce, 1 tomato (sliced), 1 cup garbanzo beans (chickpeas—okay to use canned,

just drain and rinse to reduce sodium), 2 tablespoons low-fat dressing
1 ounce whole wheat pretzel sticks
1 cup vegetable or tomato juice

Dinner
Honey Glazed Carrots and Parsnips with Chicken Thighs (page 298)
2 apricots (or 4 canned apricot halves packed in water)
1 cup skim milk

Evening Snack
½ cup ice cream

1886 calories, 99 g protein, 34 g fiber, 33 g total fat (16% of calories), 11 g saturated fat (5% of calories), 1244 mg calcium, 2652 mg sodium

Supplies more than 120% of the (adult) RDA for the following nutrients: vitamin A, thiamin, riboflavin, niacin, vitamin B_6, vitamin B_{12}, vitamin C, folate, magnesium, manganese and selenium.

DAY THREE

Breakfast

Creamy Breakfast Barley with Bananas
and Dried Cranberries (page 247)

1 cup apple juice

Lunch

Peanut butter and jelly sandwich:

2 tablespoons peanut butter, 1 tablespoon jam, 2 slices whole wheat bread

1 orange

6 baby carrots

1 cup skim milk

Afternoon Snack

2 fig bars

½ cup skim milk

Dinner

Lentil Vegetable Soup (page 371)

Salad: 2 cups romaine lettuce, ½ tomato
(chopped), 2 tablespoons dressing

1 cup skim milk

Evening Snack

1 cup fresh or frozen raspberries with
½ cup milk and a sprinkle of sugar if
you desire

*1855 calories, 80 g protein, 43 g fiber, 34 g total fat (17% fat), 7 g saturated fat (3% of calories),
1640 mg calcium, 1605 mg sodium*

*Supplies more than 120% of the (adult) RDA for the following nutrients: vitamin A, thiamin, riboflavin,
niacin, vitamin B$_6$, vitamin B$_{12}$, folate, magnesium, manganese and selenium.*

DAY FOUR

Breakfast

1 poached egg

2 slices whole wheat toast

1 teaspoons margarine

1 cup skim milk

Morning Snack

1 cup cantaloupe pieces

1 cup vegetable or tomato juice

Lunch

Favorite Tuna Pasta Salad (page 275)

5 whole grain rye crisp

1 cup skim milk

Afternoon Snack

1 chocolate chip cookie

1 peach

½ cup skim milk

Dinner

5 ounces grilled salmon

1 medium sweet potato, baked

1 teaspoon margarine

1 cup steamed broccoli

Evening Snack

1 cup nonfat frozen yogurt

1756 calories, 121 g protein, 29 g fiber, 39 g total fat (27% of calories), 9 g saturated fat (6% of calories)

*Supplies more than 120% of the (adult) RDA for the following nutrients: vitamin A, thiamin, riboflavin,
niacin, vitamin B$_6$, vitamin B$_{12}$ (578%), vitamin C (505%), folate, magnesium, manganese and selenium.*

DAY FIVE

Breakfast

Oatmeal: Mix ½ cup oats with 1 cup
skim milk. Microwave on high 2 minutes; stir and microwave for 2 minutes

more. Or combine in a heavy pot and
simmer for 7 minutes.

1 sliced banana

1 cup orange juice

Lunch

Turkey sandwich: 3 ounces lean turkey,
2 slices whole wheat bread, 1 slice
American cheese, 2 leaves romaine
lettuce, 2 slices tomato, 1 tablespoon
light mayonnaise

1 orange

1 cup skim milk

Afternoon Snack

10 thin pretzel sticks

1 cup peach or apricot nectar

Dinner

Chicken and Zucchini Spaghetti
(page 283)

1 peach

1 cup skim milk

Evening Snack

1 cup ice cream

*1849 calories, 102 g protein, 19 g fiber, 44 g total fat (21% of calories), 18 g saturated fat (9% of calories),
1415 mg calcium, 1850 mg sodium*

*Supplies more than 120% of the (adult) RDA for the following nutrients: vitamin A, thiamin, riboflavin,
niacin, vitamin B$_6$, vitamin B$_{12}$, folate, magnesium, manganese and selenium.*

Day Six

Breakfast

½ cup nonfat cottage cheese

1 whole wheat English muffin

1 tablespoon jam

1 cup skim milk

Morning Snack

1 peach

Lunch

Barley and Bacon Soup (page 370)

6 baby carrots

1 cup skim milk

Afternoon Snack

1 chocolate chip cookie

½ cup skim milk

Dinner

Hamburger: 3 ounces very lean
ground beef, 1 hamburger bun,
1 slice tomato (ketchup and mustard
as desired)

Salad: 2 cups chopped romaine
lettuce, 1 tomato (chopped), ¼ cup
grated carrot, ½ red bell pepper
(chopped), 2 tablespoons fat-free salad
dressing

1 cup skim milk

Evening Snack

1 orange

1 cup vegetable or tomato juice

*1877 calories, 118 g protein, 32 g fiber, 37 g total fat (17% of calories), 13 g saturated fat (6% of calories),
1882 mg calcium, 4100 mg sodium*

*Supplies more than 120% of the (adult) RDA for the following nutrients: vitamin A, thiamin, riboflavin,
niacin, vitamin B$_6$, vitamin B$_{12}$, vitamin C (600%), folate, magnesium, manganese, selenium and zinc.*

Day Seven

Breakfast

1 poached egg

2 slices whole wheat toast

1 tablespoon jam

½ cup skim milk

Morning Snack

1 cup orange juice

Lunch

Cream of Broccoli Soup (page 368)

1 sliced tomato, sprinkled with balsamic
vinegar and basil (dried or fresh)

1 whole wheat bagel
2 teaspoons margarine
1 cup skim milk

Afternoon Snack
2 fig bars
½ cup skim milk

Dinner
5 ounces grilled tuna
1 baked potato

2 tablespoons nonfat sour cream
½ cup frozen peas and carrots, steamed in microwave
1 cup apricot nectar

Evening Snack
½ cup nonfat frozen yogurt with a sliced banana

1946 calories, 116 g protein, 27 g fiber, 36 g total fat (17% of calories), 12 g saturated fat (6% of calories), 1297 mg calcium, 1872 mg sodium

Supplies more than 120% of the (adult) RDA for the following nutrients: vitamin A, thiamin , riboflavin, niacin, vitamin B$_6$, vitamin B$_{12}$ (965%), folate, magnesium, manganese and selenium.

References

Burrall, B., et al. "Psoriasis Therapies: Old, New, and Borrowed." *Patient Care* 29(17) (1995): 38–51.

Camisa, C., et al. *Psoriasis.* Boston: Blackwell, 1994.

Collier, P.M., et al. "Effect of Regular Consumption of Oily Fish Compared with White Fish on Chronic Plaque Psoriasis." *European Journal of Clinical Nutrition* 47 (1993): 251–54.

Fitzpatrick, T.B. "Effective Treatment of Psoriasis." *Fitzpatrick's Journal of Clinical Dermatology* 3(6) (1995): 12–16.

Greaves, M.W., and G.D. Weinstein. "Treatment of Psoriasis." *Drug Therapy* 332(9) (1995): 581–88.

Mayfield E. "Psoriasis Treatments: Relieving That Miserable Itch." *FDA Consumer* (April 1995): 12–15.

Murray, M.T. "Treating Psoriasis Naturally." *American Journal of Natural Medicine* 3(9) (1996): 8–11.

Naldi, L., et al. "Dietary Factors and the Risk of Psoriasis: Results of an Italian Case-Control Study." *British Journal of Dermatology* 134 (1996): 101–06.

National Psoriasis Foundation. *Your Diet and Psoriasis.* Pamphlet, 1995. 503/244-7404.

National Research Council. *Recommended Daily Allowances.* 10th ed. Baltimore: National Academy Press, 1989.

Prystowsky, J.H., et al. "Update on Nutrition and Psoriasis." *International Journal of Dermatology* 32(8) (1993): 582–86.

Shils, M.E., et al. *Modern Nutrition in Health and Disease.* Philadelphia: Lea-Febiger, 1994. 8th ed., vol. 1.

Sjögren's Syndrome   22

Pronounced "show-grins," Sjögren's Syndrome is a chronic inflammatory disorder in which the mucus-secreting glands (called exocrine glands) in the body don't work properly because of autoimmune destruction—the immune system working against the body's own tissues. Most noticeably, this causes dry eyes and dry mouth, with the severity of symptoms varying from patient to patient and even in the same patient. Some people with this disease also suffer from skin, nose and/or vaginal dryness. About four million Americans have this disease, with nine out of ten patients being women.

Sjögren's Syndrome can occur alone or in association with other autoimmune diseases such as rheumatoid arthritis and lupus. About 50 percent of people with Sjögren's have another disease, and are said to have secondary Sjögren's disease. Sjögren's can cause just dry eyes and dry mouth, or it can also damage the vital organs in the body. For example, it can affect the gastrointestinal tract, kidneys, blood vessels, liver, pancreas and brain. In addition, people who have the systemic version of the disease can experience debilitating fatigue and joint pain which can seriously impair quality of life.

When it comes to nutrition, Sjögren's Syndrome can have many negative effects, including:

➤ The inability to eat drier foods, due to the lack of saliva.

➤ Tooth decay and earlier tooth loss, which decreases the ability to chew and eat.

➤ The proper absorption of nutrients, thereby increasing the need for some nutrients.

➤ The need for increased nutrient intake to recover from mouth infections, which are a common concern for people with Sjögren's Syndrome.

In addition, because Sjögren's Syndrome is an autoimmune system disease, everyone with this condition should eat for a healthy immune system.

Eat for a Healthy Immune System

The immune system is the body's way of fighting off foreign invaders, such as bacteria, viruses and allergens. In people with autoimmune diseases, though, the immune system somehow goes awry. While taking large amounts of certain nutrients isn't a way to boost the immune system, making sure you are well nourished in general is an excellent way to make sure the immune system is as healthy as it can be. Some of the nutrients that are especially important to a healthy immune system (as well as foods high in that nutrient) include:

- → PROTEIN: Milk, cheese, meat, legumes (such as lentils).
- → ZINC: Good sources include seafoods, meats, whole grains, legumes.
- → IRON: Red meat (the best source), fish, poultry, legumes, nuts and seeds, whole grains.
- → MANGANESE: Whole grains.
- → COPPER: Legumes, meats, seafood, shellfish, whole grains, nuts and seeds.
- → MAGNESIUM: Foods that are a good source of protein are generally a good source of magnesium; in addition, whole grains, legumes, nuts and seeds, green vegetables, avocados, bananas are good sources.
- → SELENIUM: Protein-rich foods such as lean meat, poultry, fish, eggs, lentils, split peas and other legumes, milk, tofu and cheese are a good source of selenium, as are whole grains. One of the richest sources is Brazil nuts.
- → VITAMIN B_6: Chicken, fish, pork, eggs, liver, whole grains, legumes, avocados, bananas.
- → RIBOFLAVIN: Meat, poultry, fish, eggs, and dairy products.
- → FOLIC ACID: Dark green leafy vegetables, such as romaine lettuce and spinach; orange juice.
- → VITAMIN B_{12}: This vitamin is found only in foods of animal origin, including meats, seafood, dairy products and eggs.
- → THIAMIN: Whole grains, legumes, seeds, pork and brewer's yeast.
- → VITAMIN C: Citrus fruits, tomatoes, broccoli, cantaloupe, berries, cabbage, asparagus, green and red sweet peppers.
- → VITAMIN A: Sweet potatoes, carrots, evaporated skim milk, apricot nectar, liver, part skim ricotta cheese, cantaloupe, tomatoes, squash, spinach.
- → VITAMIN E: Asparagus, beet greens, broccoli, cabbage, mustard greens, soybeans, spinach, tomatoes, hams, almonds, peanut butter, sunflower seeds, blueberries, papaya, quinoa, wheat germ, tuna steak, salmon, sole, shrimp.
- → FATTY ACIDS: The human body needs a certain amount of special fats called essential fatty acids; most people get enough fatty acids if they get just fifteen grams of fat per day. On the other hand, diets that have too much fat are thought to suppress the immune system. Therefore, it is suggested that people with autoimmune diseases eat a low-fat diet, or one in which no more than 20 to 30 percent (with the low end more commonly recommended) of calories as fat.

As you can see, the list of nutrients important to the immune system is quite long! That's why it is so important to eat a diet that supplies all essential nutrients, including plenty of whole grains, fruits, vegetables, protein foods and dairy foods.

A word to the wise: just because some is good, it doesn't mean that a little more is better. While you may be tempted to load up on vitamins in an attempt to "boost" your immune system, consider the results of studies with zinc. Researchers know that zinc is an essential ingredient in a healthy immune system. In one study, research subjects were given high doses of zinc (many times the Recommended Dietary Allowance). Instead of boosting the immune system, these high doses actually suppressed it (as measured by the population of lymphocytes in the bloodstream; lymphocytes are one type of white blood cell). Similarly, in animal studies, the right amount of manganese helped study animals have a normal immune response, but an overdose suppressed their immune system. The best advice? Stick to the Recommended Daily Allowance (RDA) for nutrients, concentrating on getting these nutrients from a healthy diet rather than from supplements.

Not Enough Saliva

While most people don't even think about it, saliva is absolutely necessary for the ability to eat. It's nearly impossible, for example, to chew meat or bread without producing saliva to moisten it. This is how it is, though, for people with Sjögren's Syndrome. Sometimes, the problem is very severe, making a normal eating style difficult to impossible. Saliva is important for another reason: it contains substances that begin the food digestion process, especially of carbohydrates. Sometimes, it is difficult for Sjögren's patients to consume a balanced diet, simply because they must have such moist foods, making many food choices inappropriate.

Here are some suggestions to compensate for the lack of saliva:

➤ Keep your mouth moist by sipping sugar-free liquids, especially water, frequently (see below for more information about maintaining healthy teeth and why sugary liquids are a problem).

➤ Eat moister foods, such as soups, stews, meat with gravy and sauces. Some foods that you may want to emphasize are custards (see the recipes on pages 399–402); macaroni and cheese (page 278); creamy cooked cereals, but cook them with milk to increase the protein content (pages 247–50); soups (pages 364–74). In addition, try the recipes on pages 306, 323, 326, one-pot meals that are quite moist and also loaded with lots of great nutrition.

➤ Avoid spicy spices such as pepper, chili powder, nutmeg and cloves. People who have dry mouths often develop sores or infections in their mouths, and these spices can be very irritating.

➤ Avoid orange and grapefruit juices when you have sores in your mouth or if your mouth is just always so dry that these things bother you consistently.

➤ Dip dry foods such as cookies and crackers in milk, coffee or tea to help you chew and swallow them.

➤ When eating drier foods, drink fluids frequently to aid in chewing and swallowing.

Tooth Decay and Early Tooth Loss

In addition to being a critical aid in chewing and swallowing, saliva is necessary to clean the teeth. Saliva also contains minerals that help keep the teeth hard and to resist decay. Lacking enough saliva, the teeth become especially vulnerable to decay and loss. In addition, the gums can be affected, causing periodontal disease, which you'll recognize by red, swollen gums that bleed easily. This, too, can cause tooth loss: the more affected the gums, the more likely the gum line is to shrink away from the teeth. When more of the tooth surface is exposed, the possibility of decay is greater. In addition, the bone holding the teeth in place, the jawbone, can become infected if it becomes exposed; this in turns causes teeth to loosen and fall out.

Without your own teeth, chewing and swallowing can be especially difficult, making eating a nutritionally balanced diet very difficult. While good dental hygiene is important for everyone, it is especially critical for people with Sjögren's.

➤ Brush teeth after every meal. If you can't, at least rinse with plenty of water.

➤ Use dental floss daily.

➤ Polish teeth with a cotton swab at least once daily.

➤ Ask your dentist if applying a daily fluoride treatment can help you. While this can be a tremendous help in protecting teeth from decay and also making them less sensitive to hot and cold substances, do so only under a dentist's guidance.

➤ Also ask your dentist about other special (and usually prescription) substances with which to rinse your mouth to help reduce the bacteria population, and thereby reduce the chance of decay and gum disease.

➤ Yet another substance to ask the dentist about is something that helps harden your teeth, just as the minerals in saliva are supposed to.

➤ Reduce consumption of sugary foods. The bacteria that live in the mouth use the sugar in food and their own food; a by-product of their "consuming" this sugar is an acid. It is the acid produced by the combination of bacteria and sugar that causes tooth decay. This is why it is important to cut down on your consumption of sugary foods, especially sticky sugary foods such as honey, syrup, caramels and raisins.

➤ Keep your mouth as moist as possible by chewing on sugarless gum and eating sugarless candy or drinking sugar-free beverages between meals.

Nutrient Malabsorption

When Sjögren's affects the large and small intestine, it can result in malabsorption, or a condition in which the intestinal tract fails to absorb all the nutrients in food. Even if the disease process itself doesn't cause malabsorption, eating poorly and taking in too little of certain nutrients can cause a malabsorption syndrome. Whatever the cause, when this happens, the intestine becomes less efficient at absorbing nutrients, and instead shuttles them through the body unabsorbed. In addition, people may not absorb as many calories, causing them to lose excessive amounts of weight.

To counteract nutrient malabsorption:

➤ Take a multivitamin and mineral supplement daily, which might actually improve absorption.

➤ Try not to eat empty-calorie foods, opting instead for nutrient-rich foods. For example, instead of eating relatively low nutrition ice cream, opt instead for yogurt into which you've sliced fresh fruit such as a banana. Instead of white rice, choose brown rice; substitute a sweet potato for a white potato. If you mash potatoes, mash in some cottage cheese or low-fat cream cheese (low fat because it is higher in protein).

➤ Ask your doctor if you should avoid any particular food. For example, if you have severe malabsorption, you may temporarily lose the ability to digest the sugar in milk and milk products, causing a temporary lactose intolerance. As a result, you can suffer even worse malabsorption. When this occurs, it may be necessary to cut back or eliminate milk from the diet temporarily.

Fighting Mouth Infections

When the mouth becomes so dry, the tissues can become more fragile and tear. Because the bacteria population in the mouth is generally higher in people who have Sjögren's Syndrome, these sores may become infected. To help sores heal without becoming infected and also to help infected sores clear up more quickly:

➤ Increase protein intake: protein is a very necessary ingredient in healing tissues. Milk, cottage cheese, yogurt, cheese and meats all contain excellent types and quantities of protein; in addition, lentils and other legumes (which you can make up into stews and soups that are easy to swallow) are an excellent source of protein. Aim to get around sixty to a hundred grams of protein if you have an infection to heal (as long as you don't have any other condition for which protein is a problem, such as kidney disease).

➤ Get enough zinc: this mineral is also essential in fighting infections. Good sources of zinc include seafoods, meats, whole grains and legumes (such as lentils).

➤ Get enough vitamin A. Soon after its discovery, vitamin A was dubbed the anti-infective vitamin, because of the important role it has in healing. The best way to get vitamin A is to increase the amount of red/orange and dark green fruits and vegetables in your diet. However, don't overdose on vitamin A. Because it's fat soluble, the body stores excesses, which quickly become toxic. Getting vitamin A from fruits and vegetables, by the way, helps you avoid the possibility of getting toxic amounts of vitamin A. In these foods, vitamin A is found as the water-soluble building blocks, which the body converts into vitamin A as needed, secreting the excess. Foods high in vitamin A include sweet potatoes, carrots, evaporated skim milk, apricot nectar, liver, part skim ricotta cheese, cantaloupe, tomatoes, squash and spinach.

Menus

SJÖGREN'S SYNDROME

These seven days of menus meet the nutritional needs of Sjögren's patients who are experiencing a dry or infected mouth: they're loaded with good nutrition (they contain at least 100 percent of the RDA for most nutrients, with most having upward of 200 to 300 percent of the RDA). In addition, they are high in protein, to help prevent and battle mouth infections, a common concern. Finally, I've made a point of leaving out recipes with spicy flavors, as such foods might trouble people with sore mouths. I've also paid special attention to working in plenty of vitamin A and zinc—both thought to be important to individuals who live with Sjögren's Syndrome. All the recipes here are exceptionally easy to prepare, and will take you through the week!

DAY ONE

Breakfast
Creamy Oatmeal (page 249) with
   1 banana, sliced
   1 cup apple juice

Morning Snack
   1 cup vanilla yogurt with ½ cup sliced
   strawberries

Lunch
Sandwich: ½ can tuna (packed in oil);
   2 slices whole wheat bread;
   1 tablespoon mayonnaise

2 peach halves (canned in juice)
1 cup skim milk

Dinner
Chicken Pot Pie (page 310)
1 cup steamed spinach with 1 teaspoon
   margarine
1 cup pear nectar

Evening Snack
½ cup chocolate pudding (instant, made
   with skim milk) with 2 tablespoons
   frozen whipped topping

1919 calories, 97 g protein, 25 g fiber, 37 g total fat (12 g saturated fat), 1696 mg calcium, 2521 mg sodium, 4795 mg potassium, at least 100% of RDA for all nutrients

DAY TWO

Breakfast
Creamy Scrambled Eggs (page 250)
½ cup applesauce
1 cup skim milk

Lunch
Beef Stew (page 338)
1 cup peach nectar

Afternoon Snack
   1 cup vanilla ice cream with 2 tablespoons hot fudge

Dinner
White Cheddar Macaroni and Cheese
   (page 278)
1 cup steamed broccoli
1 cup skim milk

1906 calories, 94 g protein, 19 g fiber, 64 g total fat (32 g saturated fat), 1477 mg calcium, 2007 mg sodium, 3645 mg potassium, at least 100% of RDA for all nutrients

DAY THREE

Breakfast
Cream of Wheat★
1 cup skim milk

★Prepare with skim milk instead of water for additional creaminess and nutrition.

Morning Snack
½ cup 2% cottage cheese
1 sliced banana

Lunch
Grilled cheese sandwich: place 2 slices American cheese on 1 slice whole wheat bread and microwave; top with additional slice whole wheat bread

1 can Cream of Tomato soup★

Dinner
Lemon Fresh Salmon Patties with Creamed Peas (page 350)
The Best Mashed Potatoes (page 394), with 2 teaspoons margarine
5 spears asparagus, steamed with 1 teaspoon margarine
1 cup pear nectar

Evening Snack
1 cup low-fat yogurt with 2 tablespoons wheat germ blended in

1933 calories, 112 g protein, 21 g fiber, 48 g total fat (20 g saturated fat), 2140 mg calcium, 3843 mg sodium, 4507 mg potassium, at least 100% of the RDA for all nutrients

DAY FOUR

Breakfast
Apple Custard (page 401)
1 cup skim milk
2 peach halves (canned in juice)

Lunch
Chicken Pot Pie (leftover from day one)
1 cup peach nectar

Afternoon Snack
½ cup ice cream with ½ cup sliced strawberries

Dinner
Fettuccine Alfredo (page 279)
1 cup spinach with 1 teaspoon margarine
1 cup skim milk

Evening Snack
2 fig bars
1 cup skim milk

1922 calories, 94 g protein, 18 g fibers, 48 g total fat (21 g saturated fat), 2138 mg calcium, 2273 mg sodium, 3738 mg potassium, at least 100% of RDA for all nutrients

DAY FIVE

Breakfast
Cream of Wheat★
1 sliced banana
1 cup apricot nectar
★Prepare with skim milk instead of water.

Morning Snack
Apple Custard (leftover from day four)
1 cup apple juice

Lunch
Beef Stew (leftover from day two) served over mashed potatoes (leftover from day three) with 2 teaspoons margarine

Afternoon Snack
Chocolate pudding (leftover from day one) with 2 tablespoons frozen whipped topping

Dinner
Chicken Noodle Casserole (page 281)
1 cup steamed broccoli with 1 teaspoon margarine
1 cup skim milk

2032 calories, 105 g protein, 27 g fiber, 39 g total fat (11 g saturated fat), 1537 mg calcium, 2969 mg sodium, 5719 mg potassium, at least 100% of RDA for all nutrients

DAY SIX

Breakfast
Cheese omelette: 2 eggs plus 2 ounces cheddar cheese, cooked in a nonstick pan coated with vegetable oil spray
1 slice whole wheat toast
1 teaspoon margarine
1 cup skim milk

Morning Snack
1 cup pear nectar

Lunch
Lemon Fresh Salmon Patties with Creamed Peas (leftover from day three)

1 cup cooked seashell pasta with 1 teaspoon margarine
1 cup skim milk

Dinner
1 serving Fettucine Alfredo (leftover from day four)
1 cup steamed carrots
1 cup steamed broccoli with 1 teaspoon margarine
1 cup skim milk

Evening Snack
2 fig bars
1 cup skim milk

1935 calories, 113 g protein, 23 g fiber, 48 g total fat (21 g saturated fat), 2508 mg calcium, 2281 mg sodium, 3666 mg potassium, at least 100% of RDA for all nutrients

DAY SEVEN

Breakfast
Apple Custard (leftover from day four)
1 cup skim milk

Morning Snack
1 cup apricot nectar

Lunch
Chicken Noodle Casserole (leftover from day five)

5 spears steamed asparagus with 1 teaspoon margarine
1 cup skim milk

Dinner
Beef Stew (leftover from day two)
1 cup white rice
1 cup peach nectar

Evening Snack
1 cup ice cream
2 tablespoons hot fudge

2030 calories, 94 g protein, 21 g fiber, 49 g total fat (20 g saturated fat), 1217 mg calcium, 2337 mg sodium, 4126 mg potassium, at least 100% of RDA for all nutrients

References

Anaya, J.M., et al. "Sjögren's Syndrome in Childhood." *Journal of Rheumatology* 22(6) (1995): 1,152–58.

Baudet-Pommel, M., et al. "Early Dental Loss in Sjögren's Syndrome." *Oral Surgery, Oral Medicine and Oral Pathology* 78 (1994): 181–86.

Muller, K., et al. "Abnormal Vitamin D3 Metabolism in Patients with Primary Sjögren's Syndrome." *Annals of the Rheumatic Diseases* 49 (1990): 682–84.

Palma, R., et al. "Esophageal Motility Disorders in Patients with Sjögren's Syndrome." *Digestive Diseases and Sciences* 39 (1994): 758–76.

Sheikh, S.H., and T.A. Shaw-Stiffel. "The Gastrointestinal Manifestations of Sjögren's Syndrome." *American Journal of Gastroenterology* 90 (1995): 9–14.

Weiffenbach, J.M., et al. "Taste Performance in Sjögren's Syndrome." *Physiology and Behavior* 57 (1995): 89–96.

Recipes

How to Use These Recipes

All of the recipes in this section are prepared with several thoughts in mind:

1. They are exceptionally easy to prepare, most using one pot or one bowl. If you follow the directions, you will reap the benefits of this one-pot or one-bowl preparation.
2. Their ease of preparation often comes from using frozen foods or other convenience foods. If you have more energy, don't hesitate to substitute fresh vegetables for the frozen.
3. They are loaded with good nutrition: most of the main dishes are complete meals so that you don't have to think about adding a vegetable or grain—all the guesswork is done for you.
4. They are low in fat and sodium, nutritional concerns of many people with chronic illness. Some of the recipes, however, give instructions on how to change to a high-calorie food for people who simply cannot keep weight on. While this isn't the best way for some people to gain weight, simply because most of these recipes also become very high in fat, sometimes it's the only alternative (such as for people with AIDS).
5. The nutrition information is for one serving, so pay attention to how many servings the recipe makes and tally your calories and other nutritional facts accordingly.
6. Some of the recipes make larger quantities than you'd usually make, but that's the whole idea of this book: learn to make your effort in the kitchen do double and triple duty, freezing extra portions for those days when your energy is low.

Eggs, Pancakes and Breakfast Foods

Breakfast Bulghur

SERVES 2

Eat half today and reheat the remainder tomorrow—for an exceptionally easy, high-fiber breakfast with a wonderfully chewy texture.

> ½ cup bulghur, uncooked
> 1 cup apple cider (okay to substitute
>   apple juice)
> ½ teaspoon cinnamon
> 1 apple with peel, quartered and then sliced
> 10 dates, chopped

1. Mix all ingredients in microwave bowl. Microwave on high for 3 minutes, stir. Microwave another 3 minutes, stir again. Let sit for 5 minutes. Serve.
2. Alternatively, place in heavy saucepan, bring to boil. Reduce heat and simmer covered over low heat for 15 minutes, stirring occasionally.

Per serving: 334 calories; 5 g protein; 83 g carbohydrate; 11 g fiber; 1 g fat; 0.2 g saturated fat; 11 mg sodium.

Tip

Even if you're in a wheelchair, find a way to strengthen whatever muscles you can to keep strong. For example, get a rubber ball and squeeze it repeatedly throughout the day. You might be able to lift your body up by placing your hands on the wheelchair arms and lifting yourself up and down—sort of like a "sitting-down" push-up. Perhaps you can extend your lower leg up and down from the knee (after you've gotten sufficiently strong, try adding an ankle weight to the good leg). You can even try raising your bad leg or arm provided that it's okay with your doctor. You might be surprised at how well you do.

Nutty Breakfast Bulghur

SERVES 2

Start your day with a high-fiber meal like this one—it will hold your appetite for hours.

> ½ cup bulghur, uncooked
> 1 cup apricot nectar
> 1 ounce dry-roasted sunflower seeds
>   (about 3 tablespoons)
> ¼ cup dried apricots, diced

1. Mix all ingredients in microwave bowl. Microwave on high for 3 minutes, stir. Microwave another 3 minutes, stir again. Let sit for 5 minutes. Serve.
2. Alternatively, place in heavy saucepan, bring to boil. Reduce heat and simmer covered over low heat for 15 minutes, stirring occasionally.

Per serving: 311 calories; 8 g protein; 58 g carbohydrate; 9.3 g fiber; 8 g fat; 1 g saturated fat; 12 mg sodium.

Tip

Does your skin tend to be dry in the winter? Drink plenty of water to keep it well hydrated.

Creamy Breakfast Barley with Bananas and Dried Cranberries

SERVES 1 (MAY DOUBLE)

If time is short in the morning, cook breakfast the night before while you're making dinner, and then heat in microwave in the morning. Add ¼ cup milk when you reheat.

> ¼ cup medium barley, uncooked
> 1 cup skim milk
> 1 teaspoon brown sugar
> 2 tablespoons dried cranberries (Craisins)
> ½ teaspoon vanilla
> 1 banana, sliced

1. Combine barley, skim milk and brown sugar in heavy saucepan. Simmer over low heat for 30 minutes.
2. Add cranberries; simmer an additional 15 minutes.
3. Remove from heat; stir in vanilla and sliced banana. Serve.

Per serving: 408 calories; 15 g protein; 85 g carbohydrate; 11 g fiber; 2 g fat; 0.7 g saturated fat; 135 mg sodium.

Tip

If you have trouble sleeping, get out of bed and read or watch television with a cup of warm milk. Avoid staying in bed, as "trying" to fall asleep generally back-fires and you end up growing more anxious. Getting out of bed and doing something else often helps you fall asleep.

Power Porridge

Serves 1 or 2

Eat the whole batch if you're hungry or have a busy morning planned; split it if you're not very active or have a small appetite.

⅓ cup old-fashioned oats
2 tablespoons flaxseed
1 ¼ cup skim milk
2 tablespoons dried cranberries (Craisins)
2 tablespoons raisins

1. Mix all ingredients in 1-quart microwave container. Cook on 80 percent power for 5 minutes. Stir and microwave on full power for 1 minute.
2. Alternatively, combine all ingredients in heavy saucepan and cook covered over low heat about 8 minutes.

Per serving: 395 calories; 18 g protein; 67 g carbohydrate; 7.3 g fiber; 7.3 g fat; 1.2 g saturated fat; 166 mg sodium.

Tip

If you have severe drug allergies or a condition, such as diabetes, that could cause you to lose consciousness and that would demand special treatment, consider wearing an emergency notification bracelet.

Breakfast Rice and Raisins

Serves 2

Cooking rice with milk not only raises the protein content, but also makes for a richer, chewier rice.

1¾ cups skim milk
½ cup uncooked brown rice
1 tablespoon brown sugar
½ teaspoon cinnamon
¼ cup raisins

Combine all ingredients in heavy saucepan. Simmer on low heat for 40 minutes. Serve. (All of liquid will not be taken up by the rice.)

Per serving: 326 calories; 12 g protein; 67 g carbohydrate; 2.6 g fiber; 1.9 g fat; 0.6 g saturated fat; 118 mg sodium.

Tip

> While most people think of osteoporosis as a woman's disease, it can also affect men—especially if they take corticosteroid medications. Men should be concerned about getting enough calcium and vitamin D, too. This recipe is an excellent way to work more milk into the diet.

Creamy Oatmeal

SERVES 1

A great way to get extra protein into someone with a poor appetite, as well as an excellent-tasting protein boost for anyone. Notice that I've left out the sodium, even though the oatmeal package calls for adding salt. You won't miss it.

> 1 cup skim milk
> ½ cup old-fashioned oats
> 2 tablespoon skim milk powder
> 1 teaspoon brown sugar (optional)

1. Mix all ingredients in saucepan and cook over medium heat for 7 minutes.
2. Alternatively, combine all ingredients in medium microwave-safe bowl (mixture puffs up during cooking, so use a larger bowl than a serving size one). Microwave 3 minutes on high power; stir. Microwave 1 more minute. Stir and let stand 1 minute before serving.

Per serving: 280 calories; 18 g protein; 46 g carbohydrate; 4.2 g fiber; 3 g fat; 0.7 g saturated fat; 176 mg sodium.

Tip

> Although 25 percent of Americans believe they are allergic to at least one food, just 1 to 2 percent of all adults have a true food allergy. If you suspect a food allergy, see a physician for a definitive diagnosis.

Tip

> Taking antibiotics for an infection? You may be able to avoid gastrointestinal upset, such as diarrhea and loose stools, by having a container of yogurt daily (with active yogurt cultures) during your antibiotic therapy.

Creamy Oatmeal with Bananas and Walnuts

SERVES 2

A fiber-loaded, hearty and slightly crunchy breakfast that will keep you going strong all morning. Note that I've left the sodium out of this oatmeal recipe, too. You won't notice with all the other great flavors.

2 cups skim milk
1 cup old-fashioned oats
1 large banana, sliced
2 tablespoons chopped walnuts
(about 1.5 ounces)

1. Mix all ingredients in saucepan and cook over medium heat for 7 minutes.
2. Alternatively, combine all ingredients in medium microwave-safe bowl (mixture puffs up during cooking, so use a larger bowl than a serving size one). Microwave 3 minutes on high power; stir. Microwave 1 more minute. Stir and let stand 1 minute before serving.

Per serving: 339 calories; 17 g protein; 53 g carbohydrate; 5.8 g fiber; 7.7 g fat; 1.1 g saturated fat; 128 mg sodium.

Tip

If you have food allergies and you're allergic to cats, take special precautions to avoid dining with a cat in the house. Cat dander—if you're allergic to it—can prime the immune system and instigate more severe food allergy symptoms than usual.

Creamy Scrambled Eggs

SERVES 1

This recipe is great for someone with a limited appetite, as it's loaded with protein. Or try these eggs for someone who has a hard time eating solid food. It's also a great meal for people who need a protein boost—such as after surgery.

2 eggs (or the equivalent in liquid egg
substitute)
¼ cup 2% fat cottage cheese

1. Heat small nonstick pan sprayed with vegetable oil spray over medium heat.
2. In mug, beat eggs with fork; blend in cottage cheese. Transfer to hot pan. Scramble uncovered.

Per serving: 200 calories; 20 g protein; 3 g carbohydrate; 0.0 g fiber; 11 g fat; 3.8 g saturated fat; 355 mg sodium.

Tip _____

In addition to improving flexibility and agility, exercise may also help prevent cancer—several studies now show a decreasing risk of cancer with increasing activity.

Breakfast Cheese Sandwich

SERVES 1

A high-protein way to start your day—especially welcome when you expect a long and demanding morning schedule.

> 1 English muffin
> ½ cup nonfat ricotta cheese
> 1 teaspoon brown sugar
> ¼ teaspoon cinnamon
> One-half of an 11-ounce can mandarin
>   oranges, drained

1. Toast English muffin.
2. Divide ricotta cheese between muffin halves; spread evenly.
3. Mix together brown sugar and cinnamon; sprinkle evenly over ricotta cheese.
4. Divide mandarin orange sections between muffin halves and place on top.
5. Broil 5 minutes, or until cheese has heated through.

Per serving: 318 calories; 15 g protein; 49 g carbohydrate; 2.4 g fiber; 1.6 g fat; 0.3 g saturated fat; 371 mg sodium.

Tip _____

Antioxidant nutrients compounded with herbs may be trouble for women with allergies, especially those who have ragweed allergy. These preparations can cause abdominal cramps, itching and hives in sensitive people. In addition, avoid anti-oxidants compounded with bee pollen if you are allergic to bee stings. These can cause the serious, life-threatening reactions caused by a bee sting in allergic people.

Tip _____

Are you a bagel lover? Be aware that bagels from bagel shops often weigh four or five ounces, which is the equivalent of eating four to five slices of bread. Ask the server to cut it in half, and save half for tomorrow.

Eggs Goldenrod

SERVES 4

This is an old family favorite, one of Aunt Goldie's creations, which I've defatted. It's a great special breakfast food, or even an easy dinner. Just a hint of egg yolk gives this dish special color and flavor.

1 tablespoon margarine
1¼ cups skim milk
2 tablespoons flour
⅛ teaspoon salt
⅛ teaspoon black pepper
2 teaspoons sugar
10 hard–boiled egg whites, sliced
4 whole wheat English muffins
2 hard–boiled egg yolks, mashed with fork

1. Melt margarine in skillet over medium heat.
2. Combine milk and flour in jar; shake until smooth. Pour milk/flour mixture into skillet. Stir until mixture has thickened.
3. Stir in salt, pepper, sugar and egg whites.
4. Serve creamed egg whites over English muffins. Top with egg yolk ("goldenrod").

Per serving: 245 calories; 18 g protein; 30 g carbohydrate; 5 g fiber; 6.3 g fat; 1.5 g saturated fat; 716 mg sodium.

Tip

If you have a difficult time finding comfortable shoes, remember that feet change in size as we age and as we gain and lose weight. Have your feet sized periodically before you buy shoes.

Eggs for Brunch

SERVES 4

This dish is a great way to use leftover whole wheat bagels or bread. If you don't have whole wheat, substitute white or rye. Another plus—any leftovers are great served cold.

3 slices whole wheat bread (or 9 grain),
cut into 1-inch squares
2 ounces Canadian bacon, diced
½ cup chopped red pepper
½ cup chopped green pepper
1 onion, chopped
1 cup liquid egg substitute (the equivalent of 4 eggs)
1 cup skim milk

¼ teaspoon salt
⅛ to ¼ teaspoon black pepper
1 ounce sharp cheddar cheese, grated

1. Combine bread, Canadian bacon, red pepper, green pepper and onion in one quart casserole sprayed with vegetable oil spray.
2. In small bowl, mix egg substitute, skim milk, salt and pepper. Pour over bread/ vegetable mixture.
3. Cover and refrigerate for at least 1 hour; overnight is okay.
4. Bake 45 minutes at 350°. Sprinkle cheese over casserole. Bake another 15 minutes.

Per serving: 211 calories; 18 g protein; 21 g carbohydrate; 2.7 g fiber; 6.7 g fat; 3 g saturated fat; 660 mg sodium.

Tip

If you have to follow a salt-restricted eating plan, be aware that many salt alternatives still have sodium in them. Also, don't forget to substitute garlic powder for garlic salt—the latter is loaded with sodium.

Tex-Mex Scrambled Eggs

SERVES 4

These scrambled eggs also make a great dinner, and are great for someone looking for a little kick in his meal.

1 onion chopped
1 cup chopped green pepper (okay to use frozen)
4 eggs (or the equivalent in liquid egg substitute)
½ cup cottage cheese
2 ounces shredded taco cheese
4 tablespoons salsa

1. Spray nonstick skillet with vegetable oil spray. Heat over medium low heat. Add onion and green pepper, sauté briefly, 2 to 3 minutes.
2. Beat eggs slightly; blend in cottage cheese. Pour over vegetable mixture. Scrambled as you would scrambled eggs, being sure to leave pan uncovered to allow extra moisture to evaporate.
3. When eggs are just about cooked, sprinkle taco cheese over top; allow cheese to melt. Serve with salsa.

Per serving: 183 calories; 14 g protein; 8 g carbohydrate; 1 g fiber; 10.4 g fat; 5.8 g saturated fat; 382 mg sodium.

Scrambled Eggs for Dinner

SERVES 4

For one of those last-minute meals, turn eggs into a full meal with a little help from some interesting ingredients. These eggs are also great for brunch.

1 onion, chopped
8 ounces oriental blend vegetables
    (without added sauce), thawed
2 ounces Canadian bacon, diced
4 eggs
½ cup 2% fat cottage cheese
black pepper to taste

1. Spray nonstick skillet with vegetable oil spray. Heat over medium low heat. Add onion, sauté briefly, 2 to 3 minutes. Add vegetables and Canadian bacon, sauté 1 to 2 minutes.
2. Beat eggs slightly; blend in cottage cheese. Pour over vegetable/ham mixture. Scramble as you would scrambled eggs, leaving pan uncovered to allow extra moisture to evaporate. Add black pepper; serve.

Per serving: 154 calories; 15 g protein; 8 g carbohydrate; 1.8 g fiber; 6.6 g fat; 2.2 g saturated fat; 379 mg sodium.

Tip

Americans are drinking less milk than ever, which is bad news for bones (and possibly blood pressure). If you don't drink milk, make sure you get enough supplemental calcium and vitamin D.

Whole Grain Pancakes

SERVES 4

¾ cup extra-calcium cottage cheese
2 eggs (or the equivalent in liquid egg
    substitute)
3 tablespoons sugar
1 tablespoon olive oil
¾ cup skim milk
½ cup white flour
¼ cup whole wheat flour
2 tablespoons wheat germ
¼ cup milled or ground flaxseed
2 teaspoons baking powder

1. Puree cottage cheese in food miniprocessor.
2. In small mixing bowl, beat egg slightly. Add sugar, olive oil, pureed cottage cheese, skim milk; blend well.
3. Stir in flours, wheat germ, flaxseed and baking powder.
4. Cook on nonstick griddle or fry pan sprayed with vegetable oil spray. Serve with maple syrup, hot cinnamon applesauce or all-fruit spread.

Per serving: 284 calories; 15 g protein; 36 g carbohydrate; 3.4 g fiber; 9.5 g fat; 2 g saturated fat; 441 mg sodium.

Beefed-Up Pancakes

SERVES 4

Turn pancakes into a high-protein meal with this easy recipe.

¾ cup extra-calcium cottage cheese
1 egg
3 tablespoons sugar
3 teaspoons olive oil
¾ cup skim milk
1 cup plus 2 tablespoons flour
1½ teaspoon baking powder

1. Puree cottage cheese in food miniprocessor.
2. In small mixing bowl, beat egg slightly. Add sugar, olive oil, pureed cottage cheese, skim milk; blend well.
3. Stir in flour and baking powder. (If you like thinner pancakes, add more milk.)
4. Cook on nonstick griddle or fry pan sprayed with vegetable oil spray. Serve with hot cinnamon applesauce or maple syrup.

Per serving: 260 calories; 12 g protein; 41 g carbohydrate; 1.2 g fiber; 5.4 g fat; 1.3 g saturated fat; 362 mg sodium.

Tip

Keep some low-fat, high-calcium cottage cheese on hand in the refrigerator. It makes an easy, high-protein meal in itself, or you can use it in recipes like this one as a last-minute solution when you haven't planned dinner. It generally keeps for a couple of weeks in the refrigerator.

Dinner Pancakes

SERVES 4

Adding vegetables turns my high-protein pancakes into an easy, fast—and complete—dinner.

¾ cup extra-calcium cottage cheese
2 eggs (or the equivalent in liquid egg
    substitute)
3 tablespoons sugar
1 tablespoon olive oil
½ cup skim milk
½ cup white flour
¼ cup whole wheat flour
2 tablespoons wheat germ
2 teaspoons baking powder
¼ cup milled or ground flaxseed
1 carrot, grated
1 zucchini (small), grated

1. Puree cottage cheese in food miniprocessor.
2. In small mixing bowl, beat egg slightly. Add sugar, olive oil, pureed cottage cheese, and skim milk; blend well.
3. Stir in flours, wheat germ, baking powder and flaxseed. Fold in grated vegetables.
4. Cook on nonstick griddle or fry pan sprayed with vegetable oil spray. Serve with cold applesauce or mashed strawberries.

Per serving: 287 calories; 15 g protein; 37 g carbohydrate; 3.9 g fiber; 9.5 g fat; 2 g saturated fat; 440 mg sodium.

Tip

Find ways to work more fruit into your diet—such as using mashed or pureed fruit as a topping on pancakes or waffles, substituting the fruit for syrup or other empty-calorie condiments.

Cinnamon French Toast

SERVES 4

This is the perfect recipe for slightly dried-out bread; in fact, the drier the bread, the more of the mixture it soaks up.

> 6 eggs (or the equivalent in liquid egg
>   substitute)
> 2 tablespoons sugar
> 1 teaspoon cinnamon
> 1 teaspoon vanilla extract
> 8 slices whole wheat bread

1. In 9 × 13-inch cake pan, beat eggs, sugar, cinnamon and vanilla until well blended.
2. Add bread, forming one continuous layer and coating both sides. Cover and refrigerate 1 hour (overnight is fine), allowing bread to soak up all of the egg mixture.
3. Heat nonstick griddle over medium heat; spray with vegetable oil spray. Transfer bread soaked with egg mixture with a pancake turner (so that it doesn't break up) to hot griddle. Cook each side until browned, about 5 minutes per side.

Per serving: 312 calories; 16 g protein; 40 g carbohydrate; 4.7 g fiber; 10.5 g fat; 3 g saturated fat; 464 mg sodium.

Tip

Many people with chronic illness—along with their physicians—tend to forget about preventive health maneuvers. Don't forger that all adults should have a rectal exam every year after age forty.

Muffins, Breads and Bakery Treats

Kris's Better Morning Muffins

MAKES 24 MUFFINS

These muffins freeze well, so don't hesitate to make the whole batch. Or cut the recipe in half and make just twelve.

1½ cups flour
½ cup wheat germ
1¼ cups brown sugar
2 teaspoons baking soda
2 teaspoons cinnamon
3 eggs (or the equivalent in liquid egg substitute)
½ cup olive oil or canola oil
¾ cup applesauce
1 teaspoon vanilla extract
⅔ cup angel flake coconut
20 dates, chopped (or 1 cup raisins)
4 carrots, peeled and finely grated (about 2 cups—okay to use food processor to grate)

1. If you have a stand mixer, add ingredients to mixing bowl in order on the list down to, and not including, the carrots, mixing on low until well blended. Then add coconut and dates and mix until well blended. Stir in carrots.
2. If you have a hand-held mixer, combine all ingredients down to, and not including, carrots and then mix with hand-held mixer until well blended. Add coconut and dates and mix just until well blended. Stir in carrots.
3. Spray 24 muffin tins with vegetable oil spray. Divide batter between 24 muffin cups. Bake 20 to 25 minutes at 350°, or until knife inserted in the middle comes out clean.

Per serving: 154 calories; 3 g protein; 23 g carbohydrate; 1.6 g fiber; 6.3 g fat; 1.5 g saturated fat; 127 mg sodium.

Oat Muffins

MAKES 24 MUFFINS
These muffins freeze very nicely.

2 cups oats (dry, not instant)
1½ cups buttermilk
2 tablespoons olive oil
½ cup applesauce
¾ cup brown sugar
3 tablespoons molasses
2 eggs
2 teaspoons baking soda
1 tablespoon cinnamon
¼ teaspoon salt
1 cup white flour
⅓ cup wheat germ
2 cups grated zucchini (about 2 small)
1 cup raisins

1. Mix all ingredients except zucchini and raisins in stand mixer, or with any other mixer. Add zucchini and raisins; mix briefly.
2. Spray 24 muffin tins with vegetable oil spray. Fill muffin tins about ⅔ full.
3. Bake 20 minutes at 350°, or until thin knife comes out clean.

Per serving: 121 calories; 3 g protein; 23 g carbohydrate; 1.5 g fiber; 2.4 g fat; 0.5 g saturated fat; 153 mg sodium.

Tip

This recipe uses applesauce for part of the oil in the original recipe—which greatly reduces the fat grams per muffin. In some recipes, substitute pureed prunes for part of the oil—they work particularly well in recipes that have chocolate or cinnamon.

Pumpkin Muffins

MAKES 7 DOZEN MINIMUFFINS, 3 DOZEN REGULAR-SIZED MUFFINS,
OR 2 LARGE LOAVES

These muffins are so moist and rich you'd think they were loaded with fat—but they're not. Freeze and take out as you need them. They will be a favorite treat for kids—they are in my house! The wheat germ and flaxseed add extremely rich taste and moisture. Don't be afraid to add them.

⅓ cup applesauce
⅓ cup canola or light olive oil
2⅔ cup sugar
1 cup liquid egg substitute (the equivalent
    of 4 eggs)
One 16-ounce can pumpkin
⅔ cup buttermilk (can substitute ⅔ cup
    plain, nonfat or low-fat yogurt)
2⅔ cups white flour
⅔ cup wheat germ
½ cup milled flaxseed
2 teaspoons baking soda
½ teaspoon baking powder
1 teaspoon ground cinnamon
1 teaspoon ground cloves
⅔ cup raisins (optional)

1. Combine applesauce, oil, sugar, egg substitute, pumpkin, buttermilk, flour, wheat germ and flaxseed in large mixing bowl; mix on medium until well blended.
2. Add remaining ingredients (except raisins if you're adding them) and mix just until flour is blended in. Stir in raisins.
3. Spray minimuffin or regular tins with vegetable oil spray. Fill muffin cups ⅔ full or split batter between two large loaf pans.
4. Bake at 350° for about 70 minutes for loaves (until knife inserted into middle comes out clean); about 10 to 15 minutes for minimuffins; or about 20 to 25 minutes for regular muffins.

Per minimuffin: 59 calories; 1.3 g protein; 11 g carbohydrate; 0.6 g fiber; 1.4 g fat; 0.2 g saturated fat; 41 mg sodium.

Per regular muffin: 138 calories; 3 g protein; 25 g carbohydrate; 1 g fiber; 3 g fat; 0.4 g saturated fat; 95 mg sodium.

Per bread slice: 165 calories; 4 g protein; 30 g carbohydrate; 2 g fiber; 4 g fat; 0.5 g saturated fat; 114 mg sodium.

Have trouble controlling snacking? Plan some healthy snacks at the beginning of the day, and you'll end up eating a more appropriate number of calories by the end of the day.

Banana "Nut" Bread Muffins

MAKES 36 MUFFINS (OR 2 LARGE LOAVES)

So rich in flavor that even finicky kids will love them, these muffins are loaded with whole grain goodness. The flaxseed lends an excellent nutty taste and texture, but not a lot of excess fat. This recipe can also be cut in half.

½ cup olive oil
½ cup applesauce
1½ cups sugar
2 eggs (or the equivalent in liquid egg substitute)
4 ripe bananas, mashed (about 1¼ cup mashed)
½ cup nonfat plain yogurt
2 cups white flour
1¾ cups whole wheat flour
¼ cup wheat germ
1 teaspoon baking soda
1 teaspoon baking powder
¼ teaspoon salt
½ cup milled or ground flaxseed

1. Cream together olive oil, applesauce, sugar, eggs and mashed bananas.
2. Add remaining ingredients; mix well.
3. Spray muffin tins with vegetable oil spray. Place scoop of batter in muffin tins.
4. Bake at 350° for 15 to 20 minutes (about 40 to 50 minutes for loaves) or until knife inserted into middle is clean.

Per serving: 134 calories; 3 g protein; 23 g carbohydrate; 1.6 g fiber; 4.2 g fat; 0.6 g saturated fat; 71 mg sodium.

Tip _____

Take pride in your appearance daily—especially on days when illness keeps you at home.

Totally Decadent Sticky Buns

> 4 tablespoons butter
> ½ cup brown sugar
> ½ cup light corn syrup
> 2 tablespoons nonfat sour cream
> 1 tablespoon plus 1 teaspoon cinnamon
> ½ cup packed dark raisins
> One 1-pound loaf frozen bread dough,
>   thawed

1. Melt butter. Whisk in brown sugar, corn syrup, sour cream and cinnamon.
2. Pour brown sugar mixture into deep dish pie plate sprayed heavily with vegetable oil spray. Sprinkle raisins evenly over brown sugar mixture
3. Break up bread dough into 12 pieces and roll into balls. Place balls evenly throughout mixture.
4. Cover and refrigerate overnight. In morning, remove cover and place in a cold oven. Turn oven on bake, at 350°. Bake 30 to 40 minutes, or until buns are slightly browned.
5. Alternatively, cover and let stand at room temperature for 1 to 2 hours, or until dough has risen.
6. Turn pie plate upside down on a serving platter, scraping sauce over what is now the top of the buns.

Per serving: 205 calories; 4 g protein; 37 g carbohydrate; 1.8 g fiber; 5.6 g fat; 2.4 g saturated fat; 274 mg sodium.

Tip

Plan the occasional treat—such as these sticky buns! No matter what type of special diet you're on, you can still fit in foods like this. Also check out the brownies that follow.

The Fudgiest Brownies

> 1 cup sugar
> ½ cup liquid egg substitute
> ¼ cup margarine
> ¼ cup applesauce
> ½ cup flour
> 2 squares baker's chocolate, melted
> 1 tablespoon vanilla

1. Combine sugar, egg substitute and margarine in mixing bowl; cream until smooth.
2. Add applesauce, flour; blend with mixture until smooth.
3. Add melted chocolate and vanilla; blend until well mixed.
4. Spray 9×9-inch pan with vegetable oil spray. Spread mixture in pan.
5. Bake at 325° for 25 minutes.

Per serving: 179 calories; 2 g protein; 22 g carbohydrate; 0.9 g fiber; 9.6 g fat; 2.8 g saturated fat; 79 mg sodium.

Tip

Before a doctor's visit, write down all of your questions and the medications for which you need refills.

Peanut Butter Oat Bars

MAKES 30 BARS

Enjoy this highly nutritious snack or dessert frequently! It even makes a great breakfast food.

1 cup packed brown sugar
½ cup applesauce
1 cup peanut butter
¾ cup liquid egg substitute (or 3 eggs)
1 cup flour
1 tablespoon plus 1 teaspoon cinnamon
¾ teaspoon baking soda
3½ cups old-fashioned oats
⅓ cup skim milk
1 tablespoon plus 1 teaspoon vanilla
1 cup packed raisins

1. In stand or other mixer, combine brown sugar, applesauce, peanut butter and egg substitute; cream. Add remaining ingredients, except raisins; blend well.
2. Stir in raisins.
3. Spray 9×9-inch pan. Press mixture into pan.
4. Bake 20 to 30 minutes at 350°. Cool before cutting.

Per serving: 146 calories; 5 g protein; 21 g carbohydrate; 2 g fiber; 5.2 g fat; 1 g saturated fat; 88 mg sodium.

Tip

Keep foods like this on hand in the freezer for those hungry moments when you're also looking for something a little sweet.

Bread Pudding

SERVES 6

Serve this satisfyingly delicious bread pudding as breakfast food, dessert or a snack. It's just as great cold as it is hot.

> 2 eggs
> 2¼ cups skim milk
> ¼ cup skim milk powder
> ¼ cup brown sugar
> 1 teaspoon cinnamon
> 2 teaspoons vanilla
> 4 slices 9-grain or whole wheat bread
> ¾ cup raisins

1. Spray shallow glass baking dish with vegetable oil spray.
2. Crack eggs into dish; beat slightly with fork.
3. Add skim milk, milk powder, brown sugar, cinnamon and vanilla. Mix with fork.
4. Break bread into bite-size pieces, dropping into milk mixture. Mix with fork.
5. Sprinkle raisins on top.
6. Bake uncovered at 300° for 1 hour 30 minutes.

Per serving: 213 calories; 9 g protein; 40 g carbohydrate; 2.4 g fiber; 2.9 g fat; 0.9 g saturated fat; 212 mg sodium.

Tip

Looking for a sweet treat? Try a tall, ice cold glass of orange juice. For a special treat, add some chopped mint to a container of orange juice, and let it "steep" overnight. Excellent, and for a just a few calories!

Blueberry Crisp

SERVES 9

I've trimmed down this delightful old family favorite dessert of ours to make it healthy enough for a breakfast food, yet still sweetly satisfying for dessert. Add reduced-fat dairy topping or low-fat vanilla frozen yogurt for a creamy finish.

> ½ cup margarine
> ¾ cup packed dark brown sugar
> 1 cup old-fashioned oats
> 1 cup flour
> 2 teaspoons cinnamon
> 4 cups blueberries (fresh or frozen)

1. In 4-cup microwave container, melt margarine.
2. Stir brown sugar, oats, flour and cinnamon into melted margarine (a fork works best).
3. Spray 9×9-inch pan with vegetable oil spray. Spread half of oat mixture in bottom of pan and pack down with spoon or rubber spatula.
4. Pour blueberries evenly over oat crust. Sprinkle remaining oat mixture over blueberries.
5. Bake at 350° for 45 to 60 minutes, or until blueberries are bubbling.

Per serving: 257 calories; 3.4 g protein; 37.5 g carbohydrate; 3.1 g fiber; 11.1 g fat; 1.9 g saturated fat; 95 mg sodium.

Tip

When was the last time you bought yourself a new outfit? Sure, you don't work outside the home, but nice clothes make a tremendous difference in how you feel about yourself.

Fruit Pizza

SERVES 15

One 18-ounce package sugar cookie dough (buy from dairy section of the grocery store)
6 ounces nonfat cream cheese
4 ounces low-fat lemon yogurt
2 tablespoons powdered sugar
2 cups strawberries, sliced
4 kiwis, sliced
1 can mandarin oranges, drained well and patted dry
2 cups blueberries

1. Spread sugar cookie dough in the shape of a rectangle on 9×13-inch cookie sheet. Bake in 350° oven for 10 minutes, or until slightly browned.
2. In small food processor blend cream cheese, yogurt and powdered sugar.
3. Spread cream cheese mixture over baked cookie dough.
4. Arrange fruit in an interesting pattern. Chill and serve.

Per serving: 224 calories; 4 g protein; 35 g carbohydrate; 2.2 g fiber; 8.2 g fat; 2 g saturated fat; 221 mg sodium.

Tip

If you're looking for nutrition advice from a professional, always check the credentials of the person you are consulting. While anyone can call himself a nutritionist, only registered dietitians have the appropriate training. Look for the initials *R.D.* to make sure the person you consult is a registered dietitian.

Mom-Lady's Chocolate Cake

SERVES 24

It's important to have absolutely delicious recipes for special celebrations—birthday parties, anniversaries, graduations. This is our family's very favorite chocolate cake. I've never had another like it. Mom-Lady was my husband's brother's baby-sitter. She was so much like a mom to him that he dubbed her "Mom-Lady," a name that has stuck for thirty-three years.

½ cup margarine

2 cups sugar

2 eggs

2 cups flour

2 teaspoons baking soda

2 squares baker's chocolate, melted

8 ounces sour cream

1 cup boiling water

1 tablespoon vanilla

FROSTING

1 cup whole milk

5 tablespoons flour

1 cup butter

1 cup sugar

2 teaspoons vanilla

1. Cream margarine, sugar, eggs, flour and baking soda with electric beater.
2. Add melted chocolate, beating for 2 minutes.
3. Add sour cream and beat 1 minute.
4. Add boiling water and beat 1 minute; stir in vanilla.
5. Spray 2 round cake pans or one 9×13-inch cake pan with vegetable oil spray; spread batter evenly into pan or pans.
5. Bake round pans 35 minutes or 9×13-inch pan 40 to 45 minutes at 350°, or until a knife inserted in the middle comes out clean.

FROSTING

1. In small jar, shake milk and flour until all lumps are dissolved. Pour this mixture into a heavy saucepan and cook over low heat, stirring constantly until mixture forms a stiff paste. Chill in refrigerator.
2. In mixing bowl, beat butter, sugar and vanilla. Add milk/flour paste and beat until smooth.

Per serving: 252 calories; 2.8 g protein; 27 g carbohydrate; 0.8 g fiber; 14.7 g fat; 7.8 g saturated fat; 229 mg sodium.

Tip

While Mom-Lady's Chocolate Cake is slightly high in fat, remember that you won't have it daily. Reserve special treats like this for special occasions and then have no guilt about enjoying one reasonably sized piece. That's part of the pleasure of life.

Easy as Pie Apple Pie

SERVES 8

Anyone can make this pie in ten minutes flat, and impress even the most sophisticated cook. Also, because it's short on fat and long on fiber, it's a little healthier than most apple pies. Remember, apples are high in those excellent disease-fighting substances called flavonoids.

> 2 refrigerator pie crusts
> 3 Granny Smith apples, cored and
>   quartered (peel stays on)
> 3 Gala apples (or some other sweet
>   cooking apple), cored and quartered
> 3 tablespoons brown sugar
> 1 teaspoon cinnamon
> 2 tablespoons flour

1. Place first crust in bottom of deep-dish pie plate. Slice apples into crust.
2. Sprinkle brown sugar, cinnamon and flour over apples.
3. Place top crust over apples. Pinch together top and bottom crusts at edge. Cut 4 slits in top crust.
4. Bake at 350° for 1 hour, or until you see juice bubbling through top slits. Cool slightly before cutting.

Per serving: 236 calories; 2 g protein; 34 g carbohydrate; 2.8 g fiber; 10.6 g fat; 3.4 g saturated fat; 206 mg sodium.

Tip

Did you wake up today with more energy than usual? Still, remember to pace yourself. Forging full-speed ahead is always tempting, but you may be tired out by noon. Pacing yourself will spread out that fabulous energy throughout the day—and you'll accomplish far more in the long run.

Cold Pasta Salads

Basil Tomato Pasta Salad

SERVES 6

4 tablespoons olive oil

½ cup finely chopped basil

4 to 6 cloves garlic, minced

½ teaspoon salt

¼ teaspoon pepper

4 cups cooked pasta ruffles

One 16-ounce bag frozen baby corn blend
    (corn, broccoli, carrots), thawed

4 tomatoes, chopped

Tops of 8 scallions, chopped

8 ounces cooked chicken, diced

8 cups chopped fresh spinach

1. In serving bowl, mix olive oil, basil, garlic, salt and pepper. Add pasta and toss.
2. Add vegetables, tomatoes, onions and chicken; toss.
3. Divide spinach between 6 plates; top with pasta salad.

Per serving: 331 calories; 21 g protein; 44 g carbohydrate; 6.4 g fiber; 12 g fat; 1.8 g saturated fat; 289 mg sodium.

Tip

Smoking doubles your risk of stroke and triples your chance of certain kinds of hemorrhage from an aneurysm. If you smoke, stop today, or at least investigate a method to help you stop.

Lemon-Oregano Pasta Salad

SERVES 2

Enjoy this cool and easy pasta salad in the heat of summer when the produce is at its peak.

> 2 tablespoons extra-virgin olive oil
> ¼ cup lemon juice
> 1 teaspoon dried oregano
> ¼ teaspoon salt
> ¼ teaspoon ground black pepper
> 2 teaspoons sugar
> 2 cups cooked seashell pasta
> One 6-ounce can tuna (packed in water),
>   drained
> 1 large tomato, chopped (or 2 medium)
> 1 large green pepper, chopped

1. In serving bowl combine olive oil, lemon juice, oregano, salt, pepper and sugar. Add pasta and toss.
2. Add tuna, tomato and green pepper and toss to mix.

Per serving: 475 calories; 33 g protein; 47 g carbohydrate; 3.6 g fiber; 17 g fat; 3 g saturated fat; 675 mg sodium.

Tip

Tuna is a great source of omega-3 fatty acids, the type of fat found in fish that is thought to help protect against artery-clogging heart disease.

Creamy Basil Pasta

SERVES 4

This defatted basil pesto binds this tasty pasta salad together beautifully.

3 cups cooked seashell pasta

20 cherry tomatoes, quartered

6 scallions, chopped

One 7¾-ounce can garbanzo beans
(chickpeas), drained and rinsed

8 ounces 50% reduced-fat cheddar cheese,
cut into small squares

SAUCE

⅔ cup fat-free sour cream

8 large fresh basil leaves

2 tablespoons balsamic vinegar

¼ teaspoon salt

½ teaspoon sugar

black pepper to taste

1. Combine pasta, cherry tomatoes, onions, garbanzo beans and cheese in serving bowl.
2. Combine sauce ingredients in food processor or blender; process until smooth. (Food miniprocessor works well.)
3. Pour sauce over pasta/vegetable mixture. Toss to mix well. Chill.

Per serving: 411 calories; 27 g protein; 55 g carbohydrate; 5 g fiber; 10.7 g fat; 6.3 g saturated fat; 748 mg sodium.

★Nutritional analysis per serving substituting regular sour cream for nonfat and regular cheese for reduced fat: 538 calories; 24 g protein; 49 g carbohydrate; 5 g fiber; 28 g fat; 21 g saturated fat; 686 mg sodium.

★Recommended for AIDS patients.

Tip

Sports medicine experts recommend polyester or acrylic socks (as opposed to cotton) to move sweat away from the feet. Why? It can help you avoid blisters.

Mozzarella and Peppercorn Ranch Pasta Salad

271

Recipes

SERVES 4

If you don't like peppercorn ranch dressing, substitute any other flavor. The extra water chestnuts offer a delightful texture to this easy recipe.

> 3 cups cooked pasta ruffles
> One 16-ounce bag frozen broccoli, carrots and water chestnuts, thawed
> 6 ounces part skim mozzarella, cut into small pieces
> One 8-ounce can sliced water chestnuts, drained
> ¼ cup plus 2 tablespoons fat-free peppercorn ranch dressing
> 3 cups chopped romaine lettuce

1. Combine all ingredients except romaine lettuce in quart-size bowl; toss to mix.
2. Divide lettuce between 4 plates. Top each with a fourth of pasta salad.

Per serving: 365 calories; 22 g protein; 52 g carbohydrate; 7.3 g fiber; 8.2 g fat; 4.8 g saturated fat; 531 mg sodium.

*Nutritional analysis substituting regular ranch dressing for fat free peppercorn dressing: 409 calories; 22 g protein; 45 g carbohydrate; 6 g fiber; 17 g fat; 6 g saturated fat; 359 mg sodium.

*Recommended for AIDS patients.

Tip

Keeping your mouth moist may help prevent bad breath. That's because a dry mouth slows the flow of saliva, which is necessary to cleanse the mouth.

Roasted Red Pepper Pasta Salad

SERVES 4

The raw broccoli lends a delightful crunch to this pasta salad. The distinctive sauce is also great as a dressing for other salads.

3 cups cooked pasta ruffles
1 pound fresh broccoli, cut into bite-size pieces
Two 8-ounce cans garbanzo beans
   (chickpeas), drained and rinsed
1 onion, chopped

SAUCE
One 7.25-ounce jar roasted red peppers
1 cup cooked white beans (cannellini)
   (canned okay) drained and rinsed
¼ teaspoon salt
2 teaspoons sugar
4 to 6 large fresh basil leaves
ground black pepper to taste

1.   In serving bowl, mix pasta ruffles, broccoli, garbanzo beans and onion.
2.   Place sauce ingredients in food processor or blender. Process until smooth. Pour sauce over pasta/vegetable mixture. Toss to mix well. Chill.

Per serving: 394 calories; 17 g protein; 76 g carbohydrate; 12.3 g fiber; 3 g fat; 0.4 g saturated fat; 827 mg sodium.

Tip

Roasting red peppers is a lot of work, so don't hesitate to use the jar variety. Just be sure to look for ones packed in water instead of oil.

3-Bean Pasta Salad

SERVES 4

The wonderfully rich olive taste lent by the extra-virgin olive oil enhances this great pasta salad. Using frozen beans reduces the sodium, and also adds another vegetable—great for nutrition and color.

2 tablespoons plus 2 teaspoons extra-virgin
   olive oil
2 tablespoons white wine vinegar
1 teaspoon oregano
¼ teaspoon salt
¼ teaspoon black pepper

1 cup chopped onion

4 cups cooked bow-tie pasta

One 15.5-ounce can dark red kidney
   beans, drained and rinsed

One bag frozen baby bean and carrot
   blend, thawed (green beans, yellow
   beans, baby carrots)

1. In serving bowl, combine olive oil, vinegar, oregano, salt, pepper and onion. Add pasta and toss.
2. Add remaining ingredients and toss to mix. Serve at room temperature to enjoy the full olive flavor.

Per serving: 420 calories; 14 g protein; 66 g carbohydrate; 12 g fiber; 10.3 g fat; 1.4 g saturated fat; 411 mg sodium.

Tip

Do you like to enjoy an occasional glass of alcohol? Make sure it mixes okay with your medication—always ask your pharmacist and physician. This goes for over-the-counter medications, too.

3-Cheese Pasta Salad

SERVES 4

Enjoy the distinctive, rich tastes of feta and blue cheeses—without going overboard on fat. These flavors blend together magically to create an outstanding pasta salad that's a complete meal.

4 cups cooked bow-tie pasta

4 ounces crumbled feta cheese

½ cup chopped green onion

20 cherry tomatoes, cut in half

2 ounces 50% reduced-fat cheddar cheese, shredded

1 cup chopped green pepper
   (can use frozen)

2 tablespoons low-fat blue cheese salad dressing

2 cups chopped romaine lettuce

2 cups chopped fresh spinach leaves

1. Mix all ingredients except romaine lettuce and spinach in serving bowl.
2. Divide romaine lettuce and spinach between 4 plates. Top each with a fourth of pasta salad. Chill and serve.

Per serving: 356 calories; 18 g protein; 49 g carbohydrate; 4.6 g fiber; 10.1 g fat; 6.8 g saturated fat; 518 mg sodium.

10-Minute Honey Dijon Pasta Salad

SERVES 4

An exceptionally easy pasta salad that's a complete meal. Serve over a bed or romaine lettuce or fresh spinach leaves to up the great nutrition of this recipe. This also stores well in the refrigerator for several days.

> 3 cups cooked tricolor pasta twists
> 1 bag frozen baby pea blend, thawed
>   (1 pound)
> 8 ounces reduced-fat mild cheddar cheese,
>   in bite-size squares
> ½ cup fat free honey Dijon dressing
> chopped romaine lettuce or fresh spinach

In serving bowl, mix all ingredients. Serve over chopped romaine lettuce or chopped fresh spinach leaves.

Per serving: 394 calories; 25 g protein; 52 g carbohydrate; 5 g fiber; 9.8 g fat; 6 g saturated fat; 736 mg sodium.

Tip

Reduced-fat cheeses, like the one in this recipe, are much better for recipes that don't call for them to be melted or otherwise cooked. While their flavor is good, their melted texture often isn't as successful.

Feta Cheese and Olive Pasta Salad

SERVES 4

Although it doesn't seem possible to make a healthy salad with feta cheese and olives, it is! The trick is in how much of everything you use. This recipe is a great lesson is using high-fat ingredients in moderation, to achieve the great taste you're looking for and yet not blow your calorie, fat and sodium budget. Enjoy!

> 2 tablespoons olive oil
> 2 tablespoons balsamic vinegar
> ⅛ teaspoon salt
> ½ cup chopped onion
> 24 black olives, chopped
> 3 cups cooked bow-tie pasta
> 4 ounces crumbled feta cheese
> 1-pound bag frozen baby broccoli blend,
>   thawed

In serving bowl, mix olive oil, vinegar, salt, onions and olives. Add remaining ingredients and toss. Serve at room temperature.

Per serving: 390 calories; 14 g protein; 40 g carbohydrate; 5.8 g fiber; 18 g fat; 6.4 g saturated fat; 643 mg sodium.

Tip

Do you often throw out fresh fruit because you couldn't finish it before it went bad? Don't hesitate to buy frozen or canned. Frozen berries are particularly excellent, and you can find them without added sugar. Look for fruits canned in their own juice or syrup.

Favorite Tuna Pasta Salad

SERVES 4

If you like a milder-tasting pasta salad, just leave out the red onion.

> 2 cups cooked elbow macaroni
> Two 6-ounce cans chunk light tuna in
>   water, drained
> 2 hard-boiled eggs, chopped
> 1 cup frozen petite peas, thawed
> ¼ cup plus 2 tablespoons light Miracle
>   Whip
> ½ cup chopped red onion
> 4 cups chopped romaine lettuce

1. Blend all ingredients except romaine lettuce in serving bowl.
2. Serve over chopped romaine lettuce.

Per serving: 331 calories; 29 g protein; 33 g carbohydrate; 4 g fiber; 8.5 g fat; 1.1 g saturated fat; 514 mg sodium.

Tip

A great appetite booster? Some fresh air and a little bit of exercise.

Tuna Pasta Salad with Sweet Red Peppers

SERVES 2

Sweet red peppers make this quick and easy pasta salad a real standout!

1 stalk celery, sliced thinly
1 sweet red pepper, chopped
1 onion, peeled and chopped
One 6-ounce can tuna, packed in water,
    drained
1 cup cooked pasta twists
⅓ cup fat-free ranch dressing
⅛ teaspoon salt
black pepper to taste (⅛ to ¼ teaspoon)
2 cups chopped fresh spinach leaves
    (or romaine lettuce leaves)

Combine all ingredients except spinach leaves in bowl and fold to mix. Chill at least 1 hour and serve over chopped spinach leaves.

Per serving: 323 calories; 29 g protein; 44 g carbohydrate; 4.7 g fiber; 3 g fat; 1 g saturated fat; 944 mg sodium.

*Nutritional analysis substituting regular ranch dressing for fat-free ranch dressing: 402 calories; 30 g protein; 31 g carbohydrate; 4 g fiber; 18 g fat; 3 g saturated fat; 705 mg sodium.

*Recommended for AIDS patients.

Tip

To protect your eyes from sun damage, wear sunglasses in winter just as you do in summer. The sun's winter rays contain the same amount of potentially harmful ultraviolet radiation as the summer sun. By the way, eye experts say that wearing sunglasses and a wide-brimmed hat provides far more protection than any nutrition supplements you can buy.

Ruffled Crab Salad

SERVES 4

This pasta salad is as pretty as it is delicious! It's also spectacularly easy to prepare.

4 cups cooked pasta ruffles
3 cups chopped red cabbage (about ½ a
    small head, 1 to 1½ pounds)
4 chopped scallions (about 1 cup)

Two 8-ounce packages imitation crab meat
6 large basil leaves, chopped finely
6 tablespoons light Miracle Whip

In serving bowl, combine all ingredients. Toss to mix well.

Per serving: 371 calories; 20 g protein; 61 g carbohydrate; 3.5 g fiber; 5 g fat; 0.7 g saturated fat; 831 mg sodium.

Tip

Adding a new medication? Make sure you ask your physician and pharmacist if it's best taken with or without food, at a certain time of the day, and if you should avoid taking it with any other of your medications.

Crab Salad Primavera

SERVES 4

This recipe uses one of those frozen vegetable blends that make cooking so easy. You can easily keep all these ingredients on hand for a quick, last-minute dinner.

2 tablespoons plus 2 teaspoons olive oil
¼ cup lemon juice
2 teaspoons oregano
1 cup chopped red onion
2 teaspoons sugar
½ teaspoon salt
2 cups cooked elbow macaroni
1-pound bag frozen baby broccoli blend, thawed
8 ounces imitation crab meat

1. In serving bowl, mix olive oil, lemon juice, oregano, onion, sugar and salt. Add macaroni and toss.
2. Add vegetables and crab meat and toss. Serve chilled.

Per serving: 343 calories; 15 g protein; 41 g carbohydrate; 5.3 g fiber; 12 g fat; 1.5 g saturated fat; 772 mg sodium.

Tip

Are you tired beyond explanation? Remember that prescription and over-the-counter sleeping aids may actually end up making you more tired because you may awake with a hangover feeling. Try other alternatives to help you sleep better.

Easy Seafood Salad

Serves 2

> 1 cup cooked seashell pasta
> ½ cup chopped onion
> 1 cup frozen green peas, thawed
> (don't use canned)
> 8 ounces imitation crab meat
> ¼ cup low-fat Miracle Whip
> ⅛ teaspoon black pepper

Place all ingredients in serving bowl. Toss to mix. Serve chilled.

Per serving: 347 calories; 21 g protein; 49 g carbohydrate; 5.8 g fiber; 7.5 g fat; 1.2 g saturated fat; 1224 mg sodium.

Tip

Massage therapy can be a great pain reliever. It is thought to break the pain cycle by relieving muscle spasms that impair circulation and cause more pain.

Hot Pasta Dishes

White Cheddar Macaroni and Cheese

Serves 2 (may double)

This high-protein, lower fat version of another comfort food tastes so great you won't miss the fat. It's so nutritious that you can have it every day!

> 2 cups cooked small seashell macaroni
> ½ cup extra-calcium 1% fat cottage cheese
> 2 ounces shredded sharp white cheddar
> cheese
> ¼ cup skim milk
> white pepper to taste, about ⅛ teaspoon

1. Bring water to a boil. Add macaroni, reduce heat and simmer 5 minutes. Drain and return to kettle.
2. Puree cottage cheese in small food processor or blender (if you use a blender, add a tablespoon or two of milk). Add pureed cottage cheese, cheddar cheese and milk; stir well over low heat until cheddar cheese has melted and mixture has warmed through. Add pepper and serve.

Per serving: 363 calories; 22 g protein; 44 g carbohydrate; 2 g fiber; 11 g fat; 7 g saturated fat; 378 mg sodium.

Going out gardening? Don't forget a wide-brimmed hat and a tall water sipper. You'll feel much better and last longer if you don't get overheated and if you stay well hydrated.

Fettucine Alfredo

SERVES 4

The traditional recipe for this famous dish has been called "heart attack on a plate." My version is considerably slimmed down, but is rich in flavor. This dish is great as a leftover; just add a little skim milk when you reheat.

> 1 teaspoon margarine
> 2 cloves garlic
> 1 to 1½ cups skim milk
> 3 tablespoons flour
> 4 ounces nonfat cream cheese
> 4 ounces freshly shredded Parmesan
> ½ pound box fettucine noodles, cooked
>   (about 4 cups cooked noodles)
> salt and pepper to taste

1. Melt margarine over low heat in large fry pan; add garlic and sauté for 5 minutes.
2. Combine milk and flour in jar and shake to mix well. Increase heat to medium low; add milk/flour mixture, cream cheese and Parmesan cheese; stir with whisk to break up cream cheese. Mixture will thicken and cheese will melt.
3. When mixture is uniformly smooth, fold in pasta.

Per serving: 416 calories; 27 g protein; 52 g carbohydrate; 2.3 g fiber; 10.5 g fat; 5.8 g saturated fat; 722 mg sodium.

Nutritional analysis, substituting whole milk for skim milk and regular cream cheese for nonfat cream cheese: 513 calories; 24 g protein; 51 g carbohydrate; 2 g fiber; 23 g fat; 14 g saturated fat; 666 mg sodium.

Tip

Don't tempt your willpower when you are trying to watch your weight. Remove cookie jars and bread baskets from the counter—you'll be surprised what a tremendous help it is in avoiding temptation.

Fontinella-Mushroom Spaghetti

SERVES 6

Fontinella is an Italian hard cheese; if you can't find it, substitute Romano.

> 1 teaspoon margarine
> 2 cloves garlic, minced
> 6 scallions, chopped finely
> ⅛ teaspoon salt
> ⅛ teaspoon ground black pepper
> 2 tablespoons flour plus 2½ cups skim
>   milk, blended well
> 4 ounces nonfat cream cheese
> 5 ounces grated fontinella cheese
> 3 ounces freshly grated Parmesan cheese
> 4 cups sliced mushrooms; buy sliced from
>   grocery store (portobello are best)
> 6 cups cooked spaghetti

1. In a large nonstick skillet melt margarine over low heat. Add garlic and scallions; sauté 3 to 5 minutes. Stir in salt and pepper. Place flour and milk in a small jar and shake to mix. Pour milk/flour mixture over margarine, whisking until mixture starts to thicken. Whisk in cream cheese until mixture is smooth. Whisk in fontinella and Parmesan cheeses, stirring until cheese melts. Stir in mushrooms.
2. Cover. Heat mushrooms through 5 to 7 minutes. Serve over cooked spaghetti.

Per serving: 431 calories; 27 g protein; 52 g carbohydrate; 3.1 g fiber; 12 g fat; 6.5 g saturated fat; 697 mg sodium.

Tip

Buying cut-up vegetables is a great way to save energy. Just make sure you use them fairly quickly, as they don't last as long in the refrigerator as uncut vegetables do.

Spinach Fettuccine

SERVES 4

Try this recipe to get even the most stubborn spinach hater to love spinach!

> ½ pound (8 ounces) uncooked fettucine
>   noodles, or about 5 cups cooked
> 2 teaspoons margarine
> ¾ cup to 1 cup skim milk

4 ounces shredded Swiss cheese
One 9-ounce package frozen creamed
    spinach, thawed
One 10-ounce package frozen spinach, thawed
ground black pepper to taste

1.   Cook pasta according to directions. Drain, lightly rinse and set aside. Return pot to burner, reducing heat to low.
2.   Melt margarine in pan; add ¾ cup milk and Swiss cheese, stirring until cheese has melted. Stir in spinach, heating through until vegetables are piping hot. Stir in pasta, tossing to mix well. Add additional ¼ cup milk to make a thinner consistency, if you desire.

Per serving: 454 calories; 23 g protein; 52 g carbohydrate; 6 g fiber; 16.8 g fat; 7.5 g saturated fat; 375 mg sodium.

Tip

Unlike other cheeses, Swiss cheese is quite low in sodium; one ounce only has about seventy-three milligrams of sodium.

Chicken Noodle Casserole

SERVES 6

It's helpful to have a quick version of chicken noodle casserole , especially when you have leftover roasted chicken or turkey. This one is easy as well as great tasting.

6 ounces dry flat noodles (egg noodles)
2 cans cream of chicken soup
¼ teaspoon ground black pepper
1 onion, minced
2 cups frozen carrots
12 ounces cooked chicken, in chunks

1.   Cook pasta according to package directions, being careful not to over cook; drain.
2.   In quart casserole, mix soup, pepper, onion, carrots and chicken. Fold in noodles.
3.   Bake at 350° for 30 minutes.

Per serving: 271 calories; 22 g protein; 24 g carbohydrate; 3 g fiber; 9 g fat; 3.2 g saturated fat; 808 mg sodium.

Tip

Think twice about buying food from a street vendor. Remember that they have no way of washing their hands.

Chicken Parmesan and Linguine

SERVES 4

This recipe is also great substituting veal, or even eggplant, for the chicken.

1 tablespoon olive oil
2 to 3 cloves garlic, sliced thinly
12 ounces boneless, skinless chicken breasts
   (4 breast halves)
⅓ cup low-fat buttermilk
2 medium onions, chopped
½ cup nonfat Parmesan cheese
Two 8-ounce cans no-salt-added tomato sauce
4 cups sliced mushrooms
¼ teaspoon ground black pepper
¼ teaspoon salt
2 ounces low-moisture, part-skim
   mozzarella cheese, shredded
3 cups cooked linguine

1. Heat oil over low heat; add garlic and sauté for 3 to 4 minutes.
2. While garlic is sautéing, dip chicken breasts in buttermilk. After garlic has sautéed, increase heat to medium-high. Add onions and chicken breasts. Sprinkle ¼ cup of the Parmesan cheese on top of chicken breasts. After chicken has browned for 2 to 3 minutes, flip and sprinkle remainder of the Parmesan cheese on chicken. Sauté second side for 2 to 3 minutes.
3. Reduce heat. Add tomato sauce, mushrooms, pepper and salt. Blend sauce into vegetables. Cover and simmer 20 minutes.
4. Remove cover; add mozzarella cheese. Cover and simmer just until cheese has melted. Serve with hot linguine.

Per serving: 475 calories; 42 g protein; 49 g carbohydrate; 5 g fiber; 10 g fat; 3.1 g saturated fat; 436 mg sodium.

Tip

If you get your exercise by bicycling, don't forget a helmet. A 2½-year study of seven emergency departments in Seattle-area hospitals showed that bicycle helmets, regardless of type, provide substantial protection against head injuries for cyclists of all ages.

Chicken and Zucchini Spaghetti

SERVES 4

Turn chicken into a complete meal with a jar of pasta sauce, zucchini and a box of pasta.

> 1 teaspoon light olive oil
> 2 medium onions, chopped
> 4 boneless, skinless chicken thighs,
>   cut into chunks
> ½ pound zucchini (about 1 medium)
> ½ pound yellow summer squash
>   (about 1 medium)
> 2 cups spicy red pepper pasta sauce
> ⅛ teaspoon salt
> 4 cups cooked thin spaghetti

1. Heat olive oil over medium-high heat; add onions and chicken, sauté just until slightly browned.
2. Reduce heat; add vegetables, pasta sauce and salt. Simmer covered 20 minutes, or until vegetables are tender. Serve over spaghetti.

Per serving: 416 calories; 24 g protein; 55 g carbohydrate; 6.5 g fiber; 10.5 g fat; 2.4 g saturated fat; 388 mg sodium.

Tip

This recipe, like many others in this book, uses light olive oil for sautéing and stir-frying. I use olive oil whenever recipes call for oil because I like the fact that it's high in monounsaturated fats (see chapter 3) and it also has a nice complement of phytochemicals that are probably helpful in preventing cancer and heart disease. I also use this variety of olive oil when I'm using fairly high heat, for several reasons. It's light on the olive taste, so it doesn't take over the flavor in recipes. Also, it doesn't break down as easily as virgin olive oil under high temperatures. Another plus? It's also less expensive than extra-virgin olive oil.

Tuna Casserole

SERVES 6

This tuna casserole recipe has a slightly tangy taste, owing to the mayonnaise.

Two 6-ounce cans tuna packed in water,
with liquid
1 cup frozen peas
1 onion, chopped
1 can cream of mushroom or cream of
celery soup
¼ cup low-fat mayonnaise
4 cups cooked egg noodles
(about 6 ounces dry)
½ cup Chinese rice noodles

1. In 2-quart casserole, mix tuna, peas, onion, mushroom soup and mayonnaise. Fold in pasta.
2. Bake at 350° for 25 minutes. Top with rice noodles and bake 5 minutes more.

Per serving: 337 calories; 23 g protein; 41 g carbohydrate; 3.4 g fiber; 9 g fat; 2 g saturated fat; 720 mg sodium.

Tip

Natural foods (such as eggs and nuts) are far more often a source of food allergies than are food additives and coloring. That helps you appreciate how rare reactions are to food additives!

Tuna Casserole in 15 Minutes

SERVES 4

Here's a very easy version of an old favorite that is high on flavor and nutrition and low on fat. I've eliminated the need to bake this dish, so it's ready faster.

1 tablespoon margarine
2 stalks celery, chopped
1 small onion, chopped
2 teaspoons 33% reduced-sodium chicken
bouillon
1 cup skim milk
2 tablespoons flour
Two 6-ounce cans chunk white tuna
(okay to use very low sodium version)

1 cup frozen peas
⅛ teaspoon ground black pepper
4 cups cooked egg noodles (about
    6 ounces dry)

1. In large nonstick skillet, melt margarine over medium-low heat. Add celery, onion and chicken bouillon; sauté 3 to 5 minutes.
2. Put milk and flour into a jar; shake until all flour is dissolved. Pour milk/flour mixture into celery and onions, stirring constantly. Cook until sauce has thickened. Reduce heat
3. Stir in tuna (with liquid) and peas, cooking until peas have warmed through. Stir in black pepper and cooked pasta. Serve.

Per serving: 432 calories; 35 g protein; 54 g carbohydrate; 5 g fiber; 7 g fat; 1.6 g saturated fat; 755 mg sodium.

Tip

Food irradiation is an important means of eliminating harmful organisms on food. Contrary to popular belief, no radiation residue is left on the food. There is absolutely no evidence that irradiating food increases cancer risk.

Penne Pasta with Tuna in a Garlic Cream Sauce

SERVES 2

Blending tuna, garlic and broccoli into a simple white sauce creates a subtle flavor that you'll love with penne pasta.

2 teaspoons margarine
2 cloves garlic, sliced thinly
1 cup skim milk
2 tablespoons flour
One 6-ounce can tuna
8 ounces frozen broccoli
2 cups cooked penne pasta
¼ teaspoon salt
⅛ teaspoon pepper

1. Melt margarine over low heat; add garlic and sauté 3 to 4 minutes.
2. In small jar, mix milk and flour; shake to combine. Pour milk mixture into margarine/garlic; stir until mixture has thickened.
3. Add tuna (with liquid) and frozen broccoli. Cover and heat through on low heat for 5 to 7 minutes. Fold in cooked penne pasta, salt and pepper.

Per serving: 452 calories; 38 g protein; 59 g carbohydrate; 5.5 g fiber; 7 g fat; 1.5 g saturated fat; 726 mg sodium.

Salmon Spaghetti

SERVES 2

Create a new spaghetti taste sensation with this fabulously easy recipe—frozen vegetables make this recipe a snap. Feel free to leave out the capers if you don't like them.

1 tablespoon margarine
1 onion, chopped
1 teaspoon regular chicken bouillon
    granules
1 teaspoon very low sodium chicken
    bouillon granules
¾ cup skim milk
1 tablespoon plus 1 teaspoon flour
8 ounces baby pea blend frozen vegetables
    (petite peas, baby whole carrots, snow
    pea pods, baby whole cob corn)
One 6-ounce can salmon packed in water
1 tablespoon capers
2 cups cooked spaghetti

1. Melt margarine over medium low heat; add onion and chicken bouillon and sauté briefly.
2. Place milk and flour in jar; shake until mixture is smooth. Add to margarine and onions, stirring until mixture has thickened.
3. Add vegetables, salmon (with liquid) and capers. Mix well; cover and cook over low heat until mixture begins to bubble. Serve over spaghetti.

Per serving: 510 calories; 30 g protein; 65 g carbohydrate; 6 g fiber; 13.8 g fat; 2.9 g saturated fat; 1075 mg sodium.

Tip

Salmon is one of the all-time great sources of omega-3 fatty acids, those great heart disease–fighting fats. Canned salmon is just as good a source as fresh.

Italian Sausage Spaghetti

SERVES 4

This recipe is for the Italian sausage lover. Yes, the real thing is high in salt and fat—but this recipe uses the low-fat version. The flavor is so excellent that you only need a little, which keeps the salt down. This freezes extremely well.

 1 teaspoon light olive oil
 1 medium onion, chopped
 6 ounces turkey Italian sausage
 One 28-ounce can no-salt-added crushed
    tomatoes
 1 teaspoon dried oregano
 1 teaspoon dried parsley
 1 teaspoon dried basil
 ¼ pound sliced mushrooms
 4 cups cooked spaghetti

1. Heat olive oil over medium-high heat; add onion and sausage and sauté until onion is transparent.
2. Add tomatoes and herbs; simmer 15 minutes.
3. Add mushrooms; simmer 5 more minutes. Serve over pasta.

Per serving: 351 calories; 17 g protein; 57 g carbohydrate; 6 g fiber; 5.6 g fat; 1.5 g saturated fat; 383 mg sodium.

Tip

When you're feeling well, make double of your favorite recipe and freeze it. That way, you'll have food on hand for days when you're not feeling up to cooking

Vegetable Lasagna

SERVES 8

I've cut the sodium in this recipe using a unique combination of tomato and spaghetti sauces. This recipe is a little more work, but you can have it as frequently as you wish because it's healthy in every way!

3 cups extra-calcium 1% fat cottage cheese
¾ grated nonfat Parmesan cheese, divided
½ cup liquid egg substitute (the equivalent
   of two eggs)
1½ teaspoons garlic powder
4 cups thawed and drained frozen spinach
   (two 10-ounce packages)
1 cup chopped onions
2 cups sliced mushrooms
One 8-ounce can no-salt-added tomato
   sauce
3 cups of your favorite spaghetti sauce
   (I like spicy red pepper)
12 uncooked lasagna noodles
8 ounces grated part-skim mozzarella cheese

1. Preheat oven to 350°. Spray a 13×9-inch baking pan with nonstick cooking spray.
2. In large bowl, combine cottage cheese, ½ cup Parmesan cheese, eggs, garlic powder and spinach; blend well with fork.
3. Fold in onions and mushrooms; set aside.
4. Spray pan with vegetable oil spray.
5. In bottom of pan, with spatula, evenly spread can of tomato sauce; arrange 4 lasagna noodles over sauce. Spread with half of the vegetable mixture; top with 1½ cups of the spaghetti sauce. Sprinkle with 3 ounces of mozzarella cheese.
6. Repeat lasagna noodles, cottage cheese/vegetable mixture, sauce and cheese.
7. Place remaining lasagna noodles and sauce. Sprinkle with remaining ¼ cup Parmesan cheese and 6 ounces remaining mozzarella cheese. Bake 1 hour at 350°. Let stand 15 to 20 minutes before cutting.

Per serving: 417 calories; 32 g protein; 50 g carbohydrate; 6.4 g fiber; 10.5 g fat; 4.6 g saturated fat; 1126 mg sodium.

Tip

Don't worry about pesticide residues on fruits and vegetables. The health consequences of not eating fruits and vegetables are far, far greater than the potential risk of residues, which might not even be present.

No-Boil Lasagna

SERVES 8

I often avoid making lasagna because it's so much work. This no-boil recipe takes one huge step out of the preparation. You'll want to make this again and again, even on low-energy days. Don't hesitate to buy preshredded cheese, as shredding cheese is so labor-intensive; the shredded version isn't that much more expensive.

> 1 pound very lean ground beef
>   (such as sirloin)
> 1 or 2 medium onions, chopped
> One 28- or 30-ounce jar of your favorite
>   spaghetti (pasta) sauce
> Three 8-ounce cans no-salt-added tomato sauce
> 8 uncooked lasagna noodles
> 7½ ounces low-fat ricotta cheese
> ¼ cup nonfat Parmesan cheese
> 8 ounces 50% reduced-fat mozzarella
>   cheese, shredded
> 8 ounces part-skim mozzarella cheese,
>   shredded

1. Crumble and brown beef with onions. Drain grease; add jar of spaghetti sauce.
2. Pour tomato sauce in bottom of 9×13 pan. Place 4 uncooked lasagna noodles on top of sauce.
3. For next layer, spread half of meat sauce over noodles; top with all the ricotta, sprinkle with all of the Parmesan. Mix together both types of mozzarella, then sprinkle half of mozzarella mixture over top.
4. Place 4 uncooked lasagna noodles on top of cheese; spread remainder of meat sauce and then sprinkle with remaining mozzarella cheese.
5. Bake 45 minutes covered tightly at 350°. Uncover and bake 15 minutes more.
6. Let stand 15 minutes before cutting.

Per serving: 445 calories; 40 g protein; 29 g carbohydrate; 3.9 g fiber; 15.8 g fat; 8 g saturated fat; 471 mg sodium.

*Nutritional analysis substituting whole milk for skim milk and regular cream cheese for nonfat cream cheese: 513 calories; 24 g protein; 51 g carbohydrate; 2 g fiber; 23 g fat; 14 g saturated; 666 mg sodium.

*Recommended for AIDS patients.

Tip

Trying to watch your weight? Remember to shop for groceries on a full stomach—you're less likely to buy tempting treats.

Chicken and Turkey

Apricot Chicken with Walnuts

SERVES 1

This is my favorite chicken dish. Feel free to double, triple or quadruple as you wish.

> 1 teaspoon light olive oil
> 3 ounces chicken breast (half a breast)
> ½ medium onion, chopped
> 1 teaspoon 33% reduced-sodium chicken
>   bouillon
> ⅛ teaspoon ground black pepper
> ¾ cup apricot nectar
> 4 dried apricot halves, chopped
> ¼ cup uncooked brown rice
> ½ cup chopped frozen green pepper (fresh
>   is okay)
> ½ ounce chopped walnuts (about 1 table-
>   spoon)

1. Heat olive oil over high heat. Add chicken breast, onion, bouillon and pepper, sautéing chicken just 2 minutes per side or until lightly browned.
2. Reduce heat. Add apricot nectar, apricots and rice. Simmer covered 25 minutes.
3. Stir in chopped green pepper and walnuts. Simmer uncovered 5 minutes more.

Per serving: 663 calories; 37 g protein; 92 g carbohydrate; 9 g fiber; 17.8 g fat; 2.3 g saturated fat; 677 mg sodium.

Tip

Use brown rice whenever you'd use white rice. Although enriched white rice has had the B vitamins added back, it's nutritionally bankrupt in comparison to brown rice. Go for the brown rice and get more fiber, magnesium, vitamin E, vitamin B_6, copper, zinc—as well as the phytochemicals found in whole grains.

Pineapple Chicken

SERVES 4

This chicken with an oriental flair is distinctively different, but so very easy.

> 1 pound boneless, skinless chicken breast
>   (4 halves)
> One 20-ounce can pineapple tidbits, in
>   own juice
> ½ teaspoon ginger
> ⅛ to ¼ teaspoon black pepper
> 1 tablespoon 33% reduced-sodium chicken
>   bouillon
> 2 cups chopped green pepper (can use
>   frozen)
> ¼ cup cold water
> 2 teaspoons cornstarch
> 4 cups cooked brown rice

1. Spray large nonstick skillet with vegetable oil spray, heat to medium-high. Sauté chicken breasts 3 to 4 minutes per side, until lightly browned.
2. Add pineapple, pineapple juice, ginger, pepper and bouillon. Reduce heat to low, and simmer 15 minutes.
3. Add green pepper and simmer 5 more minutes.
4. Blend cornstarch into cold water until smooth with no lumps.
5. Increase heat to high; when mixture is bubbling, add cornstarch paste. Stir constantly until mixture is thickened.
6. Serve over rice.

Per serving: 515 calories; 41 g protein; 74 g carbohydrate; 6 g fiber; 5.9 g fat; 1.5 g saturated fat; 539 mg sodium.

Tip

Fire can do two things: melt butter and make steel. When adversity strikes, try always to find the good side to it—it's there.

Sweet and Sour Chicken and Onions

SERVES 4

This is one of my favorite one-pot meals. The onions, brown sugar and apples work together to create a unique, rich and luscious sauce.

1 tablespoon plus 1 teaspoon light olive oil
4 split chicken breasts, skin removed, about
    1 pound
¼ cup buttermilk (okay to substitute
    regular milk)
6 tablespoons flour
1 large red onion, peeled and in chunks
2 tablespoons balsamic vinegar
2 tablespoons red wine vinegar
3 tablespoons packed brown sugar
1 tablespoons dried rosemary (or about
    2 to 3 tablespoons fresh rosemary)
1 tablespoon 33% reduced-sodium chicken
    bouillon granules
2 large red cooking apples, in chunks
4 small red potatoes, scrubbed and halved
    (skin on)
pepper to taste

1. Heat olive oil in large nonstick skillet over high heat. Dip chicken breasts in buttermilk and then flour. Place in hot oil and brown (meaty side down) for 5 to 7 minutes.
2. Reduce heat. Add onion, vinegars, brown sugar, rosemary, bouillon, apples, potatoes and pepper. Cover and simmer 45 minutes, or until all vegetables are tender. Baste occasionally, and add a tablespoon of water as necessary (the apples will give up water to provide some liquid). Allow onions and apples to break up into small chunks.

Per serving: 446 calories; 31 g protein; 62 g carbohydrate; 5.3 g fiber; 8.4 g fat; 1.7 g saturated fat; 543 mg sodium.

Tip

Do you grow your own herbs? You can dry them quite easily in the microwave. Place a layer of herbs on a paper towel and microwave on high for about one minute. Flip and microwave for one more minute, or until dry. Store them for about six months in a dark, cool place.

Stir-Fry Chicken with Asparagus and Mushrooms

SERVES 2

Although this one-pot meal has a few more ingredients than some of the other recipes, most of them require no work. You'll love the light and refreshing orange-lemon sauce, especially with the asparagus.

2 teaspoons olive oil

2 cloves garlic, peeled and sliced

6 ounces boneless, skinless chicken breasts
cut for stir-fry

½ pound asparagus, cleaned and sliced on
the diagonal in about 1-inch pieces

1 teaspoon grated orange rind

2 teaspoons lemon juice

¼ pound sliced mushrooms

1 tablespoon plus 1 teaspoon frozen
orange juice concentrate

¼ cup water

2 teaspoons cornstarch

2 cups cooked brown rice

1. Heat olive oil and garlic slices over low heat; sauté about 3 to 4 minutes.
2. Increase heat to medium-high; add chicken breasts, asparagus, orange rind and lemon juice. Sauté 5 minutes. Add mushrooms and sauté an additional 5 minutes.
3. Mix orange juice concentrate, water and cornstarch in a small cup. Add to chicken-vegetable mixture, stirring until thickened.
4. Serve over rice.

Per serving: 472 calories; 36 g protein; 61 g carbohydrate; 6.9 g fiber; 10 g fat; 2 g saturated fat; 80 mg sodium.

Tip

In a research study involving 84,000 female nurses, adding three hours of brisk walking per week lowered the risk of heart attack by an amazing 54 percent. Those who walked more leisurely still had a significant reduction—32 percent.

Barley, Chicken and Okra in a Spicy Red Pepper Sauce

SERVES 4

If you haven't discovered okra, give it a try in this great recipe. It's distinctive yet mild, and is a powerhouse of good nutrition.

> 2 teaspoons light olive oil
> 8 skinless, boneless chicken thighs
> 1 onion, minced
> 2 cups spicy red pepper pasta sauce (or
>   another favorite of yours)
> 1 cup barley
> 2 cups water
> 2 cups frozen cut okra

1. Heat olive oil in large nonstick skillet over medium-high heat. Add chicken thighs and onions; sauté each side 2 to 3 minutes, just to brown.
2. Reduce heat. Add pasta sauce, barley and water. Simmer covered 25 minutes.
3. Add okra and simmer covered another 10 minutes.

Per serving: 504 calories; 37 g protein; 50 g carbohydrate; 12.9 g fiber; 17.5 g fat; 4.3 g saturated fat; 374 mg sodium.

Tip

Do you buckle your seat belt every time you get in the car?

Jamaican Chicken

SERVES 4

Take just five minutes to throw these ingredients into a pan and you'll have a wonderful taste treat. The teriyaki sauce does great things for Brussels sprouts, which otherwise tend to be strong tasting.

> 2 medium onions, chopped
> 8 boneless, skinless chicken thighs
> 1 cup low-sodium teriyaki sauce
> 2 cups frozen Brussels sprouts
> 4 whole wheat dinner rolls

1. Spray large nonstick skillet with vegetable oil spray. Place onions on bottom of pan; place chicken thighs on top of onions. Pour teriyaki sauce over chicken and onions. Simmer 15 minutes covered.

2. Uncover. Add Brussels sprouts and simmer 20 to 30 minutes more, until sauce is thickened and chicken is done. Serve with whole wheat dinner rolls.

Per serving: 347 calories; 37 g protein; 36 g carbohydrate; 6 g fiber; 7.3 g fat; 1.8 g saturated fat; 1306 mg sodium.

Tip

Be careful about accessing nutrition advice from the Internet. Anyone can create a "home page," including people who want to sell nutrition supplements—which they often do under the guise of nutrition education. You can generally find good nutrition advice on the computer from university medical center home pages.

Chicken Fajitas

SERVES 4

This excellent meal will take you ten to twelve minutes to fix. Enjoy it often!

> 1 tablespoon light olive oil
> 1 pound chicken, cut for stir-fry
> 1 pound bag of frozen pepper stir-fry
>   (frozen green, yellow and red peppers
>   and onions)
> 1 tablespoon very low sodium chicken
>   bouillon
> 2 teaspoons 33% reduced-sodium chicken
>   bouillon
> 4 flour tortillas
> reduced fat sour cream (optional)

1. Heat olive oil over high heat. Add chicken and stir-fry for 5 minutes.
2. Add frozen vegetables, bouillon and 1 to 3 tablespoons of water (one tablespoon at a time) to stir-fry. Stir-fry 5 to 8 minutes, or until vegetables are hot and chicken is done.
3. Divide mixture between 4 tortillas. Top each with 1 tablespoon of reduced-fat sour cream if desired.

Per serving: 442 calories; 41 g protein; 40 g carbohydrate; 3.4 g fiber; 11.6 g fat; 2.7 g saturated fat; 674 mg sodium.

Tip

Invest in one excellent nonstick skillet. It will make cooking and cleanup considerably easier.

Creamed Spinach and Chicken

SERVES 6

You don't have to worry about calories and fat when you create this rich and creamy dish.

1 tablespoon light olive oil
1 pound skinless chicken, cut for stir-fry
1 onion, minced
2 packages frozen spinach, thawed (but not
    drained)
1 tablespoon 33% reduced-sodium chicken
    bouillon granules
1 tablespoon very low sodium chicken
    bouillon granules
¼ teaspoon ground black pepper
½ cup nonfat sour cream
6 English muffins

1. In large nonstick skillet, heat olive oil over medium-high heat; add chicken and onion and brown, about 5 to 7 minutes.
2. Stir in spinach, bouillon and pepper; cover and simmer 5 to 7 minutes.
3. Stir in sour cream and heat through for 5 minutes over low heat.
4. Toast English muffins; serve creamed chicken and spinach over toasted English muffin halves.

Per serving: 343 calories; 32 g protein; 39 g carbohydrate; 4.4 g fiber; 6.2 g fat; 1.3 g saturated fat; 717 mg sodium.

★Nutritional analysis substituting regular sour cream for nonfat sour cream: 363 calories; 32 g protein; 36 g carbohydrate; 4 g fiber; 10 g fat; 4 g saturated fat; 713 mg sodium.

★Recommended for AIDS patients.

Tip

Reduced-fat and fat-free sour cream and cream cheese aren't made from chemicals—they just have the fat removed. Use them often to make food interesting, creamy and rich.

Creamed Chicken Over Toast

SERVES 4

Turn an ordinary can of soup into a nutrient-loaded feast in just minutes.

> 1 pound chicken, cut for stir-fry
> 1 cup frozen pearl onions
> 1 can cream of chicken soup
> 1 cup skim milk
> 1 tablespoon plus 1 teaspoon very low
> sodium chicken bouillon granules
> black pepper to taste
> ½ cup nonfat sour cream
> 2 cups frozen chopped green peppers
> 4 slices whole wheat toast

1. Spray nonstick pan with vegetable oil spray and heat to medium-high heat. Add chicken and onions and stir-fry until chicken is done.
2. Add cream of chicken soup, skim milk, bouillon, pepper and sour cream. Stir to combine; heat through over low heat; about 5 minutes.
3. Add frozen green peppers; simmer 5 minutes. Serve over toast.

Per serving: 440 calories; 46 g protein; 40 g carbohydrate; 3.9 g fiber; 10.3 g fat; 2.9 g saturated fat; 1031 mg sodium.

*Nutritional analysis substituting whole milk for skim milk and regular sour cream for nonfat sour cream: 487 calories; 45 g protein; 36 g carbohydrate; 4 g fiber; 18 g fat; 8 g saturated fat; 1,022 mg sodium.

*Recommended for AIDS patients.

Tip

Do you take calcium and iron supplements? If so, take one in the morning and one at night, as they interfere with the absorption of each other when taken at the same time.

Honey Glazed Carrots and Parsnips with Chicken Thighs

SERVES 4

Carrots and parsnips are a great vegetable duo—complementing each other in flavor as well as in color.

8 boneless, skinless chicken thighs
4 large carrots, sliced in thick (about
    1-inch) slices on the diagonal
4 large parsnips, sliced in thick (about
    1-inch) slices on the diagonal
1½ cups water
4 teaspoons 33% reduced-sodium chicken
    bouillon granules
4 teaspoons very low sodium chicken
    bouillon granules
black pepper to taste (about ⅛ to
    ¼ teaspoon)
2 tablespoons plus 2 teaspoons honey
4 cups brown rice

1. Spray large nonstick skillet with vegetable oil spray; heat to medium-high. Add chicken thighs and sauté until slightly browned.
2. Reduce heat. Add carrots, parsnips, water, bouillon, pepper and honey. Simmer over low heat (just slightly bubbling) about 30 minutes. Vegetables should be fork tender and sauce should be a thick glaze. Serve over rice.

Per serving: 579 calories; 33 g protein; 81 g carbohydrate; 8.7 g fiber; 13.3 g fat; 3.5 g saturated fat; 729 mg sodium.

Tip

If you use the cutting board to cut up chicken, don't forget to wash it with hot, soapy water before you use it again. Ditto for other raw meat. Better yet, put it in the dishwasher.

Chicken and Portobello Mushrooms in a Rich Garlic Mushroom Sauce

SERVES 4

The combined flavors of portobello mushrooms and garlic make chicken something special.

> 2 teaspoons olive oil
> 2 cloves garlic, minced
> 4 boneless, skinless chicken breasts
> 4 teaspoons 33% reduced-sodium chicken
>   bouillon granules
> ⅛ to ¼ teaspoon black pepper
> ½ pound portobello mushrooms, sliced
> 1 can low-sodium cream of mushroom
>   soup
> 4 cups cooked linguine

1. Heat olive oil over low heat; add garlic and sauté 3 to 5 minutes. Increase heat; add chicken breasts, bouillon and pepper, sauté 2 to 3 minutes per side, just until slightly browned.
2. Reduce heat; add mushrooms and soup; simmer uncovered 20 to 30 minutes, stirring and basting occasionally. Serve over cooked pasta.

Per serving: 227 calories; 29 g protein; 8 g carbohydrate; 1.5 g fiber; 9.2 g fat; 2.5 g saturated fat; 681 mg sodium.

Nutritional analysis with addition of 4 cups cooked linguine: 424 calories; 35 g protein; 47 g carbohydrate; 4 g fiber; 10 g fat; 3 g saturated fat; 682 mg sodium.

Tip

Don't rely on thirst to tell you when it's time to take a drink. Most people don't feel thirsty until they're almost dehydrated. As we age, the thirst mechanism becomes even less efficient. Unless your medical condition or medications don't permit it, drink at least six 8-ounce glasses of water daily.

Rosemary Roasted Chicken and Vegetables

SERVES 6

Roast up a big chicken and then have the leftovers for lunch or another meal. The rosemary and balsamic vinegar work together beautifully for a rich and satisfying taste.

> 1 tablespoon olive oil
> 2 tablespoons dried rosemary (or 3 to 4
>   tablespoons fresh rosemary)
> 1 tablespoon parsley flakes
> 1 tablespoon garlic powder
> 1 teaspoon salt
> ½ teaspoon black pepper
> 1 roasting chicken (about 2½ to 3 pounds)
> 2 tablespoons balsamic vinegar
> 1 pound red potatoes, quartered
> 1 pound baby carrots
> 3 yellow onions, quartered

1. In cup, mix olive oil, rosemary, parsley, garlic powder, salt and pepper until well blended.
2. Place chicken in roaster pan, and place a third of spice/oil mixture inside cavity of chicken. Roast in 425° oven for 30 minutes.
3. While chicken is baking, place vegetables in bowl. Add balsamic vinegar to remainder of spice/olive oil mixture, blending well. Pour mixture over vegetables; stir well to coat.
4. Pour fat from roaster pan. Arrange vegetables around chicken. Cover. Reduce heat to 375° and bake for 1½ to 2 hours, or until chicken is done (until juices run clear, or until chicken reaches an internal temperature of 185°) and vegetables are tender.

Per serving: 338 calories; 31 g protein; 29 g carbohydrate; 4.6 g fiber; 10.5 g fat; 2.5 g saturated fat; 508 mg sodium.

Tip

High-fat diets have been associated with an increase in the risk of cancers of the colon and rectum, prostate and endometrium.

Oven Roasted Chicken Legs and Sweet Potatoes

SERVES 4

Buttermilk and cornflakes add a new flavor dimension to chicken legs. Keep powdered buttermilk on hand for recipes like this one. Serve with steamed broccoli or green beans for a complete meal.

> 8 skinless chicken legs
> 1 cup buttermilk (okay to substitute
> regular milk)
> 2 cups cornflakes, crushed after measuring
> 4 sweet potatoes
> salt and pepper to taste

1. Coat chicken legs with buttermilk; dip in cornflakes. Repeat, coating chicken twice. Add salt and pepper to taste. Place on one end of cookie sheet sprayed with vegetable oil spray.
2. Place in oven at 375° for 30 minutes.
3. While chicken bakes, peel sweet potatoes and slice into ¼-inch-thick slices. After chicken has baked 30 minutes, remove from oven. On other end of cookie sheet (spray again with vegetable oil spray), spread out sweet potato slices. Spray top of sweet potatoes with vegetable oil spray. Salt lightly.
4. Return cookie sheet to oven and bake an additional 30 minutes.

Per serving: 320 calories; 30 g protein; 36 g carbohydrate; 2.8 g fiber; 5.7 g fat; 1.7 g saturated fat; 463 mg sodium.

Tip

Unless otherwise restricted by your physician, take all medications with a full glass of water. Just a sip may cause the pills to become stuck in your esophagus, the muscular tube that carries food from the mouth to the stomach.

Italian Chicken and Rice

SERVES 4

A fabulously easy one-pot meal loaded with exceptional nutrition and phenomenal taste.

> 1 pound boneless, skinless chicken breasts
> ½ cup chopped onion
> One 28-ounce can no-salt-added crushed tomatoes
> ¾ cup uncooked brown rice
> 1¼ cups water
> 1½ teaspoons oregano
> 1 teaspoon garlic salt
> 1 teaspoon parsley flakes
> 2 cups frozen cut okra
> 2 cups sliced mushrooms

1. Spray large nonstick skillet with vegetable oil spray. Heat to medium-high. Sauté chicken breasts and onions, 2 minutes per side, just to sear meat.
2. Add crushed tomatoes, rice, water, oregano, garlic salt and parsley flakes. Stir well. Reduce heat to low and simmer 20 minutes, covered.
3. Add frozen okra and mushrooms, cover and simmer an additional 15 minutes.

Per serving: 435 calories; 44 g protein; 52 g carbohydrate; 8 g fiber; 5.6 g fat; 1.5 g saturated fat; 334 mg sodium.

Tip

Although you may find fat-free mayonnaise objectionable, give the low-fat version a try. It's far more acceptable!

Everyone's Favorite Chicken and Rice Casserole

SERVES 4

This is a trimmed-down version of creamy, distinctive chicken casserole. The lemon juice shows through just enough to lend a fresh flavor.

> 12 ounces cooked chicken, diced
> 4 stalks celery, sliced
> 1 onion, chopped finely
> 2 cups cooked rice
> 1 can condensed cream of chicken soup
> 3 tablespoons lemon juice
> ¼ cup low-fat mayonnaise
> 1 tablespoon margarine
> 1 cup cornflakes

1. Combine chicken, celery, onion, rice, soup, lemon juice and mayonnaise. Mix well.
2. In small microwavable bowl, melt margarine. Add cornflakes, and then toss to coat. (Alternatively, melt margarine in small fry pan, and then coat cornflakes with melted margarine.)
3. Sprinkle cornflakes over top of casserole. Bake uncovered 25 minutes at 350°.

Per serving: 417 calories; 32 g protein; 40 g carbohydrate; 2 g fiber; 13.4 g fat; 3.2 g saturated fat; 878 mg sodium.

Tip

Suspect that you have a food allergy? Don't diagnose it yourself and place yourself on an overly restricted diet. Instead, consult an allergist for a proper diagnosis and treatment.

Chicken and Rice in a Roasted Red Pepper Sauce

SERVES 2

Grab a jar of roasted red peppers and turn ordinary chicken and rice into a flavor sensation.

> One 7.25-ounce jar roasted red peppers
> (not oil packed)
> 6 basil leaves
> 1 teaspoon light olive oil
> 1 clove garlic
> 2 boneless, skinless split chicken breasts
> ½ cup uncooked brown rice
> ⅔ cup water
> ¼ teaspoon salt
> ⅛ teaspoon ground black pepper
> 1 red pepper, cut in strips

1. Puree red peppers and basil in a blender or food processor; set aside.
2. Heat oil over low heat; add garlic and sauté 3 to 5 minutes. Increase heat slightly, add chicken breasts and sauté each side 2 to 3 minutes.
3. Reduce heat; add rice, water, pureed red peppers, salt and pepper. Simmer 25 minutes. Place red pepper strips on top of chicken and rice; cover and simmer 5 to 7 minutes, just until red pepper strips are crisp tender.

Per serving: 379 calories; 32 g protein; 44 g carbohydrate; 3 g fiber; 7.4 g fat; 1.6 g saturated fat; 734 mg sodium.

Tip

It's a good idea to keep canned fruit on hand for days when you run out of fresh fruit. Just choose the varieties packed in their own juice, as the syrup packed ones contain lots of calories, too. For example, one cup of canned pineapple pieces contains seventy-seven calories, but one cup packed in heavy syrup contains 199 calories.

Orange Ginger Chicken and Rice

SERVES 2 (DOUBLE OR TRIPLE AS NECESSARY)

Using tea bags to flavor rice, as I have in this recipe, is a great low-fat trick. Try it with other grains, too.

2 teaspoons olive oil

2 cloves garlic, minced

2 boneless, skinless chicken breast halves
    (6 to 8 ounces)

1½ cups water

2 teaspoons 33% reduced-sodium chicken
    bouillon granules

¼ teaspoon ground black pepper

¾ teaspoon ground ginger

2 orange spice tea bags

1 tablespoon reduced-sodium soy sauce

½ cup brown rice (uncooked)

1 cup chopped green peppers (okay to use
    frozen)

¼ cup water plus 1 tablespoon cornstarch,
    blended into a paste

2 teaspoons frozen orange juice
    concentrate

One 11-ounce can mandarin oranges,
    drained

1. Heat olive oil on low heat, add garlic and sauté briefly.
2. Increase heat, add chicken breasts and sauté 2 minutes each side to lightly brown.
3. Add water, bouillon, pepper, ginger, tea bags, soy sauce and brown rice. Reduce heat and simmer 25 minutes.
4. Remove tea bags. Add green peppers and simmer 5 minutes.
5. Stir in cornstarch paste, stirring constantly until mixture has thickened.
6. Remove from heat. Stir in orange juice concentrate and fold in oranges.

Per serving: 234 calories; 16 g protein; 32 g carbohydrate; 1.7 g fiber; 4.6 g fat; 0.9 g fat; 469 mg sodium.

Tip

Using very low sodium bouillon granules instead of 33% reduced-sodium lowers the amount of sodium per serving from 469 milligrams to 169 milligrams.

Tip

Homebound for a prolonged period? Change your surroundings if you can't leave them. Move pictures around, bring in an inexpensive bouquet of flowers from the grocery store once per week.

Chicken, Rice and Mushroom Casserole

SERVES 4

The velvety rice created by this combination of ingredients is a winner. The mushrooms and onions flavor this dish gently, yet richly. This recipe takes only ten minutes of preparation time—you'll want to make it frequently.

> 1 cup rice (not instant)
> 2½ cups skim milk
> 1 can cream of chicken soup
> 2 teaspoons very low sodium chicken
>   bouillon
> 2 onions, chopped finely
> ½ pound sliced mushrooms
> 4 split chicken breasts, skin removed

1. Spray 9×9-inch baking dish with vegetable oil spray. Combine rice, milk, soup and bouillon in baking dish; stir together with spoon or fork. Stir in onions and mushrooms.
2. Lay chicken breasts on top of rice mixture (meaty side down).
3. Cover tightly with aluminum foil and bake at 350° for 1 hour.

Per serving: 483 calories; 39 g protein; 60 g carbohydrate; 2.8 g fiber; 8.5 g fat; 2.5 g saturated fat; 749 mg sodium.

Tip

If cooking, shopping and cleanup are difficult, make them family chores—and make them fun. For instance, when you go the grocery store, give everyone his or her own list and then meet at the register.

One-Pot Chicken and Rice

SERVES 2

This fabulous one-pot meal freezes well for another day.

2 teaspoons light olive oil
1 onion, diced
2 split chicken breasts, skin removed,
 about ½ pound
One 14.5-ounce can no-salt-added
 crushed or pureed tomatoes
½ cup uncooked brown rice
1 cup water
2 bay leaves
2 teaspoons garlic powder
2 teaspoons 33% reduced-sodium chicken
 bouillon granules
2 teaspoons low-sodium chicken bouillon
 granules★
¼ teaspoon black pepper
1 cup frozen peas

1. Heat olive oil in large nonstick skillet over medium-high heat; add onion and chicken breasts and sauté until chicken is browned and onions are transparent.
2. Reduce heat; add remainder of ingredients, except peas, cover and simmer 30 minutes.
3. Add peas; simmer an additional 10 minutes.

Per serving: 535 calories; 39 g protein; 72 g carbohydrate; 10.7 g fiber; 9.3 g fat; 1.8 g saturated fat; 738 mg sodium.

★Substituting low-sodium chicken bouillon for the 33% reduced-sodium chicken bouillon significantly decreases the amount of sodium per serving from 1060 mg to 460 mg.

Tip

Adding herbs to your therapeutic regimen? Make sure you discuss them with your doctor, as some can interact with medications. Also, never add herbs and subtract conventional medications without discussing it with your physician.

Minted Chicken Salad

SERVES 4

The sauce for this chicken salad is an absolute explosion of flavor—and so easy, too. The mint complements the vegetables splendidly, but if you don't have fresh mint, just leave it out. The sauce still make a great chicken salad.

1 pound cooked chicken (or turkey)
   breast, diced
4 stalks celery, sliced thinly
12 cherry tomatoes, cut into quarters
1 cup petite frozen peas, thawed
½ cup low-fat sour cream
3 tablespoons lemon juice
¼ cup mint leaves, minced
¼ teaspoon salt
⅛ to ¼ teaspoon black pepper
4 cups chopped romaine lettuce leaves

1. Combine chicken, celery, tomatoes and peas in mixing bowl.
2. In small bowl, mix together well sour cream, lemon juice, mint, salt and pepper.
3. Pour sauce over chicken mixture; toss to coat well. Serve over chopped romaine lettuce leaves.

Per serving: 287 calories; 40 g protein; 27 g carbohydrate; 4 g fiber; 8.1 g fat; 3.5 g saturated fat; 177 mg sodium.

Tip

Although it's sometimes a bother to pick up unusual ingredients such as the fresh mint this recipe calls for, you'll enjoy a new flavor so much. Unique and distinctive flavors such as the fresh mint in this recipe help make low-fat, lower sodium cooking interesting.

Chicken Salad in a Pineapple Sauce

Serves 4

SERVES 4

If you make up this dish according to the directions, you'll only use one bowl—making cleanup a cinch.

SAUCE

¼ cup plus 2 tablespoons low-fat sour cream

¼ cup plus 2 tablespoons pineapple juice
   (from drained pineapple)

1 tablespoon dried cilantro (or 2 tablespoons fresh cilantro, minced)

¼ teaspoon salt

⅛ to ¼ teaspoon black pepper

TO CONTINUE RECIPE

8 ounces cooked chicken, diced

1 cup chopped green pepper

1 cup chopped red pepper

One 20-ounce can pineapple tidbits,
   drained, with liquid reserved for sauce

4 cups chopped romaine lettuce

1. In medium mixing bowl, whisk together sauce ingredients.
2. Add chicken, green pepper, red pepper and pineapple tidbits. Mix well.
3. Divide romaine lettuce between 4 plates, top with chicken salad and serve.

Per serving: 237 calories; 21 g protein; 27 g carbohydrate; 5 g fiber; 5 g fat; 2.3 g saturated fat; 215 mg sodium.

Peanut and Poppy Seed Chicken Salad

SERVES 4

Fruit, vegetables and nuts make for a distinctive chicken salad. Serve with whole wheat rolls for a complete meal.

12 ounces cooked chicken breast, diced

One 11-ounce can mandarin oranges, drained

¼ cup honey-roasted peanuts

¼ cup raisins

1 red onion, peeled and chopped

¼ cup fat-free poppy seed dressing

4 cups chopped romaine lettuce

1. Combine all ingredients except lettuce in quart-size bowl. Toss to mix well.
2. Divided romaine lettuce between 4 plates; top with chicken salad. Serve with whole wheat rolls for a complete meal.

Per serving: 298 calories; 31 g protein; 27 g carbohydrate; 2.9 g fiber; 7.8 g fat; 1.5 g saturated fat; 254 mg sodium.

Waldorf Chicken Salad

Serves 4

My variation of an all-time favorite salad is a meal in itself—it's also lean!

> 6 stalks celery, sliced
> 2 red apples (Gala works best, but not essential)
> 8 ounces cooked chicken breast, diced
> 20 dates, chopped
> 2 ounces walnuts, chopped
>
> ### SAUCE
> ¼ cup plus 2 tablespoons low-fat mayonnaise
> 2 tablespoons lemon juice
>
> ### SALAD
> 4 cups chopped romaine lettuce

1. Combine first 5 ingredients in quart-size bowl.
2. In cup, blend together sauce ingredients. Pour sauce over vegetable/chicken mixture. Toss to coat. Chill.
3. Divide lettuce between 4 plates; top with vegetable/chicken mixture.

Per serving: 409 calories; 23 g protein; 51 g carbohydrate; 8 g fiber; 15.2 g fat; 2 g saturated fat; 213 mg sodium.

Tip

Apples are loaded with flavonoids, a phytochemical thought to help fight cancer, heart disease and infections.

Chicken Pot Pie

SERVES 6

Using frozen vegetables and a prepared pie crust makes this an exceptionally easy dish. Substitute left-over roasted turkey if you have it on hand.

> 1 teaspoon margarine
> 1 onion, chopped
> 3 tablespoons flour
> 1½ cup skim milk
> 1 tablespoon 33% reduced-sodium chicken
>   bouillon granules
> ⅛ teaspoon ground black pepper
> 12 ounces cooked chicken, diced (about 2
>   whole chicken breasts)
> 1 cup frozen carrot slices
> 1 cup frozen peas
> ½ cup frozen corn
> 2 frozen deep dish pie crusts

1. Melt margarine over medium heat. Add onion and sauté briefly.
2. Mix flour, milk, bouillon granules and pepper in glass jar; shake to make a smooth paste. Pour paste over onions, stirring constantly. Cook 2 to 3 minutes, just until mixture has started to thicken.
3. Place chicken and vegetables in pie crust. Pour onion/sauce mixture evenly over the top of chicken and vegetables. Put top crust over, pinching together the top and bottom crusts at the edge. Make 4 slits in crust.
4. Bake 1 hour at 350°.

Per serving: 406 calories; 24 g protein; 39 g carbohydrate; 3.8 g fiber; 16.8 g fat; 5.2 g saturated fat; 693 mg sodium.

Tip

Avoid kitchen sponges—they are sources of germs in the kitchen. While these germs aren't a problem for most people, they can be a problem for people who are weakened by disease and/or who take certain medications. Instead, use a dishcloth that you wash daily.

Chicken Enchilada Pie

SERVES 6

This dish is a great way to use leftover chicken or turkey. If you like it zestier, just use hotter enchilada sauce. This dish freezes well.

One 20-ounce can mild enchilada sauce
3 large flour tortillas
½ pound chicken, cooked and diced
One 16-ounce can fat-free refried beans
1 cup chopped green pepper (can use frozen)
1 cup chopped onion (about 1 medium)
4 ounces shredded taco cheese

1. Spray deep dish 9-inch pie pan with vegetable oil spray. Place 2 tablespoons sauce in bottom of pan; spread to coat.
2. Put one tortilla on bottom of pan. Spread half of chicken and half of refried beans on tortilla. Sprinkle with ½ cup green pepper, and ½ cup chopped onion. Drizzle with one-third of remaining sauce and sprinkle with half of cheese. Repeat, except for cheese.
3. Place remaining tortilla on top; press edges down into sides. Spread with remaining sauce and sprinkle with remaining cheese.
4. Bake covered for 30 minutes at 350°. Uncover and bake additional 15 minutes.
5. Let stand 15 minutes before cutting.

Per serving: 347 calories; 22 g protein; 36 g carbohydrate; 4.4 g fiber; 12.4 g fat; 5 g saturated fat; 860 mg sodium.

Tip

Is your physical energy or ability limited? How long has it been since you tried swimming? Perhaps you feel you've grown too out of shape to pile all of you into a little spandex. But you won't start on the path to better physical fitness—and pride in your appearance—unless you start doing something physically active today. No matter what your figure, people will think you are brave for trying.

Creamy Chinese Cabbage and Chicken

SERVES 6

If you don't like mushrooms, substitute reduced-fat cream of chicken soup for the mushroom soup and leave out the mushrooms; it's just as tasty.

1 head Napa cabbage, also called Chinese
    cabbage (about 1½ pounds)
1 pound boneless, skinless chicken breast,
    in chunks
2 cans reduced-sodium cream of
    mushroom soup
1 pound sliced mushrooms (purchased
    already sliced)
2 cups regular rice, uncooked
2 cups water
2 tablespoons low-sodium chicken bouil-
    lon granules
½ cup cornflakes

1.   Shred cabbage with a knife.
2.   Place all ingredients but cornflakes in 2-quart casserole; toss to mix.
3.   Cover and bake 25 minutes at 350°.
4.   Uncover and bake an additional 20 to 25 minutes, or until cabbage is fork tender.
5.   Add cornflakes and bake 10 minutes more.

Per serving: 454 calories; 32 g protein; 63 g carbohydrate; 4 g fiber; 8.5 g fat; 2.6 g saturated fat; 779 mg sodium.

Tip

Keep your upper body strong by lifting two soup cans over your head, repeating five to ten times. These convenient cans turn you into a weight lifter!

Turkey-Spinach Loaf

SERVES 6

This "meat loaf" is almost a meal in one as it's loaded with lean protein, folate, fiber and minerals. Bake up a big loaf, even if you're cooking for one, and freeze in individual portions for up to one month. Bake a sweet (or regular) potato, pour a glass of milk and add an apple for a complete meal.

> 1 cup low-sodium vegetable juice
> ½ cup minced onion
> ¼ cup dried parsley flakes
> 1 teaspoon salt
> 1 pound extra-lean ground turkey
> One 10-ounce package frozen chopped
>   spinach
> 2 eggs, beaten, or the equivalent in liquid
>   egg substitute
> 1 cup oatmeal (not instant)
> ¾ cup nonfat sour cream
> 2 tablespoons bottled lemon juice

1. Place vegetable juice in 2-quart bowl. Stir in onion, parsley and salt.
2. Place remaining ingredients except sour cream and lemon juice in bowl with vegetable juice mixture; mix well with fork.
3. Spray 9-inch loaf pan with vegetable oil spray; transfer mixture into loaf pan.
4. Bake at 350° 45 minutes.
5. In small bowl, mix together sour cream and lemon juice.
6. Serve topped with lemon-flavored sour cream.

Per serving: 202 calories; 25 g protein; 18 g carbohydrate; 3 g fiber; 3.3 g fat; 1 g saturated fat; 580 mg sodium.

Tip

Don't hesitate to accept professional psychological help. I firmly believe that everyone with chronic illness should have some mental health professional with whom they can unload the burden of their illness. While family members are great for this, even they need a break from the demands of your illness. Accepting help is not giving in, it is having the strength to go forward.

Orange Glazed Turkey Cutlets with Parsnips and Sweet Potatoes

SERVES 4

Although a great source of lean protein, turkey cutlets are often dry. This is the first of several recipes that solve the problem! Keep turkey cutlets in the freezer for quick recipes like this one.

> 1 teaspoon olive oil
> 4 turkey cutlets (2 to 3 ounces each)
> 1 large sweet potato, peeled and sliced
>   thinly
> 4 parsnips, peeled and sliced
> 2 tablespoons honey
> ½ cup water
> 1 tablespoon 33% reduced-sodium chicken
>   bouillon
> 1 tablespoon grated orange rind
> black pepper to taste

1. Heat olive oil over medium heat in large nonstick skillet. Add turkey cutlets; brown on each side. Remove cutlets.
2. Add sweet potato slices, parsnips, honey, water, bouillon and orange rind. Reduce heat so that this mixture simmers (uncovered) until sweet potatoes and parsnips are tender and liquid has thickened; about 10 to 15 minutes.
3. Add cutlets back to mixture; cover and let simmer 5 minutes. Add pepper to taste and serve.

Per serving: 306 calories; 26 g protein; 32 g carbohydrate; 4.5 g fiber; 8.2 g fat; 2.1 g saturated fat; 513 mg sodium.

Tip

Use fat-free and low-fat foods with caution—substituting them for the regular fat variety in the same serving size you would normally have. Fat-free cookies and coffee cakes, for example, can have just as many calories as the regular fat counterpart, and you can end up gaining lots of weight on fat-free foods if you eat more of them.

Turkey Cutlets in an Apple Raisin Sauce with Sweet Potato Slices

SERVES 4

Warm up your soul and fill your home with rich aromas when you cook up this recipe on a cold winter day.

1 tablespoon olive oil
4 turkey cutlets (2 to 3 ounces each)
1 sweet potato, sliced
½ cup raisins
2 apples, cored and chopped coarsely
¾ cup water
1 teaspoon salt
black pepper to taste (about ⅛ to
    ¼ teaspoon)
¼ teaspoon cinnamon

1. Heat olive oil over medium heat in large nonstick skillet. Add turkey cutlets; brown and then remove.
2. Add sweet potato slices, raisins, apples, water, salt, pepper and cinnamon. Cover and simmer 10 to 15 minutes until sweet potatoes are tender and apples have started to break apart.
3. Add turkey cutlets and simmer 5 minutes uncovered.

Per serving: 327 calories; 26 g protein; 34 g carbohydrate; 3 g fiber; 10.5 g fat; 2.5 g saturated fat; 637 mg sodium.

Tip

Steam fresh vegetables rather than boiling them. Overcooking vegetables that have soluble fiber (such as asparagus and broccoli) breaks the soluble fiber down to sugars—meaning that you can lose about half the soluble fiber with overcooking.

Tomatoes with Turkey Cutlets
in a Chunky Parmesan Tomato Sauce

SERVES 2 (MAY DOUBLE OR HALVE)
Jarred pasta sauce jazzes up turkey—and is even more interesting with a touch of Parmesan cheese.

2 teaspoon light olive oil
1 clove garlic, sliced thinly
2 turkey cutlets (2 to 3 ounces each)
2 small onions, peeled and cut into chunks
1 cup spicy red pepper pasta sauce
2 cups cooked penne pasta
2 tablespoons fat-free grated Parmesan cheese

1. Heat olive oil over low heat with sliced garlic, about 3 to 4 minutes.
2. Increase heat to medium; add turkey cutlets and onions. Sauté about 5 minutes.
3. Add pasta sauce; decrease heat and simmer about 5 minutes.
4. Place half of turkey/tomato mixture on 1 cup of penne pasta; sprinkle with one tablespoon Parmesan cheese per serving.

Per serving: 511 calories; 36 g protein; 54 g carbohydrate; 5 g fiber; 14.8 g fat; 3.2 g saturated fat; 383 mg sodium.

Tip

Sneak more fiber (and vitamins and minerals) into your family's diet by adding a little wheat germ to meat loaf and casseroles.

Turkey Cutlets and Broccoli
in a Rich Cheese Sauce

SERVES 2
Garlic and cheddar cheese combine to liven up turkey cutlets and broccoli.

2 turkey cutlets (2 to 3 ounces each)
1 teaspoon margarine
2 cloves garlic, thinly sliced
1 cup skim milk
2 tablespoons flour
2 ounces sharp cheddar cheese, grated
8 ounces frozen broccoli
½ teaspoon salt
black pepper to taste
2 cups cooked egg noodles

1. Spray large nonstick skillet with vegetable oil spray; heat to medium heat. Brown cut-lets on both sides and remove from pan.
2. Add margarine and garlic, sauté over low heat 2 to 3 minutes.
3. In small jar, shake milk and flour until well dissolved. Pour over margarine and garlic; add salt and pepper. Add cheese, and stir all until mixture has thickened and cheese has melted.
4. Add broccoli, cover and heat through 5 minutes. Add turkey cutlets back, cover and heat through an additional 5 minutes.
5. Serve over egg noodles.

Per serving: 615 calories; 48 g protein; 59 g carbohydrate; 5.4 g fiber; 20.6 g fat; 9 g saturated fat; 934 mg sodium.

Tip

Using spices instead of sodium can have many unexpected advantages besides decreasing sodium: one teaspoon of chili powder, for examples, supplies 18 percent of the U.S. Recommended Daily Allowance for vitamin A in the form of beta-carotene.

Turkey Cutlets with Sliced Potatoes in a Celery Sauce

SERVES 2

The celery and onions give this easy dish a rich flavor. While the sodium in this dish is a little higher than most, you can still fit it nicely into a day, if you're on a sodium-restricted diet, by planning ahead.

> 2 teaspoons olive oil
> 2 turkey cutlets (2 to 3 ounces each)
> 2 small onions, in small chunks
> 2 potatoes, washed and sliced thinly (leave peel on)
> 2 carrots, peeled and sliced thinly
> 1 stalk celery, sliced in thick slices
> 1 can cream of celery soup
> ½ cup water
> black pepper to taste (optional)

1. Heat olive oil over medium heat in a large nonstick skillet. Add turkey cutlets and onions and brown cutlets on each side.
2. Remove cutlets, but leave onion in pan. Add potato slices, carrot slices, celery, cream of celery soup and water. Simmer for about 20 minutes, or until vegetables are tender. Add turkey cutlets back; add pepper to taste. Cover and warm through for about 5 minutes before serving.

Per serving: 508 calories; 31 g protein; 56 g carbohydrates; 7.2 g fiber; 18.4 g fat; 4.3 g saturated fat; 1260 mg sodium.

Kielbasa and Barley with Maple Syrup

SERVES 4

Low-fat turkey kielbasa flavors this dish richly, and because it's here in just the right proportions, it doesn't add too much sodium. This kielbasa is also low fat, so you don't have to worry about the fat grams either!

2 teaspoons light olive oil

12 ounces low-fat turkey kielbasa

2 onions, chopped

1 cup uncooked barley

3 cups water

1 tablespoon real maple syrup

1-pound bag baby pea blend frozen vegetables
    (petite peas, baby whole carrots, snow pea
    pods, baby whole cob corn)

1. Heat olive oil over high heat. Slice kielbasa into thin rounds. Cook kielbasa and onion briefly over high heat, just to brown both.
2. Reduce heat. Add barley, water and maple syrup. Simmer 25 minutes. Add vegetables and simmer 5 to 10 minutes more, until vegetables are warmed through.

Per serving: 400 calories; 23 g protein; 55 g carbohydrate; 11.6 g fiber; 10.3 g fat; 2.9 g saturated fat; 767 mg sodium.

Tip

Hippocrates said, "Let your food be your medicine; let your medicine be your food." Indeed, try to plan nutritious food for every day to give yourself the nutrition advantage.

Roasted Sausage and Vegetables

SERVES 4

You'll be delightfully surprised at how the beets and vinegar flavor everything so uniquely and wonderfully. The dill adds great color to this dish that cooks itself.

12 ounces low-fat turkey kielbasa, sliced
    into ½-inch rounds

1 head cauliflower (about 1 pound), in flowerettes

4 large beets (about 1 pound), peeled and
    cut into small chunks

4 medium red potatoes, quartered with skin on

2 tablespoons balsamic vinegar

1 tablespoon extra-virgin olive oil

¼ cup fresh chopped dill

salt and pepper to taste

1. Place sausage and vegetables in clay roaster or glass baking dish sprayed with vegetable oil spray.
2. Whisk together remaining ingredients in small bowl; pour over vegetables. Toss to coat.
3. Cover; bake 45 minutes, or until vegetables are tender, stirring and basting once after 20 minutes.

Per serving: 391 calories; 21 g protein; 55 g carbohydrate; 8.5 g fiber; 11.7 g fat; 2.9 g saturated fat; 894 mg sodium.

Tip

Eat potato skins whenever you can. With a medium baked potato, this doubles the amount of fiber you'll get.

Brown Sugar Roasted Apples, Sweet Potatoes and Kielbasa

SERVES 4

Everyone will love this rich and interesting combination. It's a wonderful complete meal, especially on a cold winter day.

6 sweet potatoes, peeled and cut in chunks

4 apples, quartered

½ cup packed raisins

1 pound low-fat turkey kielbasa, sliced into thin rounds.

½ cup apple juice or cider (I prefer cider)

¼ cup packed brown sugar

2 teaspoons cinnamon

1. Place sweet potato chunks, apple pieces, raisins and kielbasa in casserole; stir to mix. Pour apple juice or cider over mixture. Sprinkle with brown sugar and cinnamon. Toss to mix. Cover.
2. Bake at 350° one hour or until sweet potatoes are tender. Stir once after 30 minutes.

Per serving: 386 calories; 14 g protein; 71 g carbohydrate; 7.1 g fiber; 6.8 g fat; 2.2 g saturated fat; 691 mg sodium.

Rich and Bubbly Main Dish Baked Beans

SERVES 4

Using just the right combination of tomato products, dried mustard and flavor-rich real maple syrup—along with smoked turkey kielbasa—makes this healthy version of baked beans irresistible. Don't hesitate to freeze the leftovers.

½ cup packed brown sugar

¼ cup vinegar

One 8-ounce can no-salt-added tomato
   sauce

One 6-ounce can no-salt-added tomato
   paste

6 tablespoons real maple syrup

1 teaspoon dried mustard

½ teaspoon ground black pepper

One 15½-ounce can white beans, drained
   and rinsed

One 15½-ounce can pinto beans, drained
   and rinsed

6 ounces smoked turkey kielbasa, sliced
   and then quartered

1. Coat 2-quart baking dish with vegetable oil spray. Combine all ingredients in baking dish; mix well.
2. Cover and bake at 350° for 45 minutes. Uncover and bake for 15 minutes.

Per serving: 474 calories; 18 g protein; 91 g carbohydrate; 12.9 g fiber; 5.1 g fat; 1.2 g saturated fat; 879 mg sodium.

Tip

Many of us think that certain foods and dishes are off-limits—in most cases, though, it's possible to find a healthier version. That's true of this baked bean dish. Enjoy it frequently, and you'll actually be improving your diet due to the high fiber content and the other great nutritional attributes in the beans.

Tip _____

When buying ground turkey, look for *extra-lean* on the package. Regular ground turkey is actually quite high in fat.

Turkey Basil Loaf

SERVES 4

This meat loaf is a an easy meal to prepare. Freeze it in portions for easy lunches or a quick dinner.

> 1 pound extra-lean ground turkey
> One 10-ounce package frozen spinach,
>   thawed
> 1 cup fresh basil leaves
> 1 egg
> 2 slices whole wheat bread
> 1 sauce packet onion soup mix
> 1 cup nonfat sour cream
> 2 to 3 tablespoons lemon juice

1. Place all turkey loaf ingredients (except sauce ingredients) in food processor. Process until mixture is well blended. Alternatively, if not using food processor: a) Beat egg with a fork in medium-sized mixing bowl. b) Blend in onion soup mix. c) Chop basil; stir in. d) Break up bread into small pieces; stir into egg mixture. e) Stir in thawed spinach and turkey with fork, mix until well blended.
2. Spray 9-inch loaf pan or square 9×9-inch pan with vegetable oil spray. Bake at 350° for 40 minutes.
3. Blend lemon juice into yogurt. Top each portion of turkey loaf with lemon-yogurt mixture.

Per serving: 266 calories; 37 g protein; 25 g carbohydrate; 4 g fiber; 3.9 g fat; 1.1 g saturated fat; 479 mg sodium.

Tip _____

Refrigerate fresh herbs without washing them. They'll last longer.

Beef, Lamb and Sausage

Stir-Fry Beef and Broccoli

SERVES 4

Using frozen vegetables and buying the meat already cut up makes this a meal ready in literally minutes.

> 2 tablespoons very low sodium beef
>   bouillon granules
> ½ cup warm water
> 1 tablespoon cornstarch
> ¼ cup warm water
> 8 ounces extremely lean beef cut for
>   stir-fry (sirloin or eye of round)
> 2 tablespoons oyster sauce
> Two 1-pound bags frozen broccoli, red
>   peppers, onions and mushrooms (or
>   another blend you like)
> 4 cups cooked brown rice

1. Blend beef bouillon granules into ½ cup water; set aside. Blend cornstarch into ¼ cup water; set aside.
2. Spray large nonstick skillet or wok with vegetable oil spray. Heat to medium–high. Add beef and stir-fry until slightly browned. Add a fourth of water/bouillon mixture and oyster sauce. Stir-fry 5 minutes.
3. Add frozen vegetables and remainder of water/bouillon mixture. Cover and simmer 5 minutes, or just until vegetables have heated through, but before broccoli pales in color.
4. Add water/cornstarch mixture, stirring constantly, until thickened. Serve immediately over rice.

Per serving: 376 calories; 73 g protein; 58 g carbohydrate; 5 g fiber; 5 g fat; 1.5 g saturated fat; 309 mg sodium.

Tip

Do you have a diagnosed food allergy? Always carry with you the medications that you need to treat it. For example, carry an oral antihistamine, and perhaps an injectable substance called epinephrine. Ask your doctor what is appropriate for you.

Tip

Intensely flavored ingredients like the dark sesame oil in this recipe add lots of flavor and dimension to food. Because they are so flavor intense, you only have to add a little, which keeps the calories down.

Chinese Cabbage and Beef in Sesame-Soy Sauce

SERVES 4

Using dark sesame oil adds tremendous flavor to this stir-fry—but just a few fat grams.

> 1 tablespoon dark sesame oil
> 2 cloves garlic, minced
> 1 pound lean beef, cut in strips for
>   stir-fry★
> 5 cups chopped raw Chinese cabbage
> 3 tablespoons reduced-sodium soy sauce
> 1 cup diced sweet red pepper (about
>   1 whole pepper)
> 1 cup chopped scallions (green portion
>   only)
> ¼ teaspoon black pepper
> 1 cup grated carrots
> 2 tablespoons sesame seeds
> 3 cups hot cooked brown rice

1. Heat oil in large nonstick skillet or wok over low heat; add garlic and sauté 3 to 4 minutes. Increase heat; add beef and black pepper. Stir-fry 5 minutes.
2. Add cabbage and soy sauce and stir-fry 2 to 3 minutes. Add pepper and scallions, stir-fry 2 to 3 additional minutes.
3. Stir in grated carrots and sesame seeds. Serve over brown rice.

  ★You should be able to buy it this way at the supermarket.

Per serving: 496 calories; 42 g protein; 47 g carbohydrate; 7 g fiber; 15 g fat; 4.7 g saturated fat; 610 mg sodium.

Tip

Find a way to get outside every day—even if it is to sit on your front porch or deck in a wheelchair. The fresh air and new sights and sounds are invigorating.

Peppered Beef and Rice

SERVES 4

This one-pot meal is exceptionally easy and full of excellent flavor. The ginger tamari in this recipe is a great condiment to keep on hand; it's a great addition to vegetable stir-fries.

1 tablespoon light olive oil
2 cloves garlic, sliced
1 large yellow onion, chopped
12 ounces very lean beef, cut up for
    stir-fry★
⅛ teaspoon ground black pepper
1¼ cups water
½ cup uncooked brown rice
1 tablespoon 33% reduced-sodium beef
    bouillon granules
1 large green pepper, cored and cut into
    strips
1 large red pepper, cored and cut into
    strips

1. Heat olive oil over low heat with garlic in large nonstick skillet or electric fry pan; sauté 3 to 5 minutes.
2. Increase heat to high; add onion, beef and black pepper. Stir-fry 3 to 5 minutes to brown.
3. Add water, rice and bouillon. Cover and simmer 20 minutes.
4. Add pepper strips; cover and simmer 5 minutes more. Pepper strips should be crisp-tender.

★You should be able to buy it this way at the supermarket.

Per serving: 303 calories; 27 g protein; 25 g carbohydrate; 2 g fiber; 10 g fat; 3 g saturated fat; 509 mg sodium.

Tip

Have you tried to find a support group for people with your illness? Check the phone book, call the library or browse the Internet. Also, check "Resources" in this book for the address and phone number of the national organization that supports people with your diagnosis.

Beef Stroganoff

SERVES 6

I've remade this old-fashioned favorite dish, which is notoriously very high fat, not only in a leaner style, but also much easier. Although you have to boil noodles in another pot, you can cook the stroganoff, start to finish, in one pot. This is one is a surefire hit!

    2 tablespoons margarine
    2 onions, chopped
    1 pound lean beef, cut up for stir-fry★
    2 tablespoons flour
    1 cup water
    1 tablespoon plus 1 teaspoon beef bouillon
        granules (or 4 beef bouillon cubes)
    1 tablespoon plus 1 teaspoon very low
        sodium beef bouillon granules
    2 teaspoons ketchup
    2 teaspoons garlic powder
    ½ pound sliced mushrooms
    ⅔ cup nonfat sour cream
    ground black pepper to taste
    6 cups cooked egg noodles

1. Melt margarine in large nonstick skillet over medium-high heat; add onions and beef; brown for 10 minutes. Add flour; brown for an additional 2 to 3 minutes.
2. Reduce heat; stir in water, bouillon, ketchup, garlic powder and mushrooms. Cover and simmer 15 minutes.
3. Stir in sour cream, add pepper to taste; simmer 5 minutes. Serve over cooked noodles.

Per serving: 447 calories; 26 g protein; 54 g carbohydrate; 3 g fiber; 13 g fat; 4 g saturated fat; 763 mg sodium.

★You should be able to buy it this way at the supermarket.

Tip

Taking the time to search out a great recipe like this one—especially when the work isn't much more than heating up an already prepared meal—is well worth the few moments it takes. You'll feel like a wizard in the kitchen again—or for the first time. It's a real confidence booster for new cooks.

Spanish Rice

SERVES 6

This one-pot, easy version of an old favorite is both fresh and rich in taste. The extra dose of tomatoes adds to its tremendous flavor and texture. This stores well in the refrigerator for a great leftover lunchtime treat.

½ pound very light lean ground beef
1 tablespoon olive oil
1 large onion, peeled and chopped
1 cup uncooked rice (not instant)
One 29-ounce can no-salt-added tomato
    puree
One 14-ounce can diced tomatoes
1 teaspoon ground cumin
2 teaspoons to 1 tablespoon garlic powder
1 teaspoon chili powder
½ teaspoon salt
2 cups frozen chopped green peppers
5 ounces shredded sharp cheddar cheese

1. Spray large nonstick pan or electric fry pan with vegetable oil spray and heat to medium heat. Brown beef, breaking up into small pieces. Remove from pan.
2. Add olive oil and onion; brown onion for 5 to 10 minutes.
3. Add rice, tomato puree, diced tomatoes, cumin, garlic powder, chili powder and salt. Cover and simmer 30 minutes.
4. Stir in green peppers, cooked beef and cheese; cover and heat through 10 minutes. Serve.

Per serving: 370 calories; 18 g protein; 45 g carbohydrate; 4.9 g fiber; 14 g fat; 7 g saturated fat; 525 mg sodium.

Tip

Go for a spin through the mall to break up long weeks. Difficult to walk? Most malls have complimentary wheelchairs—just take a friend to push you. Looking at new fashions, furniture and stopping for a frozen yogurt or a flavored decaf coffee is a great way to add a new dimension to a prolonged recovery.

Taco Salad

SERVES 4

Turn ordinary tacos into a powerhouse of good nutrition with this recipe that packs in more vegetables than you can with the average taco.

½ pound ground sirloin

1 package taco seasoning (1.25 ounce)

⅓ cup water

One 15.5-ounce can kidney beans, drained
    and rinsed

½ pound romaine lettuce, chopped

2 medium tomatoes, chopped

6 scallions, cleaned and chopped
    (approximately 1½ cups)

½ cup nonfat sour cream

4 tablespoons salsa

4 ounces shredded taco cheese
    (or cheddar)

1. Brown meat in medium nonstick skillet, breaking up into tiny pieces. Drain on paper towels. Return to skillet; add taco seasoning and water. Add kidney beans and heat through.

2. Divide lettuce, tomatoes and scallions between 4 plates. Top with a fourth of the beef/kidney bean mixture. Top with sour cream, salsa and shredded cheese.

Per serving: 403 calories; 33 g protein; 35 g carbohydrate; 10 g fiber; 14 g fat; 8 g saturated fat; 1288 mg sodium.

Tip

Whenever you can, substitute romaine lettuce for leaf or head lettuce. It has loads more nutrition. As you get your family used to the switch, mix the lettuces half and half, gradually working up to all romaine lettuce.

Stuffed Cabbage Casserole

SERVES 6

Do you love stuffed cabbage—but hate the time it takes to prepare? Then try this version, and your taste buds won't know the difference! This dish freezes well.

2 cups uncooked rice (brown or white, but
  not instant)
Two 28-ounce cans no-salt-added crushed
  tomatoes
1 teaspoon sage
3 teaspoons 33% reduced-sodium beef
  bouillon
¼ teaspoon black pepper
1 cup chopped onion
1 pound very lean ground beef (such as
  sirloin), crumbled
1 medium head cabbage, shredded (or buy about
  2 pounds cabbage shredded for coleslaw)

1. Place all ingredients in a covered roasting pan; stir well.
2. Bake covered for 1 to 1½ hours at 350°, or until cabbage is fork-tender.

Per serving: 519 calories; 33 g protein; 78 g carbohydrate; 10 g fiber; 8 g fat; 2.9 g saturated fat; 383 mg sodium.

Tip

Make a commitment to help someone less fortunate than you. It will help you in so many ways; you'll feel less restricted by your disease or handicap.

Best-Loved Ground Beef Casserole

SERVES 4

This one-skillet version of the all-time favorite beef casserole will become a standby in your household.

½ pound ground sirloin
2 onions, chopped
¼ teaspoon pepper
1 teaspoon salt
One 28-ounce can crushed tomatoes
One 14-ounce can diced tomatoes
4 ounces uncooked small seashell pasta
  (about 1½ cups uncooked)
1 teaspoon sugar

1. Spray large nonstick skillet with vegetable oil spray, heating to medium-high. Add ground sirloin, onions, pepper and salt, breaking up beef with wooden spoon. Brown briefly (about 4 minutes).
2. Reduce heat to a simmer. Add tomatoes and pasta. Cover and simmer 5 to 7 minutes, or until pasta is done. Sprinkle sugar over the top and mix thoroughly.

Per serving: 343 calories; 26 g protein; 48 g carbohydrate; 6 g fiber; 4.8 g fat; 2 g saturated fat; 791 mg sodium.

Tip

Using no-sodium-added crushed tomatoes lowers the amount of sodium per serving to 743 milligrams in this recipe.

Fran's Dinner-in-One

SERVES 6

This was a favorite dish of one of my husband's medical school buddies. Dinner-in-One got them through medical school well nourished.

> 1 pound ground sirloin
> 2 medium onions, finely chopped
> ⅛ teaspoon ground black pepper
> ¼ teaspoon salt
> 1 teaspoon garlic powder
> 4 medium potatoes, sliced in ¼-inch slices
> 6 carrots, peeled and sliced
> 1 can cream of tomato soup
> 1 cup chopped green pepper

1. In medium nonstick skillet, brown sirloin with onions, salt and garlic powder, breaking up sirloin with wooden spoon as it browns.
2. In large casserole layer half of ground beef, potatoes and carrots; repeat. Pour tomato soup over the top.
3. Sprinkle chopped green pepper over top of tomato soup. Cover.
4. Bake at 350° for 1 hour, or until potatoes and carrots are tender.

Per serving: 385 calories; 25 g protein; 38 g carbohydrate; 4.7 g fiber; 15 g fat; 5.9 g saturated fat; 456 mg sodium.

Tip

Do you have children? Teach them to cook early. Grade schoolers can learn the basics of cooking that don't involve a hot stove, and teenagers can learn to prepare first one and then several easy dishes. This will be a tremendous help for you on low-energy days—and you'll be doing them a favor.

Shepherd's Pie

SERVES 6

A great dish for leftover mashed potatoes. In fact, I always make double my mashed potatoes, purposefully creating leftovers for this family favorite. You can also make the mashed potatoes when you make the dish, as I've shown in the recipe.

> 1 pound ground sirloin
> 2 onions, chopped
> ½ teaspoon salt
> pepper to taste
> 6 potatoes
> ¾ cup skim milk
> 4 ounces nonfat cream cheese
> 3 cups frozen corn

1. In nonstick skillet, brown sirloin with onions, salt and pepper, breaking up sirloin into small pieces.
2. Boil potatoes until very tender. Drain and return them to their pot. Add milk, cream cheese, salt and pepper to taste and heat through on low heat for 2 minutes★. To mash, use a stand mixer if you have one.
3. Spray 2-quart casserole with vegetable oil spray. Place half of mashed potatoes on bottom, spreading evenly and bringing up the sides about 1 inch.
4. Spread frozen corn over mashed potatoes. Sprinkle hamburger/onion mixture over top of corn. Spoon remaining mashed potatoes on top.
5. Bake at 350° for 40 minutes, uncovered.

★Potatoes mash to a smoother consistency if you heat the milk and cream cheese first.

Per serving: 392 calories; 31 g protein; 56 g carbohydrate; 6 g fiber; 11.9 g fat; 2.5 g saturated fat, 363 mg sodium.

Tip

If you're on immunosuppressive medications, be extra careful with food safety considerations. See the section in chapter 10 regarding food safety.

Beef and Barley in a Tomato Sauce

SERVES 6

Give barley a try in this tomatoey-beef dish. It adds such great texture and flavor—far more flavor than rice does.

> 1 tablespoon light olive oil
> 1 pound lean beef chunks for stew
>   (bought cut up)
> 1 cup raw barley

2 cans cream of tomato soup
2 cups water
2 tablespoons very low sodium beef bouillon
1-pound bag frozen carrot coins

1. Heat olive oil over medium-high heat. Add beef and stir-fry until just browned, about 5 minutes.
2. Reduce heat; add barley, tomato soup, water and bouillon. Cover and simmer 30 minutes.
3. Stir in carrots and simmer 15 minutes more, or until carrots are heated thoroughly.

Per serving: 380 calories; 28 g protein; 46 g carbohydrate; 8 g fiber; 9.9 g fat; 3 g saturated fat; 666 mg sodium.

Barbecued Beef and Rice

SERVES 4

If you like barbecued beef, you'll love this low-fat, lower salt version. In this recipe, I've substituted ground mustard for prepared mustard, reducing the sodium considerably; the salt is also cut down by using some tomato sauce for part of the ketchup.

1 tablespoon light olive oil
½ pound very lean beef, in chunks for stew
2 onions, chopped
1 cup chopped celery
One 8-ounce can no-salt-added tomato sauce
½ cup ketchup
¼ cup water
2 tablespoons brown sugar
1 tablespoons ground mustard
2 tablespoons Worcestershire sauce
4 cups hot cooked brown rice

1. In large nonstick Dutch oven, heat olive oil over medium-high heat. Add beef, onions and celery. Cook until browned, about 5 to 7 minutes.
2. Add tomato sauce, ketchup, water, brown sugar, mustard and Worcestershire. Simmer covered 2 hours, uncovering for just the last 20 minutes.
3. Serve over hot cooked brown rice.

Per serving: 482 calories; 25 g protein; 73 g carbohydrate; 6.6 g fiber; 10.6 g fat; 2.6 g saturated fat; 530 mg sodium.

Tip

Ordering a hamburger out? Ask your server to tell the chef not to butter the bun—most restaurants do.

Beef and Barley in a Creamy Broccoli Sauce

SERVES 6

A excellent one-pot meal that is loaded with great nutrition and fabulous taste.

> 1 tablespoon light olive oil
> 2 cloves garlic, minced (optional)
> 1 pound lean beef chunks for stew
>   (bought cut up)
> 1 cup uncooked barley
> 2 cans cream of broccoli soup
> 2 cups water
> 2 tablespoons very low sodium beef
>   bouillon granules
> 1-pound bag frozen broccoli
> ground black pepper to taste

1. In large nonstick skillet, heat olive oil with garlic over low heat. Increase heat to medium-high, add beef and brown for 5 minutes.
2. Reduce heat. Add barley, soup, water and bouillon. Cover and simmer for 30 minutes.
3. Stir in broccoli and simmer an addition 10 to 15 minutes, or until broccoli is warmed through.

Per serving: 390 calories; 31 g protein; 36 g carbohydrate; 8.3 g fiber; 13.4 g fat; 5 g saturated fat; 708 mg sodium.

Tip

People who are allergic to avocados, bananas, kiwis, peaches, papayas and chestnuts might also be allergic to latex—the material from which surgical gloves, balloons and condoms are made. If you have these food allergies, alert any medical personnel who might touch you with surgical gloves, including the dentist.

Beef and Sweet Potatoes with Onion Confit

SERVES 4

Prepare this gourmet meal with ease. Another plus? It's a one-dish meal.

> 1 tablespoon light olive oil
> ¾ pound sirloin steak, trimmed of fat
> 3 sweet potatoes, peeled and sliced in
>   about ¼-inch slices
> 1 cup frozen pearl onions

1½ cups water

2 teaspoons 33% reduced-sodium beef
    bouillon granules

½ cup white wine

6 tablespoons dried currants

1. Heat oil in large nonstick skillet over medium-high heat; add steak and brown on both sides 2 to 3 minutes each side.
2. Combine remaining ingredients in saucepan with steak; cover and simmer over medium heat for 20 minutes.
3. Uncover and simmer over low heat for 20 minutes to reduce, basting occasionally.

Per serving: 356 calories; 27 g protein; 36 g carbohydrate; 4.2 g fiber; 9.5 g fat; 3 g saturated fat; 475 mg sodium.

Tip

Cold and flu season? Wipe down the bathroom with a cloth dipped in a weak bleach solution—especially around the sink and faucets.

Minted Lamb and Peas

SERVES 2

2 lamb chops (choose a lean variety, such
    as sirloin)

2 carrots, peeled and sliced thinly

1 onion, chopped

½ teaspoon garlic powder

salt and pepper to taste

1 cup frozen green peas

¼ cup mint sauce★

1. Spray large nonstick pan with vegetable oil spray; heat over medium-high heat. Add lamb chops, carrots and onion, cooking chops about 7 minutes per side, and stir-frying vegetables.
2. Reduce heat; add garlic powder, salt, pepper, peas and mint sauce. Cover and cook approximately 5 to 7 minutes.

★Buy in a jar in the condiment section of your supermarket.

Per serving: 214 calories; 19 g protein; 23 g carbohydrate; 7.2 g fiber; 4.9 g fat; 1.7 g saturated fat; 135 mg sodium.

Curried Lamb and Rice

SERVES 2

While you often think of lamb as a fattier meat, that's not always true. Just choose carefully and you can get a fairly lean cut. Curry is a great complement to the lamb—and to the parsnips, carrots and rice.

> 2 lamb chops (choose a lean variety, such
> as sirloin)
> 1 onion, chopped
> 2 stalks celery, sliced thinly
> 2 parsnips, peeled and sliced in ½-inch slices
> 2 carrots, peeled and sliced in ½-inch slices
> ⅔ cup uncooked rice
> 2⅔ cup water
> 1 teaspoon curry powder
> ½ teaspoon salt
> ⅛ teaspoon ground black pepper

1. Spray large nonstick skillet with vegetable oil spray; heat over medium–high heat. Add lamb chops and onion; sauté each side for 3 to 4 minutes.
2. Reduce heat. Add celery, parsnips, carrots, rice, water, curry powder, salt and pepper. Cover tightly and simmer 25 minutes.

Per serving: 440 calories; 21 g protein; 77 g carbohydrate; 7.9 g fiber; 5.3 g fat; 2.3 g saturated fat; 692 mg sodium.

Tip

New research has shown that increasing the amount of fiber-rich whole grains in your diet may help decrease the risk of developing adult-onset (type II) diabetes. Researchers think that the fiber helps slow the absorption of carbohydrates; it's also possible that the magnesium that is so plentiful in grains may help the body use insulin more efficiently to lower blood sugar. Of course, regular exercise and maintaining a trim body weight are also essential in reducing diabetes risk.

Baked Reuben

SERVES 6

This makes an absolutely beautiful dish that tastes just like the real Reuben—for a fraction of the sodium and fat—and a whole lot more nutrition.

> 1 head purple cabbage, shredded (about
> 1 to 1½ pounds)
> 1½ cups uncooked brown rice
> ¼ cup balsamic vinegar
> 3 cups water

1½ cups fat-free thousand island dressing
1 pound flank steak
3 ounces grated Swiss cheese

1. Spray a 9×12-inch baking dish with vegetable oil spray. In pan, combine cabbage, rice, vinegar, water and thousand island dressing. Mix well.
2. Place flank steak on top of cabbage-rice mixture.
3. Cover tightly with aluminum foil and bake at 350° for 1 hour.
4. Place ½ ounce grated Swiss cheese on top of each portion when served.

Per serving: 508 calories; 30 g protein; 67 g carbohydrate; 7 g fiber; 13.2 g fat; 6.1 g saturated fat; 726 mg sodium.

Tip

Settle for no less than fabulously nutritious food—especially when you're not feeling well. Make an effort to add a vegetable and a fruit to both lunch and dinner. You'll be surprised at what a difference it makes!

Basil-Roasted Vegetables and Flank Steak

SERVES 4

Mild, yet distinctive balsamic vinegar tenderizes the flank steak and lends a fabulous flavor to this meal; the basil adds even more flavor. The carrots, parsnips and leek also add rich flavor and make this meal complete and vitamin packed. Leaving the carrots and parsnips whole preserves vitamins.

4 tablespoons balsamic vinegar
1 tablespoon olive oil
2 to 3 cloves garlic, minced
4 to 6 basil leaves, chopped finely
1 pound flank steak
4 carrots, peeled
½ pound parsnips, peeled
1 leek, in chunks

1. In roasting pan, blend balsamic vinegar, olive oil, garlic and basil. Add flank steak, carrots, parsnips and leek. Toss to coat vegetables and meat with liquid.
2. Cover tightly and bake at 350° for 1 hour.

Per serving: 374 calories; 33 g protein; 26 g carbohydrate; 5.5 g fiber; 15.3 g fat; 5.5 g saturated fat; 135 mg sodium.

Tip

If you take vitamin tablets, opt for one multivitamin/mineral tablet (and perhaps a calcium supplement) instead of many different pills for each different nutrient. It's easy to overdose on vitamins, which can be dangerous. Also, keep iron supplements out of reach of children—accidental overdose of iron remains a leading cause of fatal poisoning in children under age six.

Swiss Steak with Celery, Onions and Potatoes

SERVES 4

The mushroom soup and tomatoes blend together to create a rich sauce for this lean complete beef meal.

> 1 tablespoon light olive or canola oil
> 1 pound lean sirloin, trimmed of all fat and
>   cut into 4 pieces
> ¼ cup flour
> ¼ to ½ teaspoon ground black pepper
> 2 medium onions, quartered
> 8 stalks celery, each cut in thirds
> 4 potatoes, scrubbed and quartered with peel on
> One 28-ounce can no-salt-added crushed tomatoes
> 1 can cream of mushroom soup
> 1 tablespoon low-sodium beef bouillon
> 2 teaspoons sugar

1. Heat oil in large nonstick skillet or electric fry pan on medium–high. Coat meat in flour, sprinkle with pepper and then brown.
2. Reduce heat. Add remainder of ingredients, stirring to mix well.
3. Simmer covered for 1 hour.

Per serving: 606 calories; 42 g protein; 70 g carbohydrate; 8 g fiber; 17.4 g fat; 4.9 g saturated fat; 774 mg sodium.

Tip

Occasionally, reflect on how far you have come in coping with a chronic illness— especially on "bad days." You'll no doubt be proud of how well you've built up your coping skills.

Poppy's Favorite Cash

SERVES 4

As a little boy, my husband dubbed this old family favorite hash recipe "cash." Over the years, it became known as Poppy's Favorite Cash—my father-in-law came to look forward to turning leftover roast beef and fixins into this fabulous old-fashioned food. I've eliminated the leftover fat-laden gravy, and substituted a hearty, concentrated beef bouillon that makes it moist and flavorful. This is also a great food for people who have a difficult time chewing.

> 2 to 3 medium onions, peeled and cut into
>   large chunks
> leftover roast beef (about 8 ounces), trimmed
>   of all fat and cut into large chunks
> leftover potato chunks (about 3 to 4 potatoes that
>   were baked with roast, skin on and in chunks)

leftover roasted carrots (about 4 to 6 whole
   carrots—if you don't have leftovers, cook some)
1 tablespoon very low sodium beef bouillon granules
1 tablespoon regular beef bouillon granules
black pepper to taste
garlic powder to taste
1 to 1½ cups water

1. In a food processor, in small batches, process onions, beef, potatoes and carrots just until coarsely ground. (If you don't have a food processor, dice all ingredients finely.)
2. Spray large nonstick skillet or electric fry pan with vegetable oil spray and heat to medium-high. Add processed mixture; add bouillon granules, pepper and garlic powder and water. Heat through, stirring constantly to mix seasonings. Serve piping hot.

Per serving: 297 calories; 20 g protein; 44 g carbohydrate; 6 g fiber; 4.3 g fat; 1.5 g saturated fat; 758 mg sodium.

Tip

Have you been forgoing beef in an attempt to cut down on fat and cholesterol? You don't have to. Note that chosen properly, beef can be quite lean. It's also a great source of some minerals that are in much lower quantities in chicken and fish, especially zinc and iron. Enjoy a reasonable-sized portion of lean beef twice per week without hesitation.

Crock Pot Flank Steak

SERVES 6

This dish cooks itself, creating a rich sauce. Leaving the peels on the potatoes not only makes this meal easier, but also boosts fiber intake.

1 pound flank steak, cut into 6 pieces
3 small onions, quartered
4 carrots, peeled and cut in thirds
6 potatoes, scrubbed and halved (peel on)
Two 8-ounce cans no-salt-added tomato sauce
Two 14-ounce cans diced tomatoes
1 tablespoon plus 1 teaspoon 33%
   reduced-sodium beef bouillon

Place all ingredients in slow cooker. Cook on high power for 4 hours, or until all vegetables are tender.

Per serving: 372 calories; 25 g protein; 48 g carbohydrate; 7 g fiber; 7.9 g fat; 3.4 g saturated fat; 728 mg sodium.

Beef Stew

Serves 6

Using some frozen vegetables and already cleaned baby carrots makes this beef stew so easy to prepare. You'll be delightfully surprised by the great flavor the parsnips lend to the sauce.

1 tablespoon canola or light olive oil
1 pound lean beef for stew
3 tablespoons flour
½ pound baby carrots
4 parsnips, peeled and chunked
3 small yellow onions, peeled and
    quartered
2 cups water
1 tablespoon 33% reduced-sodium beef
    bouillon
2 tablespoons very low sodium beef
    bouillon granules
1 tablespoon garlic powder
½ pound frozen peas

1. Heat oil in large nonstick skillet over medium-high heat; add beef and flour. Brown, stirring to coat beef with flour.
2. Reduce heat. Add remaining ingredients (except frozen peas); simmer for 45 minutes, or until vegetables are done.
3. Stir in frozen peas and heat an additional 5 to 10 minutes, or until peas are warmed through.

Per serving: 284 calories; 26 g protein; 27 g carbohydrate; 6.4 g fiber; 8 g fat; 2.2 g saturated fat; 406 mg sodium.

Tip

Instead of planning one vegetable for dinner, always plan two. And make sure they are different colors. That's a great way of making sure you harvest a good complement of nutrients.

Pot Roast

SERVES 4

Turn an ordinary pot roast into a feast. The balsamic vinegar helps tenderize even a tougher cut of meat; it also lends a richness—not a vinegary taste at all. Using potatoes with the peel not only saves work, but it also adds more fiber and nutrients to this meal. I always make more than we can eat, and use the leftovers to make Poppy's Favorite Cash (page 336).

1 pot roast, trimmed of visible fat
(about 1¼ to 1½ pounds)
1 cup water
1 package onion soup mix
garlic powder to taste (about 2 to
3 teaspoons)
black pepper to taste
⅓ cup balsamic vinegar
6 carrots, peeled (keep them whole)
4 potatoes, scrubbed and quartered

1.   Place roast in roasting pan. Pour water over roast. Sprinkle with onion soup mix, garlic powder and pepper. Pour balsamic vinegar over spices. Cover and bake at 325° for 2 hours.
2.   Add carrots and potatoes. Cover and bake an additional hour.

Per serving: 426 calories; 29 g protein; 48 g carbohydrate; 6 g fiber; 14.8 g fat; 6 g saturated fat; 256 mg sodium.

Tip

Try to make complete meals like this one work for two nights. Just double the recipe and serve it three or four days later with a different fruit for dessert—and no one will recognize it as leftovers. This way, you can save yourself some time in the kitchen at least two nights a week.

Pork

Pork Stir-Fry in a Gingered Orange Sauce

SERVES 4

This is another excellent and distinctive one-pot meal that you can make in just minutes by buying the meat already cut up and using frozen vegetables.

> 1 teaspoon dark sesame oil
> 2 cloves garlic, minced
> 8 ounces very lean pork, cut into chunks
>   for stir-fry
> ¼ teaspoon pepper
> 2 teaspoons beef bouillon
> Two 16-ounce bags frozen oriental blend
>   vegetables
> 2 tablespoons orange marmalade
> 1 tablespoon reduced-sodium soy sauce
> 2 tablespoons water
> ½ teaspoon ground ginger
> ¼ cup water plus 1 tablespoon cornstarch,
>   blended into a paste
> 4 cups cooked egg noodles or rice

1. Heat oil in large nonstick skillet over low heat with minced garlic, stir-frying garlic for 3 to 5 minutes.
2. Increase heat and add pork, stir-frying until pork is browned and done.
3. Add pepper, bouillon, frozen vegetables, orange marmalade, soy sauce, 2 tablespoons water and ginger; mix well, reduce heat, cover and let mixture steam for 7 to 10 minutes, or until vegetables are hot.
4. Stir in cornstarch paste, and stir until mixture has thickened. Serve over hot egg noodles (or rice).

Per serving: 458 calories; 29 g protein; 61 g carbohydrate; 7.2 g fiber; 9 g fat; 2.7 g saturated fat; 629 mg sodium.

Tip

If you don't sleep well at night, try limiting daytime naps. Also, try not to nap after two or three in the afternoon.

Pork (or Chicken or Beef) Chow Mein

SERVES 4

Using fresh sprouts not only improves the flavor, but also lowers the sodium of this recipe. This chow mein is also great made with chicken or beef.

1 teaspoon olive oil
½ pound lean pork (sirloin or tenderloin),
    cut into chunks
1½ cups chopped celery, with leaves
1 teaspoon very low sodium beef bouillon
    granules
1 cup chopped green pepper
1 cup water
¼ cup reduced-sodium soy sauce
2 cups fresh bean sprouts
One 5-ounce can sliced water chestnuts,
    drained
¼ cup cold water
1 tablespoon cornstarch
4 cups brown rice, cooked

1. Heat olive oil over medium heat. Add pork, celery and beef bouillon and cook until pork has browned, about 7 to 10 minutes.
2. Reduce heat. Add green pepper, water and soy sauce. Simmer 5 minutes.
3. Add bean sprouts and water chestnuts. Simmer 3 minutes.
4. Increase heat. Blend water and cornstarch into a paste. Stir in cornstarch paste, stirring constantly until mixture has thickened. Serve over brown rice.

Per serving: 421 calories; 25 g protein; 60 g carbohydrate; 6.5 g fiber; 9 g fat; 2.6 g saturated fat; 600 mg sodium.

Tip

Trying to add some exercise into your daily routine? Find a friend, and agree to call each other every day when it's time for your daily walk.

Sage Simmered Pork Chops and Rice

SERVES 4

Don't hesitate to enjoy pork—just choose lean cuts, trim all fat and have a reasonable-sized portion.

4 lean pork chops, trimmed of fat (about 1 pound)
2⅔ cup water
1 cup uncooked brown rice
½ to 1 teaspoon sage
2 teaspoons regular beef bouillon granules (or 2 beef bouillon cubes)
2 teaspoons very low sodium beef bouillon granules
black pepper to taste
1 cup chopped onions
1 cup sliced mushrooms (optional)
1 cup frozen green peas (optional)

1. Spray electric fry pan or large nonstick skillet with vegetable oil spray; heat over medium-high heat. Add pork chops and brown.
2. Add water, rice, sage, bouillon, pepper and onions. Reduce heat and simmer for 30 minutes.
3. Add mushrooms and peas; simmer 10 minutes more.

Per serving: 458 calories; 40 g protein; 47 g carbohydrate; 4.7 g fiber; 11 g fat; 3.6 g saturated fat; 566 mg sodium.

Tip

What alternative ways of dealing with pain have you tried? Self-hypnosis and visualization are great ways to escape the pain without taking medication. You may also be pleasantly surprised at what regular gentle exercise, such as swimming or a gentle stroll, does to help relieve pain.

French Fried Onion and Pork Chop Bake

SERVES 4

Remember the all-time favorite recipe of canned green beans, cream of mushroom soup and french fried onions? This menu is based on that recipe, but it's been transformed into a healthier complete meal.

½ cup seasoned bread crumbs, divided
4 lean pork chops, trimmed of all fat
   (about 1 pound raw meat)
4 small red potatoes, scrubbed and thinly
   sliced
3 cups frozen cut green beans
One 10¾-ounce can cream of mushroom
   or cream of chicken soup, undiluted
½ cup skim milk
One-half a 2.8-ounce can of french fried
   onions
black pepper to taste

1. Spray 9×13-inch pan heavily with vegetable oil spray. Sprinkle 2 tablespoons of bread crumbs on bottom of pan. Lay pork chops evenly in pan. Sprinkle pork chops with 3 tablespoons bread crumbs.
2. Lay potato slices in an even layer over top of pork chops. Spray potatoes with vegetable oil spray. Sprinkle remaining 3 tablespoons of bread crumbs evenly over potatoes. Cover tightly and bake 30 minutes at 350°.
3. Uncover and sprinkle frozen green beans over top. Mix soup and milk; spoon soup mixture over top of beans (use a rubber spatula to spread out). Cover tightly again and bake additional an 30 minutes.
4. Uncover and sprinkle french fried onions over top. Bake 15 minutes uncovered.

Per serving: 485 calories; 34 g protein; 51 g carbohydrate; 6.2 g fiber; 16.2 g fat; 4.8 g saturated fat; 1010 mg sodium.

Tip

Try to work in at least three different vegetables into your eating plan daily. Don't hesitate to use frozen or already cut vegetables.

Cauliflower au Gratin

SERVES 4

A great way to get anyone to eat cauliflower—even my kids will eat it! Make this highly nutritious, yet creamy, rich dish often as a main course.

One 16-ounce bag frozen cauliflower
4 ounces Canadian bacon, chopped
2 onions, chopped
¼ cup flour
2 teaspoons margarine
½ teaspoon nutmeg
⅛ teaspoon ground black pepper
2 teaspoons 33% reduced-sodium chicken
    bouillon
2 cups skim milk
3 ounces Swiss cheese, grated

1. Place cauliflower, Canadian bacon and onions in 2-quart casserole sprayed with vegetable oil spray.
2. Sprinkle flour, margarine, nutmeg, black pepper and bouillon over cauliflower mixture. Toss to coat.
3. Add milk and cheese; mix well.
4. Bake uncovered at 350° for about 45 minutes to 1 hour or until mixture is thick and bubbly.

Per serving: 267 calories; 20 g protein; 25 g carbohydrate; 3.6 g fiber; 10.5 g fat; 5 g saturated fat; 863 mg sodium.

Tip

Research has shown that people who exercise in the morning are more likely to accomplish their exercise goal than are people who plan to exercise in the afternoon.

Scalloped Potatoes

SERVES 4

This lower fat version of an all-time favorite is rich in flavor. Leaving the peel on the potatoes increases the fiber—and decreases preparation time. Substitute any other potato for red potatoes if you don't have red potatoes.

> 1 pound red potatoes, scrubbed and sliced
> into thin slices (leave peel on)
> 6 ounces Canadian bacon, diced
> 2 medium onions, chopped
> 2 tablespoons margarine
> ¼ cup flour
> ½ teaspoon salt
> ¼ teaspoon pepper
> 2 cups skim milk
> 2 ounces cheddar cheese (the sharp variety
> is excellent)

1. Place potatoes, Canadian bacon, onions and margarine in a 2-quart casserole sprayed with vegetable oil spray.
2. Sprinkle in flour, salt and pepper; stir to coat all potatoes with flour.
3. Pour over skim milk; stir entire mixture.
4. Bake uncovered at 350° for 1 hour 15 minutes. Sprinkle cheese over hot mixture, return to oven and bake for another 15 minutes.

Per serving: 373 calories; 20 g protein; 42 g carbohydrate; 2.9 g fiber; 13.9 g fat; 5.9 g saturated fat; 1091 mg sodium.

Tip

If you take more than one medication, keep a list of all your medications and the time you take them in your wallet. It may come in handy if you see a new physician or make an unexpected trip to the hospital.

Pork and Parsnips on a Bed of Creamy Rice

SERVES 6

Pork and parsnips are one of the best food combinations. This easy meal adds carrots for sweet flavor and a colorful appearance.

> 1 pound very lean pork cutlets, trimmed
>   of all fat
> 2 onions, chopped
> 2 teaspoons beef bouillon granules
> 2 cans low-sodium cream of mushroom
>   soup
> 1 cup uncooked brown rice
> 2 cups water
> black pepper to taste
> 4 parsnips, peeled and sliced on the
>   diagonal into ½-inch-thick slices
> 4 carrots, peeled and sliced on the diagonal
>   into ½-inch-thick slices

1. Spray large nonstick skillet with vegetable oil spray and heat over high heat. Add pork, onions and beef bouillon. Sauté each side 2 minutes, or until browned.

2. Reduce heat. Add soup, rice, water, pepper, parsnips and carrots. Simmer covered for 30 minutes.

Per serving: 407 calories; 27 g protein; 46 g carbohydrate; 6 g fiber; 13.8 g fat; 4.6 g saturated fat; 394 mg sodium.

Tip

Always try to make your meals as interesting in appearance as they are in flavor. Although we don't realize it, we taste with our eyes before the food even hits our taste buds—and the "eye" test is just as important.

Pork and Pear Stew

SERVES 4

Everyone will think you're a gourmet cook when you serve this fabulously rich stew—but no one has to know it took you only minutes to prepare. Don't worry about the alcohol—it cooks off, but the taste remains to make a richer sauce. You can make this into a complete meal in one by adding red potato slices (with peel on) if you don't feel like making mashed potatoes.

> 2 teaspoons light olive oil
> 1 pound pork sirloin cubes
>   (buy it this way)
> 4 carrots, peeled and sliced thinly
> salt and pepper to taste
> 1½ cups pear nectar
> 4 just ripe pears, cut into 1-inch cubes
> 1 tablespoon dried thyme
> ¼ cup plus 2 tablespoons dry cooking
>   sherry (or brandy)
> ½ cup nonfat sour cream
> 1 recipe, The Best Mashed Potatoes
>   (page 394)

1. Heat olive oil over medium heat in large nonstick skillet; add pork cubes and carrot slices. Season with salt and pepper; stir-fry 3 to 5 minutes, until pork is browned on all sides.
2. Add pear nectar, pears, thyme and cooking sherry. Simmer (mixture should bubble slightly) for 30 minutes uncovered.
3. Stir in sour cream; simmer for an additional 5 minutes. Serve over mashed potatoes.

Per serving: 643 calories; 42 g protein; 83 g carbohydrate; 8.6 g fiber; 15 g fat; 4.6 g fat; 239 mg sodium.

Tip

Every year, Americans spend $1 billion on unproved arthritis remedies. Remember, if something promises a "cure" be wary—and save your money.

Seafood: Hot and Cold

The Absolute Best (and Easiest) Tuna Salad

SERVES 2

Turn an ordinary can of tuna into a nutritional powerhouse with carrots and romaine lettuce.

> 2 tablespoons low-fat Miracle Whip
> 2 teaspoons lemon juice
> ¼ teaspoon salt
> black pepper to taste (⅛ to ¼ teaspoon)
> One 6-ounce can tuna packed in water, drained
> 2 carrots, grated
> 1 stalk celery, cleaned and sliced thinly
> ¼ cup chopped walnuts
> 2 cups chopped romaine lettuce

1. In serving bowl, and with fork, mix together Miracle Whip, lemon juice, salt and pepper. Add tuna, carrots, celery and walnuts; blend together.
2. Serve over chopped romaine lettuce.

Per serving: 301 calories; 29 g protein; 14 g carbohydrate; 4 g fiber; 15 g fat; 2 g saturated fat; 787 mg sodium.

Tip

If you have osteoporosis, keep your back muscles strong. Research has shown that women with stronger back muscles have fewer fractures and less spinal curvature than other women with osteoporosis.

Tuna Melt

SERVES 2

This is a great recipe that's ready in just minutes. I keep shredded cheese in the freezer for recipes like this—it stays fresh and adds that special touch that makes a meal interesting.

> One 6-ounce can tuna packed in water,
>   drained
> 1 tablespoon low-fat Miracle Whip or mayonnaise
> ground black pepper to taste
> 1 green pepper or 2 stalks celery, chopped
> 1 small onion, minced
> 2 English muffins
> 1 ounce sharp cheddar cheese, shredded

1. In small bowl, mix tuna, Miracle Whip, pepper, green pepper and onion.
2. Open English muffins; divide mixture evenly between 4 halves. Sprinkle with cheese.
3. Place under broiler (or in toaster oven) and broil just until cheese starts to bubble and turns golden (about 2 to 3 minutes).

Per serving: 336 calories; 29 g protein; 33 g carbohydrate; 2.8 g fiber; 9.7 g fat; 4 g saturated fat; 762 mg.

Tip

Buying a new refrigerator? Consider a model with the freezer on the bottom. You spend far more time in the refrigerator section, and not having to bend over to look for things is considerably easier.

Tuna Patties with a Sour Cream Sauce

SERVES 2

Nonfat sour cream creates a rich sauce for these classic tuna patties. For extra interest, serve the patties with the mushroom sauce.

One 6-ounce can tuna
1 slice whole grain bread
1 egg
1 medium onion, peeled and quartered
1 tablespoon lemon juice
1 teaspoon Worcestershire sauce
⅛ to ¼ teaspoon ground black pepper

MUSHROOM SAUCE
1 cup sliced mushrooms
10 cherry tomatoes, quartered
¼ cup nonfat sour cream
1 tablespoon lemon juice
⅛ teaspoon ground black pepper

1. Place all ingredients (except those for sauce) in food processor. Using pulse setting, process just until onion is in tiny pieces.
2. Heat nonstick skillet, sprayed with vegetable oil spray, to medium heat. Form tuna mixture into two patties, and place in pan. Cook, flipping after 5 to 7 minutes. Cook on second side 5 to 7 minutes.

MUSHROOM SAUCE
1. Place mushrooms and tomatoes in same skillet after flipping the patties. When patties have cooked on second side for 5 to 7 minutes, remove them from pan.
2. Stir in sour cream, lemon juice and black pepper into skillet. Pour sauce over patties.

Per serving: 265 calories; 28 g protein; 24 g carbohydrate; 3.5 g fiber; 6 g fat; 1.7 g saturated fat; 490 mg sodium.

Lemon Fresh Salmon Patties with Creamed Peas

SERVES 6

This dish freezes well, so make it ahead of time just for yourself! This is a healthier version of an old family favorite.

PATTIES
2 eggs
One 14½–ounce can salmon, drained and
    skin removed (leave the bones in for
    extra calcium)
3 tablespoons lemon juice
2 slices whole wheat bread, broken up
2 stalks celery, chopped
1 medium onion, chopped
black pepper to taste (about ⅛ to
    ¼ teaspoon)

SAUCE
3 cups frozen green peas
3 tablespoons lemon juice
1 cup low-fat sour cream
1 teaspoon sugar
black pepper to taste, about ⅛ teaspoon

1. Crack eggs into small mixing bowl, beat briefly with a fork. Add remainder of patty ingredients and mix well with a fork.
2. Form into 6 patties. Place in large nonstick skillet or electric fry pan sprayed heavily with vegetable oil spray and heated to medium-high heat. Cook each side for about 5 to 6 minutes. Remove patties from pan.
3. Put frozen peas and lemon juice in pan; cook for about 4 minutes. Add sour cream, sugar and pepper and continue to cook for about 3 to 4 more minutes, or until peas are heated thoroughly. Divide sauce between patties.

Per serving: 279 calories; 22 g protein; 22 g carbohydrate; 4.8 g fiber; 12.8 g fat; 5 g saturated fat; 610 mg sodium.

Tip

Research has shown that pets can be extremely valuable in treating depression and loneliness. Consider getting a dog or cat to keep you company if you are home-bound.

Tip

No matter what your age, try to get a little exercise daily. Research on a group of people aged sixty and over who had osteoarthritis in one or both knees has now shown that the exercise decreased their pain and increased their mobility. In addition, it helped them sleep better at night.

Tuna in Mushroom Sauce Over English Muffins

SERVES 2

Low-sodium chicken bouillon and garlic turn bland reduced-sodium soup into a wonderful cream sauce for canned tuna.

> 1 teaspoon margarine
> 1 clove garlic, minced
> 1 cup sliced mushrooms
> 1 teaspoon 33% reduced-sodium chicken
>   bouillon
> 1 teaspoon very low sodium chicken
>   bouillon
> One 6-ounce can chunk white tuna,
>   packed in water
> 1 tablespoon cornstarch
> One 10-ounce can reduced-sodium cream
>   of mushroom soup
> 2 English muffins

1. Melt margarine in nonstick skillet over low heat; add garlic and mushrooms and sauté briefly. Stir in bouillon.
2. Stir in tuna.
3. Blend 1 tablespoon cornstarch into the mushroom soup. Add soup to tuna and mushrooms, heating briefly until mixture has thickened. Serve over English muffins.

Per serving: 361 calories; 27 g protein; 37 g carbohydrate; 3.5 g fiber; 12 g fat; 3.6 g saturated fat; 940 mg sodium.

Tip

Many people take vitamin B_6 supplements to treat carpal tunnel syndrome. The latest research, however, indicates that the B_6 may not help at all. In fact, the excessive doses people take for B_6 may cause another type of nerve damage, one that might not be reversible.

Tuna Quiche

SERVES 4

This quiche mixes up in just minutes, and is great to have in the refrigerator for the whole week, either as an easy lunch or as a quick snack. It's just as good cold as it is hot.

> 2 stalks celery, chopped (about 1 cup)
> 1 medium onion, chopped (about 1 cup)
> One 6-ounce can very low sodium
>   albacore tuna★
> 12 cherry tomatoes, quartered
> 1 deep-dish frozen pie crust
> 1 cup liquid egg substitute (the equivalent
>   of 4 eggs)
> 1 cup skim milk
> ½ teaspoon salt
> ¼ teaspoon pepper

1. In small bowl, mix together celery, onion, tuna and tomatoes. Pour into pie shell.
2. In same small bowl, whisk together egg, milk, salt and pepper. Pour over tuna mixture.
3. Bake at 325° for 60 minutes.

Per serving: 323 calories; 25 g protein; 26 g carbohydrate; 2.3 g fiber; 13 g fat; 4 g saturated fat; 690 mg sodium.

★Or use regular tuna in a can; just make sure it is water-packed.

Tip

Constipation a problem? Do you drink enough water? Coming up just a little bit short at the end of the day can cause constipation in many people.

Salmon Loaf

SERVES 2

The lemon juice highlights the salmon beautifully in this easy recipe.

> ¼ to ½ red onion, chopped
> 2 tablespoons seasoned bread crumbs
> 1 egg
> One 6-ounce can salmon packed in water
> 2 tablespoons lemon juice
> black pepper to taste
> 2 medium sweet potatoes

1. In a small mixing bowl, blend all ingredients, except sweet potatoes, with a fork, mixing well. Transfer to a miniloaf pan sprayed with vegetable oil spray.
2. Bake at 350° for 30 minutes with sweet potatoes to make a complete meal.

Per serving: 326 calories; 23 g protein; 38 g carbohydrate; 4.3 g fiber; 10 g fat; 2.5 g saturated fat; 662 mg sodium.

Tip

Are you the caregiver for someone with chronic illness? Research on caregivers of people with Alzheimer's disease found that the caregivers were able to care for some with Alzheimer's disease approximately one year more when they participated in a support program. If you're a caregiver, seek out formal or informal forms of support for your demanding job.

Citrus and Poppy Seed Salmon Salad

SERVES 2

The combination of tart and sweet ingredients makes this a most interesting cold salad. The walnuts and croutons also lend a fabulous texture. Building the salad right on the plates eliminates cooking dishes.

> 3 cups chopped romaine lettuce
> ½ cup pink grapefruit sections (buy chilled in dairy section)
> ½ cup white grapefruit sections (buy chilled in dairy section)
> 10 strawberries, sliced
> 2 scallions, chopped
> One 6-ounce can salmon, drained
> 4 tablespoons chopped walnuts (about 1 ounce)
> 4 tablespoons fat-free poppy seed dressing
> ¼ cup seasoned croutons

Divide lettuce between 2 plates. Top each plate with ½ of each of the rest of the ingredients, in the order indicated.

Per serving: 376 calories; 25 g protein; 36 g carbohydrate; 7 g fiber; 17.6 g fat; 2.6 g saturated fat; 754 mg sodium.

Tip

If you're homebound, consider having someone plant a perennial garden outside of the window in the room where you spend the most time. Plan the garden yourself from gardening books, making sure to include a combination of plants, so that something is blooming continually.

Seafood Salad

SERVES 2

Put this cold lunch or dinner together in literally minutes. Just add a whole wheat bagel or dinner roll, a piece of fruit, and you have a complete, nutritious meal.

2 tablespoons nonfat sour cream
2 tablespoons cocktail sauce
2 teaspoons lemon juice
2 teaspoons horseradish
1 teaspoon sugar
4 scallions, chopped
2 stalks celery, chopped
8 ounces imitation crab meat★
4 cups chopped romaine lettuce leaves
lemon slices

1. In small mixing bowl, combine sour cream, cocktail sauce, lemon juice, horseradish and sugar. Stir in remainder of ingredients except lettuce.
2. Arrange romaine lettuce leaves on each plate. Divide seafood salad between 2 plates. Serve, garnished with lemon slices.

★You can purchase bite-sized pieces in the frozen section of your supermarket.

Per serving: 197 calories; 18 g protein; 28 g carbohydrate; 3.6 g fiber; 2 g fat; 0.4 g saturated fat; 1222 mg sodium.

Tip

When you're using prepared foods, make sure you understand serving size. Many times, what looks like one serving is really intended for two or more people, and the nutrition information on the label is for one serving, not the whole package.

Basil Scallop Stir-Fry

SERVES 6

This scallop recipe has a slight oriental flair to it, but is still healthfully low in sodium. The purple cabbage provides an explosion of color that makes this dish even more tempting.

4 tablespoons light olive oil
1 pound scallops
1 small head purple cabbage, sliced thinly
    (about 1 to 1¼ pound)
½ pound snow peas
¼ cup ginger tamari★

12 large basil leaves, chopped

1 tablespoon sugar

2 teaspoons garlic powder

black pepper to taste

6 cups cooked brown rice

1. Heat olive oil in large skillet over medium-high heat; add scallops and cabbage and stir-fry for 5 minutes.
2. Add snow peas and ginger tamari; reduce heat, cover and simmer 5 minutes.
3. Stir in basil, sugar, garlic powder and black pepper; remove from heat. Serve over cooked rice.

  ★Buy in the oriental section of your supermarket; store in the kitchen cabinet.

Per serving: 423 calories; 20 g protein; 56 g carbohydrate; 7 g fiber; 13 g fat; 2 g saturated fat; 585 mg sodium.

Tip

If your doctor has prescribed antibiotics, make sure you finish the whole prescription, unless otherwise instructed. Not finishing the antibiotic may cause the bacteria creating the infection to become antibiotic-resistant and harder to treat.

Scallops in a Spicy Red Pepper Sauce

SERVES 2

Here's a great way to work low-fat seafood into your diet, even if you're not a seafood lover. Using frozen chopped green peppers and jarred pasta sauce makes this an exceptionally easy dish. Angel hair pasta provides just the right finishing touch. Freeze this dish for another day, if you'd like.

2 teaspoons light olive oil

½ red onion, chopped

½ pound scallops

1 cup frozen chopped green pepper (fresh OK)

1 cup spicy red pepper pasta sauce

⅛ teaspoon pepper

¼ teaspoon salt★

½ teaspoon oregano

2 cups cooked angel hair pasta

1. Heat olive oil over medium-high heat; add onion and scallops and stir-fry until onions are wilted and scallops are done (scallops will turn white and change texture).
2. Reduce heat; add green pepper, pasta sauce and spices. Simmer for 10 minutes. Serve over angel hair pasta.

Per serving: 441 calories; 28 g protein; 53 g carbohydrate; 5.7 g fiber; 11.7 g fat; 1.9 g saturated fat; 1007 mg sodium.

  ★Eliminate the salt and cut the sodium from 1007 mg per serving to 740 mg per serving.

Tuna Alfredo

SERVES 4

The cheese sauce in this recipe is incredibly rich and delicious—you'd never know it is low fat! Loaded with fast and easy frozen vegetables, this meal is ready in a snap.

½ pound box linguine, cooked (about 4
    cups cooked pasta)
1 teaspoon margarine
2 cloves garlic, minced
1 cup skim milk
2 tablespoons flour
3 ounces nonfat cream cheese
4 ounces sharp cheddar cheese, shredded
One 6-ounce can tuna packed in water
½ pound frozen broccoli, cauliflower and
    carrot medley

1. While pasta cooks, melt margarine in a large nonstick skillet over low heat; add garlic and sauté 3 minutes.
2. Combine milk and flour in a jar, and shake until mixture is smooth. Increase heat to medium-low and add milk/flour mixture, cream cheese and cheddar cheese. Using a whisk, break up cream cheese and whisk mixture until cheddar melts, cream cheese is dispersed and mixture is thickened.
3. Decrease heat to low; stir in tuna (with liquid) and frozen vegetables; cover and allow mixture to heat through about 10 minutes, or until vegetables are piping hot.
4. Divide pasta between 4 plates. Top each plate of pasta with a fourth of the tuna-cheese sauce.

Per serving: 456 calories; 32 g protein; 51 g carbohydrate; 5 g fiber; 13 g fat; 7 g saturated fat; 529 mg sodium.

Tip

Are you facing a long at-home recovery after a surgery or because of another therapy? Plan for it (if you can) by going to the bookstore or library and stocking up on a pile of your favorite reading material. Collect videos from friends and family (so you don't have to worry about acquiring and returning rental videos). Also, set up a table of projects such as pictures to put in albums. Think of using the time to catch up on projects and reading rather than as lost time. You'll be surprised at how much faster you recover.

Cutting down on caffeine? Don't forget to cut down on the chocolate, too.

Lobster Florentine

SERVES 4

This recipe makes use of another imitation seafood product. I love them because I'm allergic to shell-fish, but still enjoy the flavor of crab and lobster. Although they're higher in sodium, you can still use them in the right recipes. Another plus: this recipe tastes sinfully rich, but it's still healthy!

> Two 8-ounce packages imitation lobster
> meat (or use real lobster meat★)
> One 10-ounce package frozen chopped
> spinach, thawed
> One 9-ounce package frozen creamed
> spinach, thawed
> 4 ounces Swiss cheese, shredded
> ¼ cup seasoned bread crumbs
> ¼ cup lemon juice

1. Spray 9×9-inch baking pan with vegetable oil spray. Spread lobster meat evenly on bottom.
2. Spread thawed chopped spinach over lobster. In next layer, spread thawed creamed spinach.
3. Sprinkle Swiss cheese over spinach. Sprinkle bread crumbs over cheese. Sprinkle lemon juice over the very top.
4. Bake uncovered at 350° for 30 minutes.

Per serving: 354 calories; 24 g protein; 31 g carbohydrate; 4 g fiber; 14.6 g fat; 7.1 g saturated fat; 1396 mg sodium.

★Please note that substituting real lobster for the imitation lobster decreases the amount of sodium per serving from 1396 mg to 1013 mg.

Tip _____

Did you know that real lobster, crab and shrimp aren't high in cholesterol, as food scientists once thought? More sophisticated methods of analyzing food have revealed that these shellfish actually contain a cholesterol-like compound that passes through the body largely unabsorbed.

Lemon-Ginger Scrod and Asparagus

SERVES 2

This easy, light dinner is ready in fifteen minutes or less, from the time you step foot in the kitchen. It's high in protein and is loaded with vitamins. It's also light on calories for those days when energy expenditure is low, but nutrition needs are high. This exceptionally easy dinner also ranks high on taste.

> 1 tablespoon light olive oil
> 2 cloves garlic, sliced
> ½ pound scrod
> ½ pound asparagus spears, tough ends
>   broken off and sliced on the diagonal
>   in 1-inch slices
> 1 tablespoon lemon juice
> 2 teaspoons ginger tamari★

1. Heat olive oil in nonstick skillet over low heat; add garlic and sauté 2 to 3 minutes.
2. Increase heat to medium; add scrod and asparagus. Add lemon juice and ginger tamari; stir-fry briefly and then cover and let fish and asparagus cook for 5 minutes. Uncover briefly, 2 to 3 minutes, allowing part of liquid to evaporate and flavors to intensify. Serve with whole wheat dinner rolls and fruit for a complete meal.

★Buy in the oriental section of your supermarket; store in the kitchen cabinet.

Per serving: 185 calories; 23 g protein; 6.7 g carbohydrate; 2.5 g fiber; 7.8 g fat; 1.1 g saturated fat; 191 mg sodium.

Tip

Experts from five national medical societies concluded that the death rate from colorectal cancer could be reduced by 50 percent if people fifty years of age and older were given a test for occult blood (blood in the stool) annually and underwent a flexible sigmoidoscopy every five years. People at increased risk because of family history should begin screening at a younger age.

Cod in a Carrot-Dill Sauce with Cauliflower and Broccoli

SERVES 4

Fish is such a fabulous, low-fat protein source—but often too bland or dry for many people. Adding a fresh sauce and vegetables transforms it into a feast.

1 tablespoon light olive oil
1 pound cod (fresh or frozen), cut into
    4 pieces
½ pound carrots, peeled and cooked until
    tender
1½ teaspoons 33% reduced-sodium
    chicken bouillon granules
¼ cup skim milk
¼ cup nonfat sour cream
¼ cup chopped fresh dill, packed
⅛ teaspoon black pepper
1-pound bag of cauliflower and broccoli
    mix, thawed
4 cups cooked brown rice, hot

1. Heat olive oil over medium heat. Add cod and cook 5 to 7 minutes.
2. Meanwhile, place the following ingredients in food processor or blender: cooked carrots, bouillon, skim milk, sour cream, dill and pepper. Process until smooth.
3. After fish has cooked 5 to 7 minutes, add thawed vegetables and carrot sauce. Cover and simmer 5 minutes or until mixture is piping hot. Serve with hot rice.

Per serving: 426 calories; 31 g protein; 61 g carbohydrate; 9 g fiber; 6.5 g fat; 1 g saturated fat; 412 mg sodium.

Tip

If you must take an iron supplement, take it with a glass of orange juice or another food high in vitamin E—it helps your body absorb the iron.

Sole in a Mushroom Fontinella Sauce

SERVES 4

Substitute any mild-flavored fish for the sole, or even frozen fillets. The sauce is so wonderfully flavored that you won't mind frozen fish.

1 teaspoon margarine
2 cloves garlic, minced
2 tablespoons flour
1 cup skim milk
4 ounces nonfat cream cheese
4 ounces shredded fontinella cheese
   (if can't find, use Romano)
⅛ teaspoon salt
⅛ teaspoon ground black pepper
4 cups sliced mushrooms (portobello are best)
1 pound sole fillet (frozen okay to use)

1. Melt margarine over low heat in large skillet or electric fry pan; add garlic and sauté for 3 to 5 minutes.
2. Combine flour and milk in jar and shake to create a smooth mixture. Pour flour/milk mixture over margarine; increase heat to medium, add cream cheese and fontinella cheese, salt and pepper and whisk until mixture is smooth.
3. Add mushrooms and fish; reduce heat to low. Cover and simmer for 15 minutes.

Per serving: 293 calories; 38 g protein; 12 g carbohydrate; 1 g fiber; 9.7 g fat; 4.6 g saturated fat; 683 mg sodium.

Tip

If you walk for exercise, don't wear socks with holes in them. They increase the chances that you'll get a blister.

Sole and Asparagus in a Raspberry Chive Sauce

SERVES 4

You won't believe the flavor explosion created by raspberries, chives and orange juice until you try this recipe. This is a great way to get nonfish eaters to love fish.

1 tablespoon olive oil
1 pound fresh sole (frozen is okay, too), cut
   into 4 pieces.
1 pound fresh asparagus, ends broken off
   and sliced diagonally into 1-inch slices

1½ cups frozen raspberries, thawed (okay
    to use fresh)
2 to 4 tablespoons orange juice (depending
    on thickness desired); start with 2 table-
    spoons
1 tablespoon white wine vinegar
1 teaspoon granulated sugar
1 tablespoon orange zest
4 tablespoons chopped chives

1. Heat olive oil in large nonstick skillet over medium heat. Add sole and asparagus pieces. Cook about 5 to 7 minutes.
2. Meanwhile, place remaining ingredients in food processor or blender. After fish and asparagus have cooked 5 to 7 minutes, reduce heat and pour sauce over top. Cover and simmer 3 to 4 minutes.

Per serving: 194 calories; 25 g protein; 14 g carbohydrate; 6 g fiber; 5.3 g fat; 0.8 g saturated fat; 94 mg sodium.

Tip

Using a night-light can help prevent dangerous slips and falls in the dark.

Fish Fillets in a Creamy Mushroom Sauce

SERVES 2

An exceptionally easy main meal that's ready in just minutes. Even though frozen fish isn't as divine as fresh, this recipe works miracles. It's a great idea to keep some frozen foods like this on hand so that you can whip up a complete nutritious meal in minutes.

2 frozen grilled (not batter-coated) fish fillets
1 can cream of mushroom soup
8 ounces frozen stir-fry vegetables (such as
    broccoli, carrots and cauliflower)
2 cups cooked brown rice

1. Combine all ingredients except rice in large nonstick skillet. Cover and let simmer about 15 minutes, or until fish is done and vegetables are hot.
2. Serve over rice.

Per serving: 488 calories; 25 g protein; 63 g carbohydrate; 6 g fiber; 14 g fat; 4 g saturated fat; 1126 mg sodium.

Tip

Ask your pharmacist and physician if any of your medications make you more sensitive to the sun. If so, take appropriate precautions.

Tip

Learn how to choose healthy fast foods—those foods in the grocery store that you can transform into a complete meal in minutes, and without breaking your fat, sodium and calorie budget. Most frozen meals are terribly high in salt and/or fat, making them difficult to fit into any restricted diet. They're also generally low in fiber and light on the vegetables that are so necessary for good health.

Scallop Gumbo

SERVES 2

The okra helps thicken the rich broth of this fish gumbo. I like to keep imitation scallops on hand in the freezer for a quick meal like this one. Just add a whole wheat dinner roll or bagel and you've got a complete meal. I also like to freeze this soup for a quick and easy lunch later on.

> 1 tablespoon light olive oil
> 1 medium onion, chopped
> One 14-ounce can diced tomatoes
> 1 bay leaf
> ½ pound package imitation scallops
>   (or ½ pound regular scallops)
> ½ pound frozen okra
> 1 cup water
> 1 teaspoon garlic powder
> 1 teaspoon very low sodium chicken
>   bouillon granules
> 1 cup frozen corn

Heat olive over medium heat; add onion and stir-fry 3 to 5 minutes. Add remaining ingredients and simmer 15 minutes.

Per serving: 351 calories; 22 g protein; 53 g carbohydrate; 8 g fiber; 7.7 g fat; 1.1 g saturated fat; 1250 mg sodium.

Tip

Feeling blue because it's the middle of winter? Get some bulbs—tulips, daffodils or others—and force them. You'll have a touch of spring to brighten up your home and your life. (Ask the people at the garden store how to force bulbs.)

Jambalaya

SERVES 6

This jambalaya is gentle yet flavor packed—great for the person whose stomach doesn't tolerate a spicy hot dish. Yet, you can turn up the heat on this great one-pot meal by increasing the Tabasco. Don't like shrimp? Substitute chicken or lean pork for the shrimp.

2 tablespoons olive oil

3 onions, chopped

2 cloves garlic, chopped

½ pound shrimp (all shells removed and clean; okay to use shrimp that is cooked and then frozen)

½ cup dry white wine

One 28-ounce can diced tomatoes

½ cup water

½ teaspoon thyme

½ teaspoon basil

¼ teaspoon paprika

1 teaspoon very low sodium beef bouillon

¼ teaspoon Tabasco sauce

1 cup uncooked rice (not instant)

½ pound very low fat kielbasa (such as turkey kielbasa), sliced and quartered

1 cup frozen chopped green pepper (or fresh)

1. Heat olive oil over medium heat; add onions and garlic; stir-fry 5 minutes.
2. Add shrimp, wine, tomatoes, water, thyme, basil, paprika, bouillon, Tabasco, rice and kielbasa. Simmer covered for 30 minutes.
3. Stir in chopped pepper. Simmer an additional 10 minutes.

Per serving: 315 calories; 18 g protein; 38 g carbohydrate; 2.5 g fiber; 8.5 g fat; 1.8 g saturated fat; 625 mg sodium.

Tip

Is your appetite best in the morning? Then plan your biggest meal for that time of the day.

Meal-in-One Soups

Wild Rice and Kielbasa Soup

SERVES 6

This is my favorite soup. Perhaps it's the wild rice that reminds me of my growing up years in northern Minnesota, one place from which wild rice comes. The turkey kielbasa is rich in taste, but light on calories and fat, and flavors the soup beautifully. Go ahead and freeze this soup—it's a treat to take out of the freezer.

2 teaspoons olive oil
1 large onion, chopped
½ pound turkey kielbasa, sliced into thin
　　rounds
4 cups water
1 cup wild rice (uncooked)
2 teaspoons beef bouillon
2 tablespoons very low sodium beef
　　bouillon
1 teaspoon garlic powder
¼ teaspoon black pepper
2 teaspoons Italian seasoning
One 15½-ounce can great northern beans
　　(white beans), drained, rinsed and
　　pureed
½ pound kale, stems removed and chopped

1. Heat olive oil over medium heat in soup pot. Add onion and turkey kielbasa and brown.
2. Add water, wild rice, beef bouillon, garlic powder, black pepper, Italian seasoning and pureed great northern beans. Simmer 25 minutes.
3. Add chopped kale; simmer an additional 40 minutes.

Per serving: 231 calories; 14 g protein; 33 g carbohydrate; 5.6 g fiber; 5.2 g fat; 1.3 g saturated fat; 669 mg sodium.

Tip

Finding it hard to get out and exercise? Snag a friend, and the two of you can serve as encouragement for each other.

Tip _____

Equip your kitchen with enough freezer-to-microwave containers so that you can cook ahead meals for those days when you have just enough energy to heat up something in the microwave. Cooking up larger batches and freezing portions is also a great idea if you live alone.

Roasted Red Pepper Soup

SERVES 2

This decadently rich soup is ready in just minutes.

> 1 cup cooked white beans (canned okay,
>   just drain and rinse)
> 1 cup low-fat buttermilk
> One 7.25-ounce jar roasted red peppers
>   (packed in water), drained
> 6 to 8 large fresh basil leaves (or use dried
>   basil, about 1 tablespoon)
> ⅛ teaspoon black pepper
> 1 teaspoon sugar
> croutons

1. Combine all ingredients except croutons in food processor or blender; process until fairly smooth. You will still see some basil leaf flecks.
2. Transfer to a microwave-safe container or heavy pot. Heat microwave-safe container in microwave on high for 4 to 5 minutes, stirring once halfway through cooking. If heating on stove top, place heavy pot on stove over low heat for 5 to 10 minutes, until mixture just starts to bubble. Serve with croutons.

Per serving: 191 calories; 10 g protein; 32 g carbohydrate; 5.8 g fiber; 2.2 g fat; 0.8 g saturated fat; 773 mg sodium.

Tip _____

Get all your prescriptions at one pharmacy. That way, the pharmacist can track your drug history and check for potentially dangerous drug interactions. Most pharmacies today are computerized, and any potential interaction generally shows up on the screen when the pharmacist enters a new prescription.

Onion and Cheesy Tomato Soup

SERVES 2

A hearty, nutritious and delicious easy meal for those low-energy days. Serve with crackers and a side salad.

> 1 teaspoon olive oil
> 1 onion, sliced thinly and slices separated
> 1 can cream of tomato soup
> One 10-ounce can skim milk
> 4 ounces 50% reduced-fat cheddar cheese
>   (or 50% reduced-fat mozzarella cheese)
> 12 Ritz crackers

1. Heat olive oil over medium heat; add onion rings and sauté until brown and transparent. Remove from pan, dividing between two soup bowls.
2. In same pan, whisk together tomato soup and skim milk; heat until bubbly hot.
3. Add 2 ounces of cheese to each soup bowl. Divide tomato soup between 2 bowls. Stir to melt cheese and mix onions. Serve with crackers.

Per serving: 430 calories; 26 g protein; 45 g carbohydrate; 1.6 g fiber; 18.6 g fat; 8.2 g saturated fat; 1698 mg sodium.

★Nutritional analysis substituting whole milk for skim milk and regular cheese for reduced-fat cheese: 557 calories; 24 g protein; 44 g carbohydrate; 1.6 g fiber; 33 g fat; 21 g saturated fat; 1,641 mg sodium.

★Recommended for AIDS patients.

Tip

Yes, this meal is relatively high in sodium; unfortunately that's the "cost" of using convenience foods like canned soup. But, if you watch the sodium content of the rest of your meals for the day, you *can* fit a food like this into your diet.

Herbed Split Pea Soup

SERVES 2

Looking for something different to do with split peas besides the traditional split pea and ham soup? This is it! Feel free to double the recipe, as the soup freezes very well.

> ½ cup split peas, uncooked
> 2 carrots, diced
> 1 stalk celery, diced
> 1 medium onion, diced
> 1 beef bouillon cube
> ½ teaspoon garlic powder
> ½ teaspoon dried oregano

1 tablespoon dried parsley flakes
⅛ teaspoon ground black pepper
2 teaspoons olive oil

Place all ingredients in small soup kettle. Bring to a boil; reduce heat and simmer 45 minutes to 1 hour, or until peas are tender.

Per serving: 275 calories; 14 g protein; 44 g carbohydrate; 7 g fiber; 5 g fat; 1 g saturated fat; 504 mg sodium.

Tip

> Another hint if you're on immunosuppressive medications: don't share towels with other family members. Have a hand towel in the bathroom that's only for you, or use paper towels there. Also, wash towels daily, especially kitchen dishcloths.

Potato Soup

SERVES 4 (MAY DOUBLE)
This easy and defatted version of an old favorite is rich, hearty and loaded with good nutrition. Don't hesitate to try it, even if every other potato soup recipe is a lot of work. You'll be surprised at how easy this one is.

1 pound potatoes, peeled and quartered
2 medium onions, quartered
2 stalks celery, chunked
2 cups water
2 beef bouillon cubes★
⅛ to ¼ teaspoon black pepper
8 ounces nonfat cream cheese
1 teaspoon Worcestershire sauce
1 tablespoon dried parsley flakes

1. Place potatoes, onions, celery, water and bouillon in small soup pot. Bring to a boil; reduce heat and simmer about 30 minutes, or until vegetables are fork tender.
2. Place cooked vegetables, with cooking water, in food processor or blender with pepper, cream cheese and Worcestershire sauce. Process until perfectly smooth. Stir in parsley flakes. Serve.

Per serving: 180 calories; 12 g protein; 33 g carbohydrate; 2.8 g fiber; 0 g fat; 0 g saturated fat; 528 mg sodium.

★★Nutritional analysis substituting regular cream cheese for nonfat: 327 calories; 7 g protein; 31 g carbohydrate; 2.8 g fiber; 20 g fat; 12 g saturated fat; 214 mg sodium.

★Using low-sodium beef bouillon considerably lowers the level of sodium in this recipe from 828 mgs to 321 mgs.

★★Recommended for AIDS patients.

Tip _____

Perhaps you've heard that red wine can help decrease your risk of heart disease. While this may be true, heart disease experts discourage people from adding red wine to their diet if they don't already drink. Better to exercise and cut dietary fat, say these experts, than to add alcohol.

Cream of Broccoli Soup

SERVES 4

Serve this with a whole wheat bagel and a piece of fruit for a complete meal.

> 1 pound frozen broccoli pieces
> 8 ounces nonfat cream cheese
> 1 cup skim milk
> 2 tablespoons very low sodium chicken
>   bouillon granules
> 3 ounces cheddar or taco cheese, shredded

1. Cook broccoli per package directions.
2. Put broccoli, nonfat cream cheese, skim milk and bouillon granules in food processor or blender; process until smooth.
3. Transfer to saucepan, add cheese. Heat over low heat until warmed through well. Alternatively, place soup and cheese in microwave-safe bowl and microwave until hot, about 4 to 5 minutes, stirring once.

Per serving: 205 calories; 20 g protein; 15 g carbohydrate; 3.3 g fiber; 7 g fat; 5 g saturated fat; 465 mg sodium.

*Nutritional analysis substituting whole milk for skim milk and regular cream cheese for the nonfat adding 1 extra ounce of cheddar cheese: 502 calories; 19 g protein; 14 g carbohydrate; 3.3 g fiber; 42 g fat; 26 g saturated fat; 490 mg sodium.

*Recommended for AIDS patients.

Tip _____

If you have arthritis, test out different times of the day to find the most optimal time to exercise. If you are stiffest in the morning, for example, you might want to choose another time to exercise. Discuss with your doctor the possibility of taking aspirin or a nonsteroidal anti-inflammatory medication one hour before exercise—some people find this to be a tremendous help.

Hearty Beef Vegetable Soup in an Hour

SERVES 8

Beef vegetable soup is wonderful, but generally so much work. Using lean, precut beef saves work. I've also eliminated some of the cutting and chopping by using baby carrots and some frozen veggies. This convenient soup freezes well.

1 tablespoon olive oil
2 cloves garlic, minced
1 pound very lean beef chunks for stew
4 onions, chopped
One 28-ounce can no-salt-added crushed
   tomatoes
1 tablespoon low-sodium beef bouillon
   granules
1 tablespoon 33% reduced-sodium beef
   bouillon granules
¼ to ½ teaspoon black pepper
1 bay leaf
1 tablespoon oregano
½ teaspoon cayenne red pepper
½ pound baby carrots
¼ head cabbage, in large wedges
3 cups water
1 cup uncooked barley
One 10-ounce bag frozen chopped green
   peppers
1 pound frozen broccoli pieces

1. Heat olive oil and garlic over low heat 3 to 5 minutes in heavy soup pot. Increase heat to high. Add beef and onions, cooking just long enough to brown.
2. Reduce heat. Add remaining ingredients, except for green peppers and broccoli. Simmer 1 hour covered. Add green peppers and broccoli, and simmer 7 minutes more. Serve.

Per serving: 307 calories; 24 g protein; 39 g carbohydrate; 10 g fiber; 6.8 g fat; 1.8 g saturated fat; 302 mg sodium.

Tip

So it's been a while since you dusted the kitchen with flour or filled your soup pot with hearty warmth. Don't be afraid to get back into the kitchen. Just keep it simple yet interesting and delicious. You'll love the sense of accomplishment you'll have once again.

Barley and Bacon Soup

SERVES 4

Use great-tasting soups like this to sneak in a power vegetable such as kale. It enhances the soup, and the soup makes the vegetable quite appealing, even though you might not like it alone.

1 tablespoon light olive oil

1 large red onion, chopped coarsely

½ pound Canadian bacon, diced

1 tablespoon plus 1 teaspoon beef bouillon
    granules (or 4 cubes)

1 tablespoon low-sodium beef bouillon
    granules

2 teaspoons oregano

¼ to ½ teaspoon chili powder

¼ teaspoon ground black pepper

4½ cups water

1 cup uncooked hulled barley

1 15½-ounce can white beans, drained and
    rinsed

½ pound kale, stems removed and chopped

1. Heat olive oil over medium heat; add onion and Canadian bacon; sauté until onion has wilted and slightly browned.
2. Add bouillon, oregano, chili powder, black pepper, 4½ cups water and barley.
3. Puree beans with ½ cup water; add to soup mixture. Simmer covered 40 minutes.
4. Add chopped kale and simmer an additional 40 minutes.

Per serving: 465 calories; 28 g protein; 70 g carbohydrate; 15.6 g fiber; 9.3 g fat; 2 g saturated fat; 1749 mg sodium.

Tip

Do you know someone else who has limited energy because of an illness? Speak with her about swapping meals. Here's how it works: even if you live alone, make a big batch of soup like this and trade it for a portion of a casserole or different soup your friend makes.

Lentil Vegetable Soup

SERVES 4

This fabulously easy and rich soup is one of the most nutritious you'll have! It has a gentle, yet robust taste, thanks to the wonderful complement of flavorful vegetables. This soup also freezes well.

2 tablespoons light olive oil

3 cloves garlic, sliced (can use less)

½ red onion, chopped

4 cups water

4 carrots, peeled and sliced on the diagonal

2 medium potatoes, peeled and sliced
   thinly or diced

1 cup lentils, uncooked

1 teaspoon salt

¼ teaspoon black pepper

½ teaspoon dried sweet basil

1 bag frozen mustard greens (1 pound)

1. Heat olive oil, garlic and onion over low-medium heat. Sauté 10 minutes.
2. Add remaining ingredients, except mustard greens. Simmer covered 50 minutes. The potatoes should cook and then break up (turn to "mush") to thicken the soup.
3. Stir in mustard greens and simmer 10 minutes more.

Per serving: 350 calories; 19 g protein; 56 g carbohydrate; 12 g fiber; 8 g fat; 1 g saturated fat; 597 mg sodium.

Tip

Appetite poor, and you can't stand the thought of a whole meal? Plan six small snacks throughout the day rather than three large meals. It's much more manageable.

Spicy and Thick Lentil and Kale Soup

SERVES 2

This thick soup is almost like a stew. While the kale looks like a huge bunch, it cooks down dramatically.

½ cup lentils
2 onions, chopped
One 28-ounce can no-salt-added crushed
   tomatoes
2 cups water
2 teaspoons powdered garlic
½ teaspoon ground cumin
1½ teaspoons chili powder
½ teaspoon curry powder
2 beef bouillon cubes★
1 tablespoon Worcestershire sauce
2 teaspoons olive oil
1 teaspoons sugar
¾ pound kale, stems removed, chopped

1. In soup pot, combine lentils, onions, tomatoes, water, garlic, cumin, chili powder, curry powder, bouillon, Worcestershire sauce, olive oil and sugar. Bring to a boil; reduce heat and simmer 20 minutes.
2. Add chopped kale; simmer another 30 minutes, stirring 3 to 4 times.

Per serving: 426 calories; 26 g protein; 81 g carbohydrate; 19 g fiber; 2 g fat; 0.3 g saturated fat; 1064 mg sodium.

★Using 33% reduced-sodium beef bouillon granules lowers the sodium content per serving from 1064 mg to 764 mg.

Tip

Kale is one of the most nutritious yet underused vegetables. Get used to it in soups like this one—and then start working it into stir-fries. It has lots of nutrients in an amazingly small number of calories. Another benefit: it's one of the great cancer-fighting cruciferous vegetables.

Oriental-Style Lentil and Brown Rice Soup

SERVES 2

This soup takes only minutes to prepare. It stores well in the refrigerator or freezer, so don't hesitate to make a double batch.

½ cup lentils, uncooked
½ cup brown rice, uncooked
6 cups water
1 teaspoon ground ginger
2 tablespoons plus 2 teaspoons low-sodium
    soy sauce
⅛ to ¼ teaspoon ground black pepper
1 cup green pepper, chopped (okay to use
    frozen)
1 cup red pepper, chopped

1. In small soup kettle, blend lentils, rice, water, ginger, soy sauce and black pepper. Bring to a boil; reduce heat and simmer 35 minutes.
2. Add green and red pepper; simmer an additional 10 minutes.

Per serving: 384 calories; 20 g protein; 73 g carbohydrate; 9.8 g fiber; 2 g fat; 0.4 g saturated fat; 706 mg sodium.

Tip

Do you have medications on hand that you only take on rare occasions? For example, do you carry nitroglycerin for chest pain (angina) or injectable migraine headache medication? If so, check their dates to make sure they have not expired. Some may be dangerous if they are outdated, but others—such as life-saving nitroglycerin—simply won't be effective if they are past date.

Lentil and Brown Rice Chili

SERVES 4

This vegetarian chili cooks up fast and easy, and also freezes well. Make a big batch and freeze in individual portions for quick, microwavable lunches.

1 tablespoon light olive oil
1 onion, diced
6 ounces turkey kielbasa
½ cup lentils
½ cup brown rice
One 28-ounce can no-salt-added pureed
  tomatoes
3 cups water
1 tablespoon garlic powder
2 teaspoons cumin
1 tablespoon chili powder
2 tablespoons very low sodium beef
  bouillon granules
¼ cup lemon juice
1 pound frozen corn
5 ounces frozen green peppers
¼ teaspoon black pepper, or to taste

1. Heat olive oil over medium heat. Add onion and kielbasa; stir-fry until onion is transparent.
2. Decrease heat; add lentils, brown rice, tomatoes, water, spices, bouillon and lemon juice. Simmer 35 minutes.
3. Stir in frozen corn and green peppers; simmer 10 minutes more. Stir in ground black pepper.

Per serving: 481 calories; 23 g protein; 85 g carbohydrate; 17 g fiber; 9 g fat; 2 g saturated fat; 488 mg sodium.

Tip

Energy limited? Try serving food from the cooking pots, directly from the stove. This eliminates the energy required to transfer food to serving bowls and then to the table; it also reduces the number of dishes you have to wash. Another added benefit: you're less likely to take a second helping, which is a help in controlling weight.

One-Pot Chili

SERVES 10

This chili is spicy enough to be interesting, yet mild enough for sensitive stomachs. If you like it hotter, just add more chili powder. This bountiful recipe makes three quarts. Serve it to a crowd, or freeze the leftovers.

> 1 pound ground sirloin
> 2 onions, chopped (about 2 cups)
> 2 stalks celery, chopped (about 1 cup)
> Two 16-ounce cans dark red kidney beans
> One 28-ounce can no-salt-added crushed
>   tomatoes
> One 14½-ounce can no-salt-added whole
>   tomatoes
> 2 teaspoons sugar
> 1 teaspoon dried sweet basil
> 1 teaspoon dried oregano
> 1 tablespoon chili powder
> 1 teaspoon salt
> 1 tablespoon garlic powder
> ¼ teaspoon ground black pepper

1. Spray bottom of heavy soup kettle with vegetable oil spray. Add ground sirloin and chopped onions, and brown on medium heat.
2. Add remainder of ingredients. Reduce heat and simmer covered for 45 minutes, allowing flavors to reach their peak.

Per serving: 241 calories; 18 g protein; 32 g carbohydrate; 11 g fiber; 5 g fat; 1.7 g saturated fat; 289 mg sodium.

Tip

Do you have an intolerance to milk—lactose intolerance? Don't hesitate to try specially formulated milks available in the dairy section of your grocery store. These Lactaid milks have an added enzyme that breaks down the milk sugar that otherwise causes the uncomfortable gastrointestinal symptoms.

Clam Chowder

Serves 4

Although this version is light on calories, it's heavy on rich flavor. The nonfat sour cream steps in nicely for the cream that you usually find in clam chowder.

1 tablespoon margarine
1 large onion, peeled and chopped
3 slices bacon
3 tablespoons flour
2 cups skim milk
4 red potatoes, scrubbed and diced
   (skin on)
Two 6.5-ounce cans chopped clams
   (with liquid)
½ to 1 teaspoon thyme
ground black pepper to taste
½ cup nonfat sour cream

1. Melt margarine over medium heat in nonstick skillet or electric fry pan. Add onion and bacon; brown for 5 to 7 minutes (until bacon is crisp).
2. Blend together flour and milk (I put both in a jar and shake—a great way to get all the lumps out). Reduce heat to low and add flour/milk mixture and potatoes to onions and bacon. Add clams (with liquid), thyme and pepper; cover and simmer over very low heat for 40 minutes, or until potatoes are very tender (it's okay if they start to break up).
3. Stir in sour cream; heat through briefly.

Per serving: 332 calories; 23 g protein; 45 g carbohydrate; 3 g fiber; 6.2 g fat; 1.6 g saturated fat; 340 mg sodium.

*Nutritional analysis, substituting whole milk for skim milk and regular sour cream for nonfat sour cream: 395 calories; 22 g protein; 40 g carbohydrate; 3 g fiber; 16 g fat; 8 g saturated fat; 329 mg sodium.

  *Recommended for AIDS patients.

Tip

Try to include some fish and shellfish in your diet at least once or twice per week. It's a great way to cut the fat in your diet, and also to get a different complement of nutrients.

Kielbasa Corn Chowder

SERVES 4

Just adding some low-fat turkey kielbasa and corn to the basic potato soup recipe lends an entirely different flair.

1 pound potatoes, peeled and quartered

2 medium onions, quartered

2 celery stalks, chunked

2 cups water

2 teaspoons very low sodium beef bouillon
    granules

⅛ to ¼ teaspoon pepper

8 ounces nonfat cream cheese

1 teaspoon Worcestershire sauce

1 tablespoon dried parsley flakes

2 cups frozen cut corn

½ pound reduced-fat turkey kielbasa, sliced
    and quartered

1. Place potatoes, onions, celery, water and bouillon in small soup pot. Bring to a boil; reduce heat and simmer about 30 minutes, or until vegetables are fork tender.

2. Place cooked vegetables, with cooking water, in food processor or blender with pepper, cream cheese and Worcestershire sauce. Process until perfectly smooth. Stir in parsley.

3. Return soup to pot; stir in frozen corn and kielbasa. Heat through on low heat, about 10 minutes. Serve.

Per serving: 329 calories; 23 g protein; 51 g carbohydrate; 4.8 g fiber; 4.9 g fat; 1.6 g saturated fat; 831 mg sodium.

Nutritional analysis substituting nonfat cream cheese for regular cream cheese: 475 calories; 18 g protein; 49 g carbohydrate; 4.8 g fiber; 25 g fat; 14 g saturated fat; 724 mg sodium.

*Recommended for AIDS patients.

Tip

Always check with your doctor and pharmacist to make sure the over-the-counter medication you plan to take does not interact with your prescription medications. Even the most simple medications can cause potentially dangerous side effects.

Portobello, Barley and Wild Rice Stew

SERVES 4

This meatless stew is fabulously rich in flavor, owing to its interesting combination of seasonings. It also makes an excellent stew to freeze for another night down the road. Just add a glass of milk and a bowl of fruit, and you've got a great meal.

1 tablespoon light olive oil
1 clove garlic, minced
1 cup chopped onion
½ cup whole barley, uncooked
½ cup wild rice, uncooked
2 tablespoons Worcestershire sauce
1 tablespoon low-sodium beef bouillon
1 tablespoon 33% reduced-sodium beef
    bouillon
6 cups water
black pepper to taste
2 teaspoons dried sweet basil
1 teaspoon dried oregano
½ pound portobello mushrooms, sliced
1 tablespoon balsamic vinegar

1. In large nonstick skillet or soup pot, heat olive oil with garlic and chopped onion. Sauté for about 5 to 7 minutes, to let flavors blend.
2. Add barley, wild rice, Worcestershire sauce, bouillon, water, pepper, basil and oregano. Simmer covered for 60 minutes.
3. Stir in mushrooms and balsamic vinegar. Cover and simmer 10 minutes more.

Per serving: 227 calories; 7 g protein; 42 g carbohydrate; 6 g fiber; 4.4 g fat; 0.6 g saturated fat; 546 mg sodium.

Tip

Choosing a frozen dairy dessert can be confusing. Many people turn to frozen yogurt, assuming it's the lowest fat choice. But many frozen yogurts are exceptionally high in fat. Read labels carefully of all ice cream and frozen yogurt choices.

Black Bean and Barley Stew with Mushrooms

SERVES 4

This meatless meal is rich and hearty; it also freezes exceptionally well.

1 cup dried black beans

One 28-ounce can no-salt-added crushed
  tomatoes

One 14½-ounce can no-salt-added whole
  tomatoes

2 cups water

¼ cup lemon juice

2 to 3 teaspoons chili powder

1 tablespoon garlic powder

1 to 2 teaspoons cumin

1 tablespoons 33% reduced-sodium beef
  bouillon granules

1 tablespoon low-sodium beef bouillon
  granules

½ cup barley

½ pound turkey kielbasa, sliced, each slice
  quartered

½ pound sliced mushrooms

1. In soup pot, combine beans, tomatoes, water, lemon juice, chili powder, garlic powder, cumin and bouillon; bring to a boil. Reduce heat, simmer for 15 minutes.
2. Add barley and kielbasa; simmer 1 hour.
3. Add mushrooms, simmer 15 minutes.

Per serving: 403 calories; 25 g protein; 64 g carbohydrate; 17 g fiber; 6.3 g fat; 1.9 g saturated fat; 997 mg sodium.

Tip

Before you start a new exercise regimen, check with your doctor to make sure it's safe. This is especially true if you have not exercised in a long time.

Meatless Meals and Sides

Eat 'em Every Day Peanut Butter Sandwich

SERVES 4

Perfect for making ahead of time for yourself—the sandwich stores easily in the refrigerator. If you love peanut butter, but avoid it because of the high fat content, then here's a great way to enjoy it, and boost calcium and protein intake, too! Don't let the cottage cheese scare you off. My husband hates cottage cheese but loves this peanut butter.

> ¼ cup peanut butter
> ¼ cup fat-free cottage cheese
> 8 slices whole wheat bread
> jelly or jam, if desired

1. Place peanut butter and cottage cheese in food miniprocessor. Process until smooth.
2. Divide peanut butter mixture between 4 sandwiches, adding jam or jelly if desired (or store remainder in refrigerator for up to a week).

Per serving: 252 calories; 11 g protein; 31 g carbohydrate; 4.3 g fiber; 10.3 g fat; 2.1 g saturated fat; 433 mg sodium.

Tip

Even if you're on a restricted diet, always find things you *love* to eat—not just things that "fit into your diet." Not enjoying your food eventually leads to feelings of deprivation—and that makes it harder to eat as you should for better health.

Peanut Butter and Banana Sandwich

SERVES 2

Here's another great way to enjoy a low-fat peanut butter sandwich. Serve with a glass of skim milk and an apple for a complete lunch.

> 1 medium banana
> 2 tablespoons peanut butter
> 4 slices whole wheat bread

1. Place banana and peanut butter in food processor. Process until smooth.
2. Divide peanut butter mixture between 2 sandwiches.

Per serving: 287 calories; 10 g protein; 43 g carbohydrate; 6 g fiber; 11 g fat; 2.3 g saturated fat; 370 mg sodium.

Tip

Finding a voluntary organization that is committed to helping people with your disease (such as the Arthritis Foundation) can be a tremendous help. Consult "Resources" at the end of this book. They can help you find a support group, provide you with a list of doctors that treat people who have your disease and also help you understand current acceptable treatments.

Egg Salad Sandwich

SERVES 1

Many people have become so health conscious that they tend to avoid all eggs. But most people can handle up to four egg yolks per week. This egg salad sandwich is light and easy—and quite interesting with the red onion and touch of black pepper. Using extra egg whites makes it high in protein.

> 1 hard-boiled egg
> 2 hard-boiled egg whites
> 1 celery stalk, chopped thinly
> 2 tablespoons finely chopped red onion
> ⅛ teaspoon black pepper
> 2 tablespoons light Miracle Whip or light
>   mayonnaise
> 2 slices whole wheat bread
> romaine lettuce leaves

1. In small bowl, chop egg and extra egg whites. Add chopped celery, red onion, pepper and Miracle Whip or mayonnaise; use a fork to blend all ingredients together well.
2. Arrange egg salad on one slice whole wheat bread; top with romaine lettuce leaves. Top with second slice of bread.

Per serving: 344 calories; 21 g protein; 37 g carbohydrate; 5.6 g fiber; 13.5 g fat; 2 g saturated fat; 848 mg sodium.

Tip

Although you may not realize it, being constipated can really turn off your appetite. You'll feel much better in so many ways by bulking up your diet with more fiber.

Loaded Spinach Salad

SERVES 4

An absolute explosion of carotenoids and vitamins! The flavors in these vegetables combine phenome-nally well. If you don't like blue cheese dressing, substitute French or Catalina, both of which work very well with this salad.

½ pound fresh spinach leaves, washed,
    dried, destemmed and torn
20 cherry tomatoes, halved
2 large carrots, grated
6 scallions (top and bottom), chopped
8 ounces 50% reduced-fat mozzarella
    cheese
⅓ cup reduced-fat blue cheese dressing

Combine all ingredients in salad bowl; toss to mix.

Per serving: 220 calories; 21 g protein; 13 g carbohydrate; 4 g fiber; 9 g fat; 5 g saturated fat; 316 mg sodium.

*Nutritional analysis substituting whole milk mozzarella for reduced-fat mozzarella and regular blue cheese for reduced-fat blue cheese: 320 calories; 15 g protein; 15 g carbohydrate; 4 g fiber; 23 g fat; 10 g saturated fat; 506 mg sodium.

*Recommended for AIDS patients.

Tip

Start your day off with excellent nutrition, especially if you are not hungry. Doing so will boost your energy and keep you from turning to junk food later in the day when you become hungry.

Strawberry Spinach Salad with Garbanzo Beans and a Poppy Seed Dressing

SERVES 4

This vibrantly colored salad is a gold mine of fabulous nutrition and a meal in itself. Just add a whole wheat bagel and a glass of milk.

½ pound fresh spinach leaves, washed,
    dried, destemmed and torn
1 quart strawberries, sliced
2 ounces walnuts, chopped (about 16 walnuts)

Three 7¾-ounce cans garbanzo beans
(chickpeas), drained and rinsed
⅓ cup fat free poppy seed dressing

Combine all ingredients in salad bowl*; toss to mix.

*Dry spinach leaves well to prevent the salad from becoming soggy.

Per serving: 378 calories; 15 g protein; 60 g carbohydrate; 13.6 g fiber; 10.7 g fat; 0.8 g saturated fat; 746 mg sodium.

Tip

While nuts are high in fat, it is okay to include them in a healthy, lower fat diet—just in the right proportions.

Greens and Garbanzo Beans in a Raspberry Chive Sauce

SERVES 4

An exceptionally easy yet flavorful (and very low sodium) salad for a hot summer's day.

1½ cups frozen raspberries, thawed
2 tablespoons orange juice
1 tablespoon white wine vinegar
1 teaspoon granulated sugar
1 tablespoon orange zest
4 tablespoons chopped chives (divided)
4 cups chopped romaine lettuce
4 cups chopped fresh spinach
Three 7¾-ounce cans garbanzo beans
(chickpeas), drained
4 tablespoons chopped walnuts (about 3 ounces)

1. Process raspberries, orange juice, vinegar, sugar, orange zest and 2 tablespoons chives in food processor or blender. After all is processed, stir in remaining chopped chives.
2. Divide lettuce, spinach and garbanzo beans between 4 plates; drizzle sauce over top.

Per serving: 380 calories; 17 g protein; 51 g carbohydrate; 13.5 g fiber; 14.5 g fat; 1 g saturated fat; 521 mg sodium.

Tip

When berries are in season, freeze some for later—without washing—and they'll hold their shape when you defrost them (that's when you should wash them).

Portobello Broil

SERVES 6

Portobello mushrooms are the latest food craze. This easy recipe is a magnificent way to enjoy their taste—highlighted by basil, garlic and Parmesan cheese. Though this recipe is a little more work than many in this book, it is much easier than it looks.

1 tablespoon light olive oil
1 Vidalia onion, sliced and slices separated
    into rings
One 8-ounce can no-salt-added tomato
    sauce
1½ teaspoon oregano
1½ teaspoon dried sweet basil
1 teaspoon garlic powder
1 loaf ciabatta or Italian bread
¾ cup nonfat Parmesan cheese
12 ounces low-moisture, part-skim
    shredded mozzarella cheese
6 very large portobello mushroom caps,
    stems removed

1. Heat olive oil in small pan over medium-high heat. Add onion and sauté until it is soft and browned. Remove from heat. Stir in tomato sauce and spices.
2. Split ciabatta bread in half lengthwise (creating a top and a bottom). Cut each of those into thirds.
3. Divide sauce and onions between 6 pieces of ciabatta bread. Sprinkle Parmesan cheese over sauce and onions. Divide half of mozzarella cheese between 6 pieces, sprinkling over the Parmesan. Place a portobello mushroom cap on each. Brush top of caps with olive oil. Broil for 5 minutes.
4. Remove from oven. Sprinkle remaining mozzarella cheese over mushroom caps. Bake at 375° for 5 to 7 minutes, or until cheese is just slightly browned. Serve with a romaine lettuce salad for a complete meal.

Per serving: 419 calories; 27 g protein; 43 g carbohydrate; 3.4 g fiber; 14.5 g fat; 7.2 g saturated fat; 792 mg sodium.

Tip

Always stretch before and after you exercise—no matter what your form of exercise is. Stretching first and last can save you from suffering sore muscles.

The Cheesiest Pizza

SERVES 6

You'll feel like you're in the best deep-dish pizza restaurant when you prepare this pizza. Using frozen bread dough and frozen vegetables, though, you can toss this pizza together in just minutes.

> One 1-pound loaf frozen bread dough, thawed
> One 8-ounce can no-salt-added tomato sauce
> 2 teaspoon dried Italian seasoning
> 1 teaspoon garlic powder
> ⅛ teaspoon black pepper
> red pepper flakes to taste
> 1 cup frozen chopped green pepper
> 1 cup frozen broccoli pieces
> 1 medium onion, chopped
> 2 small tomatoes, chopped
> One 12-ounce package part skim mozzarella cheese, shredded

1. Spray 9-inch round pan with vegetable oil spray. Spread dough over pan.
2. Spread tomato sauce evenly over dough; sprinkle with Italian seasoning, garlic powder, black pepper and red pepper flakes.
3. Spread vegetables evenly.
4. Sprinkle cheese evenly over vegetables.
5. Bake at 400° for 15 to 18 minutes, or until cheese bubbles.

Per serving: 389 calories; 23 g protein; 48 g carbohydrate; 4.6 g fiber; 12.7 g fat; 5.8 g saturated fat; 702 mg sodium.

Tip

Don't be afraid of the kitchen because you're disabled or chronically fatigued. There are many fabulous things you can whip up in just a few minutes—activities that will put you back in charge of your life and on top of the world.

Spinach Pie

SERVES 6

An absolutely delicious and high-protein way to enjoy spinach, a powerhouse of nutrients and phyto-chemicals.

1 cup liquid egg substitute

1 cup 2% fat cottage cheese

One 10-ounce package frozen chopped
  spinach, thawed

½ pound baby carrots, grated in food
  processor (or buy at grocery store
  already grated)

¼ cup dried, minced onion

1 tablespoon 33% reduced-sodium chicken
  bouillon granules

2 ounces sharp cheddar cheese

1 frozen pie crust

1. Crack eggs into large mixing bowl; beat gently with fork.
2. Add remainder of ingredients to bowl; mix with fork or large spoon.
3. Pour mixture into frozen pie crust. Bake at 350° for 30 to 40 minutes, or until knife inserted into edge comes out clean.

Per serving: 250 calories; 15 g protein; 19 g carbohydrate; 2.5 g fiber; 12.5 g fat; 5 g saturated fat; 727 mg sodium.

Tip

How long has it been since you had a vacation? Like many people with chronic illness, you gave up on travel because you thought it was too difficult. Today, however, airlines and every other form of travel make it much easier for people with limited energy and with handicaps to travel. It's essential to take a break from the grind of your illness, just as it's essential to take a vacation from the demands of a career. If nothing else, check into a hotel downtown and enjoy an evening of room service and a movie on the in-room television.

Broccoli Quiche

SERVES 4

Make this wonderfully delicious and nutrition-packed quiche on Monday and then have it for several lunches during the week.

> 1 frozen deep dish–pie crust
> One 16-ounce bag frozen cut broccoli
> 1 cup liquid egg substitute (the equivalent of 4 eggs)
> 1 cup skim milk
> ¼ teaspoon salt
> ¼ teaspoon pepper
> ⅓ cup fat-free Parmesan cheese
> 5 cherry tomatoes, halved

1. Place frozen broccoli into pie crust and distribute evenly.
2. In mixing bowl, whisk together egg substitute, milk, salt, pepper and Parmesan cheese. Pour over broccoli.
3. Decorate with cherry tomato halves, cut side up.
4. Bake at 325° for 60 minutes, or until knife inserted into edge comes out clean.

Per serving: 299 calories; 17 g protein; 29 g carbohydrate; 4 g fiber; 12.7 g fat; 3.9 g saturated fat; 589 mg sodium.

*Nutritional analysis substituting whole milk for skim milk and regular Parmesan cheese for fat-free Parmesan cheese: 327 calories; 18 g protein; 26 g carbohydrate; 4 g fiber; 17 g fat; 7 g saturated fat; 662 mg sodium.

*Recommended for AIDS patients.

Tip

Try adding an extra piece of fruit to your diet each day. Once you have achieved that, try adding one extra vegetable. You might be pleasantly surprised at how much better you'll feel—and how much easier it is to control your weight.

Minute Cheese Taco

SERVES 1

You can fix this balanced meal in just minutes. Spice it up with a little salsa if you wish.

> 1 large flour tortilla
> 2 ounces 50% reduced-fat cheddar cheese,
>   shredded
> 1 small tomato, chopped
> 1 scallion, chopped (about 2 tablespoons)
> ¼ sweet green pepper, cored, chopped
> 1 tablespoon nonfat sour cream

1. Spread cheese on tortilla. Place in microwave for about 30 seconds, or until cheese has melted. Alternatively, melt cheese on tortilla in toaster oven or under the broiler.
2. Sprinkle vegetables over melted cheese. Top with sour cream.

Per serving: 370 calories; 23 g protein; 43 g carbohydrate; 3.5 g fiber; 13.3 g fat; 6.5 g saturated fat; 698 mg sodium.

Tip

Refrigerate leftover food immediately after a meal to avoid foodborne infections. Also, avoid fixing food hours ahead of a meal and leaving it on the stove. It's okay to fix dinner early in the day—just refrigerate until mealtime.

Bean Enchiladas

SERVES 4

Fix this meatless meal in a flash. Add a little salsa if you like more of a kick to your Mexican food.

> 4 large flour tortillas
> One 16-ounce can fat-free refried beans
> 3 ounces shredded taco cheese (or sharp
>   cheddar)
> 1 onion, minced
> 1 large tomato, chopped finely
> 1 cup romaine lettuce, chopped
> 4 tablespoons nonfat sour cream

1. Lay tortillas on large cookie sheet sprayed with vegetable oil spray. Divide refried beans between the 4 tortillas; spread evenly. Divide cheese between tortillas and sprinkle evenly over beans.

2. Bake at 375° for 10 to 15 minutes, or just until cheese has melted.
3. Sprinkle with onion, tomato and romaine lettuce. Top with 1 tablespoon of sour cream per tortilla and roll up!

Per serving: 409 calories; 18 g protein; 58 g carbohydrate; 8.5 g fiber; 11 g fat; 5.2 g saturated fat; 860 mg sodium.

Tip

When was the last time you had a tetanus shot? Remember that all adults need a booster every ten years.

Microwave Spicy Peanut Stir-Fry

SERVES 2

This fabulously easy and delectably delicious meal is ready in literally minutes.

> 8 ounces frozen broccoli stir-fry★
> 1 tablespoon peanut butter
> 2 tablespoons low-sodium soy sauce
> cayenne red pepper to taste (about
> ⅛ teaspoon)
> 2 tablespoons fresh cilantro, chopped
> One 7¾-ounce can of garbanzo beans
> (chickpeas), drained and rinsed
> 1 ounce peanuts (about 3 tablespoons)

1. Place frozen vegetables in microwave-safe container; cover and cook on high 2 minutes.
2. Blend together peanut butter, soy sauce, red pepper and cilantro (use a fork, or put the ingredients into a food miniprocessor or blender and process).
3. After vegetables have cooked for 2 minutes, remove from microwave. Stir in garbanzo beans, peanuts and sauce. Heat for 1 or 2 minutes in microwave until everything has warmed through.

★I use the one with broccoli, mushrooms, red peppers, mushrooms and onions.

Per serving: 282 calories; 13 g protein; 30 g carbohydrate; 9.9 g fiber; 13.2 g fat; 1.8 g saturated fat; 895 mg sodium.

Tip

Do you love croissants? Just go easy on them, as each one has at least twelve grams of fat. Better to have the plain ones, as those with fillings can have about forty grams of fat.

Sunflower Seed and Broccoli in a Honey Mustard Sauce

SERVES 2

This easy, meatless meal is both interesting and speedy.

2 teaspoons olive oil
1 bunch broccoli (about ¾ pound),
      separated into flowerettes and stems
      sliced on the diagonal
1 ounce (about 3 tablespoons) dry-roasted
      sunflower seeds
1 teaspoon 33% reduced-sodium chicken
      bouillon granules
¼ to ½ cup water
1 large sweet red pepper, seeded and cut
      into thin strips
1 tablespoon Dijon mustard
1 tablespoon honey
2 tablespoons cold water
2 teaspoons cornstarch
One 10.5-ounce package extra-firm light
      tofu, cut into ½-inch cubes
2 cups cooked brown rice

1. Heat olive oil in wok or large nonstick skillet over medium-high heat. Add broccoli, sunflower seeds and bouillon. Cook briefly, stirring constantly; about 5 minutes. Add water in tablespoons, just to keep a small amount of liquid in bottom of pan.
2. Add sweet red pepper, mustard and honey, stirring constantly for 2 to 3 minutes.
3. Mix 2 tablespoons water and cornstarch to form a paste. Stir in cornstarch paste, stirring until mixture has thickened. Remove from heat; stir in tofu. Cover and allow tofu to heat through. Serve with rice.

Per serving: 516 calories; 24 g protein; 75 g carbohydrate; 10 g fiber; 16 g fat; 2 g saturated fat; 682 mg sodium.

Tip

Tofu is another great food to keep on hand in the refrigerator for last-minute meals. Just be sure to buy the low-fat (light) version.

Garlic-Gingered Vegetables with Tofu

SERVES 6

Another unique blend of flavors that is sure to delight every palate. The tofu, as always, picks up the flavors surrounding it, in this case the garlic, sesame oil and ginger. This stores well in the refrigerator for three to four days.

2 teaspoons sesame oil
1 teaspoon reduced-sodium chicken
    bouillon granules, dissolved in ¾ cup
    boiling water
2 tablespoons minced fresh gingerroot
3 garlic cloves, crushed
2 cups frozen carrot coins
2 cups sliced zucchini
2 cups frozen chopped green bell pepper
Two 10.5-ounce packages extra-firm light
    tofu (1% fat), cut into 1-inch cubes
⅛ teaspoon freshly ground black pepper,
    or to taste
6 cups cooked egg noodles

1. In large nonstick skillet, heat oil and ¼ cup dissolved bouillon; add ginger and garlic. Cook over low heat, stirring frequently, 5 minutes.
2. Increase heat to high; add frozen carrots and zucchini. Stir-fry 3 to 4 minutes. Add green bell pepper and remainder of dissolved bouillon granules. Add tofu cubes and black pepper. Cook, stirring occasionally, 3 minutes, until vegetables are tender-crisp.
3. Serve over egg noodles.

Per serving: 311 calories; 16 g protein; 51 g carbohydrate; 4.8 g fiber; 5.3 g fat; 0.8 g saturated fat; 243 mg sodium.

Tip

Splurge on something that gives you pleasure. Is it a classical music CD? What about a bright bouquet of flowers in the dead of winter? Whatever it is, spend a few dollars occasionally to bring yourself pleasure.

Tofu Chow Mein

SERVES 4

Don't hesitate to try this meatless meal. Tofu assumes the flavor of whatever you cook it with, so you won't have to deal with a strong new taste.

1 tablespoon dark sesame oil
2 onions, chopped
2 stalks celery, chopped
2 tablespoons low-sodium chicken
 bouillon
¼ teaspoon black pepper
½ pound fresh bean sprouts
1 cup frozen chopped green pepper
¾ cup water
1 cup sliced mushrooms
¼ cup reduced-sodium soy sauce
One 8-ounce can water chestnuts, drained
1 teaspoon garlic powder
¼ cup water
1 tablespoon cornstarch
Two 10.5-ounce packages extra-firm light
 tofu, cut into 1-inch squares
4 cups hot cooked rice

1. Heat oil over medium heat; add onions and celery, cooking about 5 minutes.
2. Reduce heat. Add bouillon, pepper, sprouts, green pepper, water, mushrooms, soy sauce, water chestnuts and garlic powder. Simmer 5 to 7 minutes.
3. Mix ¼ cup water and cornstarch into a paste. Increase heat and stir in cornstarch paste, stirring until thickened. Remove from heat. Stir in tofu.
4. Serve over rice.

Per serving: 421 calories; 20 g protein; 73 g carbohydrate; 6 g fiber; 6.1 g fat; 0.7 g saturated fat; 679 mg sodium.

Tip

Tofu and other soybean products are loaded with phytoestrogens. Phytoestrogens are one type of phytochemical, nonnutrient substances in plant foods thought to confer many health benefits. Among other benefits, phytoestrogens are thought to help protect against osteoporosis by helping bones hang on to calcium.

Asparagus and Garbanzo Beans in a Roasted Red Pepper Sauce

SERVES 2

A most unusual "spaghetti" sauce that is loaded with powerful nutrition, this dish is also very easy.

One 7.25-ounce jar roasted red peppers
(not oil packed)
6 medium to large size basil leaves
(or 8 small)
1 teaspoon cornstarch
2 teaspoons margarine
1 large clove garlic, minced
½ medium onion, chopped
¼ teaspoon salt
⅛ teaspoon black pepper
½ pound asparagus, sliced into ¼-inch slices
on the diagonal
7¾-ounce can garbanzo beans (chickpeas),
drained and rinsed
2 cups cooked thin spaghetti

1. In food processor or blender, puree roasted red peppers (with juice), basil leaves and cornstarch; set aside.

2. Melt margarine in large nonstick skillet over low heat; add garlic, onion, salt and pepper and sauté 3 to 5 minutes, or until onion is slightly transparent. Add asparagus; sauté briefly, just until asparagus is tender-crisp (about 3 to 5 minutes. Add drained garbanzo beans.

3. Pour roasted red pepper mixture over top, stirring until mixture has just begun to thicken. Serve over pasta.

Per serving: 406 calories; 15 g protein; 71 g carbohydrate; 13.3 g fiber; 7.8 g fat; 0.9 g saturated fat; 957 mg sodium.

Tip

Did you know that asparagus is a member of the lily family? Asparagus is a nutrient-loaded, very low calorie vegetable. Six spears have just twenty-two calories and lots of folic acid and vitamin C.

Cream Cheese and Carrots

SERVES 4

A smooth way to enjoy carrots. Also a great way to get any kid to eat them!

> 1 pound baby carrots
> 2 tablespoons brown sugar
> 2 tablespoons nonfat cream cheese
> ¼ teaspoon cinnamon
> ⅓ cup skim milk
> 1 tablespoon brown sugar

1. Cook carrots in ½ cup water and 2 tablespoons brown sugar until tender. Drain; return to pot.
2. Add cream cheese, cinnamon, milk and remainder of brown sugar to carrots; warm 2 to 4 minutes over low heat.
3. Pour all ingredients into food processor; process until smooth. (If you don't have a food processor, use a hand-held mixer.)
4. Return carrot mixture to saucepan. Add ¼ cup skim milk and heat over low heat until completely warmed through.

Per serving: 84 calories; 3 g protein; 17 g carbohydrate; 3.7 g fiber; 0.6 g fat; 0.14 g saturated fat; 93 mg sodium.

*Nutritional analysis substituting whole milk for skim milk and regular cream cheese for nonfat cream cheese: 107 calories; 2 g protein; 17 g carbohydrate; 4 g fiber; 4 g fat; 2 g saturated fat; 74 mg sodium.

*Recommended for AIDS patients.

Tip

When you awaken each day, make plans for what you'll accomplish—especially when you're not feeling well. Perhaps you'll write some thank-you notes, or answer phone calls. Having a sense of accomplishment is critical to feeling good about yourself, especially when you're ill.

The Best Mashed Potatoes

SERVES 6

Try this defatted, higher protein version of an old comfort food. It stores well in the refrigerator for three or four days.

> 6 medium potatoes, peeled, and cut into
> small pieces
> One 4-ounce package nonfat cream cheese
> ¾ cup skim milk
> salt and pepper to taste

1. Place potatoes in pot; cover with water and bring to a boil. Reduce heat; simmer about 30 minutes, or until tender.
2. Drain and return to pot. Add cream cheese and milk; heat briefly over low heat.
3. Transfer all to food processor and whip until smooth. Alternatively, beat with an electric mixer or transfer to free-standing mixer and beat until smooth.
4. Add salt and pepper to taste.

Per serving: 144 calories; 6 g protein; 30 g carbohydrate; 2 g fiber; 0.2 g fat; 0.07 g saturated fat; 114 mg sodium.

*Nutritional analysis substituting whole milk for skim milk and regular cream cheese for nonfat cream cheese: 201 calories; 5 g protein; 29 g carbohydrate; 2 g fiber; 8 g fat; 5 g saturated fat; 78 mg sodium.

★Recommended for AIDS patients.

Tip

To make yogurt cheese—a powerhouse of protein and nutrients: Buy a yogurt strainer in the housewares section of William-Sonoma (or similar store). Allow yogurt to drain overnight, "converting" to cheese.

Gelatins and Custards

When making any of these gelatin recipes, feel free to use either regular or sugar-free, whatever best suits your calorie needs.

Creamy Gelatin

SERVES 4

A wonderfully smooth, rich and high-protein gelatin for days when appetite lags, the yogurt cheese concentrates calories, protein and calcium in less volume. And if you like a milder flavor, substitute plain yogurt for the vanilla.

> One 0.3-ounce package favorite instant gelatin
> ½ cup boiling water
> 1 quart vanilla yogurt cheese (see Tip above)

1. Dissolve gelatin in boiling water.
2. Pour dissolved gelatin over yogurt cheese; whisk together until smooth and well mixed.
3. Transfer to shallow refrigerator container. Refrigerate until mixture has gelled, about 1 to 2 hours.

Nutritional analysis per serving, using regular gelatin★: 235 calories; 14 g protein; 36 g carbohydrate; 0.0 g fiber; 3 g fat; 2 g saturated fat; 229 mg sodium.

Nutritional analysis per serving, using sugar-free gelatin: 163 calories; 14 g protein; 18 g carbohydrate; 0 g fiber; 3 g fat; 228 mg sodium.

★Recommended for AIDS patients.

Creamy Strawberry-Banana Gelatin

SERVES 4

> One 0.3-ounce package strawberry-banana
> gelatin
> ½ cup boiling water
> 2 cups fat-free frozen whipped topping
> 2 cup extra-calcium 1% fat cottage cheese
> 2 bananas, sliced

1. In mixing bowl, dissolve gelatin in boiling water. Add whipped topping and using wire whisk, blend whipped topping into gelatin.
2. Fold in cottage cheese and sliced bananas. Transfer to shallow container, cover and refrigerate until mixture is firm.

Nutritional analysis per serving, using regular gelatin★: 272 calories; 16 g protein; 48 g carbohydrate; 1 g fiber; 1 g fat; 1 g saturated fat; 448 mg sodium.

Nutritional analysis per serving, using sugar-free gelatin: 201 calories; 16 g protein; 30 g carbohydrate; 1 g fiber; 1 g fat; 1 saturated fat; 448 mg sodium.

★Recommended for AIDS patients.

Tip

Don't be discouraged because you've had to scale back your physical activity. Instead, watch your progress daily: perhaps you walked to the mailbox with a lilt in your step, or made it through the grocery store unassisted. Try doing a little more each day.

Strawberry-Mandarin Orange Gelatin

SERVES 4

A high-protein gelatin loaded with fruit—this makes a great healthy snack.

> One 0.3-ounce package strawberry gelatin
> ½ cup boiling water
> One 16-ounce container of low-fat vanilla
> yogurt, made into yogurt cheese
> (see Tip page 395)
> One 20-ounce can pineapple tidbits,
> drained, with juice set aside
> One 11-ounce can mandarin oranges,
> drained

1. Dissolve gelatin in boiling water. Add pineapple juice and mix well.
2. Whisk together yogurt cheese and gelatin mixture.
3. In bottom of shallow refrigerator container (or 9×9-inch pan), mix together the pineapple tidbits and mandarin oranges. Pour yogurt/gelatin mixture over fruit. Fold to mix well.
4. Refrigerate for 1 to 2 hours, or until mixture has set.

*Nutritional analysis per serving, using regular gelatin: 251 calories; 9 g protein; 51 g carbohydrate; 3 g fiber; 2 g fat; 1 g saturated fat; 152 mg sodium.

Nutritional analysis per serving, using sugar-free gelatin: 180 calories; 9 g protein; 33 g carbohydrate; 3 g fiber; 2 g fat; 1 g saturated fat; 151 mg sodium

 *Recommended for AIDS patients.

Tip

It's great to get extra calcium from yogurt, cheese and cottage cheese—but remember that these dairy foods are not fortified with vitamin D (they're made with milk before it's been fortified). Without enough vitamin D, your body can't absorb or use the calcium. Check with your doctor about a vitamin D supplement if you're not drinking four 8-ounce glasses of milk daily.

Raspberry Cream Gelatin

SERVES 4

 One 0.3-ounce package raspberry gelatin
 ½ cup boiling water
 1½ cups extra-calcium cottage cheese

1. Dissolve gelatin in boiling water.
2. Puree cottage cheese in food miniprocessor.
3. Whisk together dissolved gelatin and pureed cottage cheese until well blended. Refrigerate until firm, about 1 hour.

*Nutritional analysis per serving, using regular gelatin: 140 calories; 12 g protein; 22 g carbohydrate; 0.0 g fiber; 1 g fat; 1 g saturated fat; 334 mg sodium.

Nutritional analysis per serving, using sugar-free gelatin: 68 calories; 12 g protein; 4 g carbohydrate; 0 g fiber; 1 g fat; 1 g saturated fat; 334 mg sodium.

 *Recommended for AIDS patients

Tip

Most grocery stores have extra-calcium cottage cheese. This is just of many ways in which choosing food carefully can help you boost nutrients.

Apricot and Pear Gelatin

SERVES 6

One 0.3-ounce box orange gelatin

⅓ cup boiling water

⅔ cup apricot nectar

1 cup nonfat frozen whipped dairy topping

½ cup dried apricots, chopped

One 20-ounce can pears (packed in own
juice), drained and chopped

¼ cup walnut halves, coarsely chopped

1. Dissolve gelatin in water. Stir in nectar. Whisk in dairy topping.
2. In bottom of 1-quart container, place chopped apricots, pears and walnuts.
3. Pour nectar/gelatin mixture over fruit and nuts. Cover and refrigerate until mixture has jelled, about 1 hour.

*Nutritional analysis per serving using regular gelatin: 278 calories; 5 g protein; 5 g carbohydrate; 4 g fiber; 5 g fat; 3 g saturated fat; 75 mg sodium.

Nutritional analysis per serving using sugar-free gelatin: 206 calories; 4 g protein; 39 g carbohydrate; 4 g fiber; 5 g fat; 0.3 g saturated fat; 75 mg sodium.

*Recommended for AIDS patients.

Tip

Protect yourself during cold and flu season by washing your hands whenever you come in from the store or any other public place.

Carrot-Date Gelatin

SERVES 6

A great high-fiber, high-protein and vitamin-loaded snack or dessert.

One 0.3-ounce box orange gelatin

1 cup boiling water

2 cups nonfat cottage cheese

½ pound carrots, grated (in food processor)

16 dates, chopped

1. Stir gelatin into boiling water until well dissolved. Add one more cup cold water.
2. In 9×9-inch square pan, mix cottage cheese, carrots and dates.

3. Pour gelatin mixture over cottage cheese mixture; mix well. Cover and refrigerate until mixture has jelled, about 1 hour.

Nutritional analysis per serving using regular gelatin★: 275 calories; 18 g protein; 53 g carbohydrate; 4 g fiber; 0.3 g fat; 0.1 g saturated fat; 447 mg sodium.

Nutritional analysis, using sugar-free gelatin: 204 calories; 17 g protein; 35 g carbohydrate; 4 g fiber; .3 g fat; .1 g saturated fat; 447 mg sodium

★Recommended for AIDS patients.

Tip

Do you take care of your caregiver? Whether it be your spouse, your children, your parents or a dear friend, the people who sacrifice to take care of your needs have needs too. Do something nice for them, and find a way to give them a break from the grind.

Sweet Potato Custard

SERVES 4
This keeps well in the refrigerator for up to four or five days.

> 2 eggs (or the equivalent in liquid egg sub-
>   stitute)
> One 12-ounce can evaporated skim milk
> One 16-ounce can sweet potatoes, drained
>   (and rinsed if in syrup)
> 1 teaspoon cinnamon
> ¼ cup brown sugar
> 1 teaspoon vanilla

1. Place all ingredients in food processor, or mix with electric beater until smooth.
2. Spray a 2-quart casserole with vegetable oil spray. Pour custard mixture into casserole.
3. Bake at 350° for 1 hour or until a knife inserted in the middle comes out clean.

Per serving: 226 calories; 12 g protein; 38 g carbohydrate; 1.9 g fiber; 2.9 g fat; 0.9 g saturated fat; 222 mg sodium.

Tip

Cutting fat from the diet is critically important for everyone: it'll reduce heart disease and cancer risk, and also help you keep weight at a healthy level.

Pumpkin Custard

Serves 4

Whip up a batch and enjoy it for several days—it keeps well in the refrigerator for up to five days.

> One 12-ounce can evaporated skim milk
> 3 eggs (or equivalent in liquid egg substitute)
> One 16-ounce can pumpkin
> ½ cup brown sugar
> 1 teaspoon cinnamon
> ½ teaspoon ginger
> ¼ teaspoon cloves

1. Place all ingredients in food processor, or mix with electric beater until smooth.
2. Spray a 2-quart casserole with vegetable oil spray. Pour mixture into casserole.
3. Bake at 350° for 50 to 60 minutes, or until a knife inserted in the middle comes out clean.

Per serving: 171 calories; 13 g protein; 21 g carbohydrate; 5 g fiber; 3.9 g fat; 1.3 g saturated fat; 164 mg sodium.

Tip

When you eat, make sure every calorie is worth its weight in gold—or at least nutrients. Rather than have an empty-calorie candy bar, try this great pumpkin custard, for example. It's loaded with protein, calcium and beta-carotene.

Banana Custard

Serves 6

> 3 eggs (or equivalent in liquid egg substitute)
> One 12-ounce can evaporated skim milk
> ½ cup sugar
> 3 bananas

1. Place all ingredients in food processor, or mix with electric beater until smooth.
2. Spray 1-quart casserole with vegetable oil spray. Pour custard mixture into casserole. Bake at 350° for 45 minutes, or until a knife inserted in the middle comes out clean.

Per serving: 198 calories; 8 g protein; 37 g carbohydrates; 1.2 g fiber; 2.9 g fat; 0.9 g saturated fat; 97 mg sodium.

Tip

Has food become a source of entertainment for you? Because you can't leave the house very often, do you turn to comfort foods to bring you amusement and assuage feelings of boredom? Find another activity that will accommodate your energy and mobility budgets. Crossword puzzles, cruising the Internet, reading the classics, making handcrafts for charity bazaars, bringing in someone to teach you how to play the piano are just a few ideas. Find something you enjoy, and that captures your interest—your fascination with food will fade!

Apple Custard

SERVES 6

A delightful variation of a food that's great for all appetites—but higher in fiber and with a tiny little crunch for interest.

> 3 eggs or the equivalent in liquid egg substitute
> One 12-ounce can evaporated skim milk
> ½ cup sugar
> 4 apples, with skin, quartered
> 1 teaspoon cinnamon

1. Place all ingredients in food processor or blender using pulse setting, until apples are in very small pieces.
2. Spray 1-quart casserole with vegetable oil spray. Pour custard mixture into casserole. Bake at 350° for 45 minutes, or until a knife inserted in the middle comes out clean.

Per serving: 201 calories; 8 g protein; 38 g carbohydrate; 2 g fiber; 2.9 g fat; 0.9 g saturated fat; 97 mg sodium.

Tip

Find hope in the smallest of signs, and cling to it fiercely. Can you move your legs today with less pain? Perhaps you were able to shop for groceries by yourself. Whatever the accomplishment, no matter how small, find hope in it and don't let go.

Applesauce Custard

SERVES 6

Make this tempting high-protein food on days when appetite is lagging.

> 3 eggs (or equivalent in liquid egg substitute)
> One 12-ounce can evaporated skim milk
> ½ cup sugar
> 1 cup applesauce, no sugar added
> 1 teaspoon cinnamon

1. Place all ingredients in bowl; mix with spoon until well blended.
2. Spray 1-quart casserole with vegetable oil spray.
3. Pour custard mixture into casserole. Bake at 350° for 45 minutes, or until a knife inserted in the middle comes out clean.

Per serving: 165 calories; 7.5 g protein; 28 g carbohydrate; 0.7 g fiber; 2.6 g fat; 0.9 g saturated fat; 98 mg sodium.

Tip

Try bartering to accomplish activities you cannot so because you have limited energy. Can you, for example, watch your friend's school-age children while she does errands? If you can, then she could run your errands too. Be creative, figuring out what you can offer to others and then trade it for something that's difficult for you.

Hot Cinnamon Chunky Applesauce

SERVES 4

Top pancakes and waffles with this wonderfully warm and delicious applesauce—or just enjoy it as is for dessert. It's exceptionally easy because the peels are left on the apples, which also makes it higher in fiber.

> 4 cooking apples, cored and sliced (peel on)
> 2 tablespoons brown sugar
> 2 tablespoons water
> 1 teaspoon cinnamon

1. Combine all ingredients in microwave-safe bowl. Cover, leaving a steam vent in one corner.
2. Microwave on high power for 5 minutes. Transfer to food processor or blender. Using the pulse setting, process for 10 seconds at a time, repeating 3 to 4 times. The goal is to create a chunky applesauce. Serve hot or cold.

Per serving: 100 calories; 0.3 g protein; 26 g carbohydrate; 3 g fiber; 0.5 g fat; 0.08 g saturated fat; 1.9 mg sodium.

Catalogs:
Adaptive Kitchen Information

Activities for Daily Living
Smith and Nephew Rolyan
P.O. Box 1005
Germantown, WI 53022
Phone: 414/251-7840
Fax: 800/545-7758
Fax: 414/251-7758

After Therapy Catalog
NCM Consumer Products Division
P.O. Box 6070
San Jose, CA 95150-6070
Phone: 800/235-7054
Fax: 408/277-6824

Aids for Arthritis
3 Little Knoll Court
Medford, NJ 08055
Phone: 609/654-6918

Enrichments
P.O. Box 471
Western Springs, IL 60558
Phone: 800/323-5547
Fax: 800/547-4333
Fax: 708/325-4602

Self Care Catalogs
104 Challenger Drive
Portland, TN 37148-1711
Phone: 800/345-1848

Williams-Sonoma
P.O. Box 7456
San Francisco, CA 94120
Phone: 800/541-1262

Resources

Asthma/Allergy Information Sources

Allen & Hanbury's Respiratory Institute
Five Moore Drive
Research Triangle Park, NC 27709
919/248-2643

Asthma & Allergy Foundation of America
1125 15th Street N.W., Suite 502
Washington, DC 20005
Phone: 800/7-ASTHMA, in Nashville TN
202/466-7643, in Washington, DC
Fax: 202/466-8940
Web site: www.aafa.org
Publication: *Advance*
Bimonthly newsletter

Allergy & Asthma Network/Mothers of Asthmatics
3554 Chain Bridge Road, Suite 200
Fairfax, VA 22030
Phone: 800/878-4403
Fax: 703/352-4354
Publication: *The MA Report*
Monthly newsletter

American Academy of Allergy and Immunology
611 East Wells Street
Milwaukee, WI 53202
800/822-2762

American Lung Association
National Headquarters
1740 Broadway
New York, NY 10019-4374
212/315-8700
Look in the phone book for the ALA in your area.

Food Allergy Network
4744 Holly Avenue
Fairfax, VA 22030
703/691-3179

Indoor Air Quality Association
289 South Wilma Street
Longwood, FL 32750
800/557-7002

National Asthma Education Program
National Heart, Lung and Blood Institute
Information Center
P. O. Box 37105
Bethesda, MD 20824-0105
301/251-1222

National Institute of Allergy and Infectious Diseases
National Institutes of Health
Office of Communications
9000 Rockvillle Pike
Building 31, Room 7A-50
Bethesda, MD 20892
301/496-5717

National Jewish Center For Immunology and Respiratory Medicine, Lung Line
1400 Jackson Street
Denver, CO 80206
800/222-LUNG (5864)

Other Information

Alzheimer's Association
919 North Michigan Avenue, Suite 1000
Chicago, IL 60611
Phone: 800/272-3900
Fax: 312/335-1110
Web site: www.alz.org
Publication: *Alzheimer's Association National Newsletter*
Three times/year

The Arthritis Foundation
1330 West Peachtree Street N.E.
Atlanta, GA 30309
Phone: 404/872-7100
Fax: 404/872-0457
Web site: www.arthritis.org
Publication: *Arthritis Today*
Bimonthly

Fibromyalgia Alliance of America
P. O. Box 21990
Columbus, OH 43221-0990
Phone: 614/457-4222
Fax: 614/457-2729
E-mail: masaathoff@aol.com
Publication: *Fibromyalgia Times*
Quarterly newsletter

The Lupus Foundation of America
1300 Piccard Drive, Suite 200
Rockville, MD 20850
Phone: 301/670-9292
Fax: 301/670-9486
Publication: *Lupus News*
Quarterly newsletter
Note: The American Lupus Society recently merged with this organization.

The Multiple Sclerosis Foundation
6350 North Andrews Avenue
Ft. Lauderdale, FL 33309
Phone: 800/441-7055
Fax: 954/351-0630
Web site: www.msfacts.org
Publication: *FYI*
Every other month

The Muscular Dystrophy Association
3300 East Sunrise Drive
Tucson, AZ 85718
Phone: 800/572-1717

Fax: 520/529-5300
Web site: www.mdausa.org
CompuServe\GOMDA
Publication: *Quest Magazine*
Six times/year

The Myasthenia Gravis Foundation of America
222 South Riverside Plaza, Suite 1540
Chicago, IL 60606
Phone: 800/541-5454
Fax: 312/258-0461
Web site: www.med.uncedu\mgfa
Publication: *MGS Newsletter*
Once/year

National Psoriasis Foundation
6600 Southwest 92nd Avenue, Suite 300
Portland, OR 97223-7195
Phone: 800/723-9166
Fax: 503/245-0626
Web site: www.psoriasis.org
Publications: *The Bulletin*
Bimonthly

Osteoporosis and Related Bone Diseases National Resource Center
1150 17th St., NW, Suite 500
Washington, DC 20036
202/223-0344

Parkinson's Disease Foundation
710 West 168th Street
New York, NY 10032
Phone: 800/457-6676
Fax: 212/923-4778
Web site: www.parkinsons-foundation.org
Publication: *Parkinson's Disease Newsletter*
Quarterly newsletter
Note: There is a National Parkinson's Foundation in Miami, Florida at 800/327-4545.

Sjögren's Syndrome Foundation
333 North Broadway, Suite 2000
Jericho, NY 11753
Phone: 800/475-6473
Fax: 516/933-6368
Web site: www.sjogrens.com
Publication: *The Moisture Seekers Newsletter*
Nine times/year

Index